T0281071

The mind at work

The mind at work

Psychological ergonomics

W.T. SINGLETON

Emeritus Professor of Applied Psychology
University of Aston in Birmingham

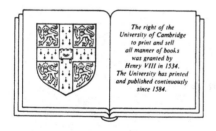

The right of the
University of Cambridge
to print and sell
all manner of books
was granted by
Henry VIII in 1534.
The University has printed
and published continuously
since 1584.

CAMBRIDGE UNIVERSITY PRESS

Cambridge

New York   Port Chester

Melbourne   Sydney

CAMBRIDGE UNIVERSITY PRESS
Cambridge, New York, Melbourne, Madrid, Cape Town, Singapore, São Paulo

Cambridge University Press
The Edinburgh Building, Cambridge CB2 2RU, UK

Published in the United States of America by Cambridge University Press, New York

www.cambridge.org
Information on this title: www.cambridge.org/9780521265799

© Cambridge University Press 1989

This book is in copyright. Subject to statutory exception
and to the provisions of relevant collective licensing agreements,
no reproduction of any part may take place without
the written permission of Cambridge University Press.

First published 1989
This digitally printed first paperback version 2005

A catalogue record for this publication is available from the British Library

Library of Congress Cataloguing in Publication data

Singleton, W.T. (William Thomas)
The mind at work : psychological ergonomics / W.T. Singleton.
    p.   cm.
ISBN 0-521-26579-7
1. Psychology, Industrial.   2. Human engineering.   3. Man–machine
systems.   I. Title.
HF5548.8.S527   1989
158.7—dc19   88-37890
CIP

ISBN-13 978-0-521-26579-9 hardback
ISBN-10 0-521-26579-7 hardback

ISBN-13 978-0-521-01750-3 paperback
ISBN-10 0-521-01750-5 paperback

To Pamela Elizabeth

Contents

Key to symbols used   page xiv

| 1 | **HUMAN RESOURCES AND SYSTEM DESIGN** | 1 |

1.1   **Concepts**   1

1.1.1 *The human contribution*   1
    The human role as a system controller   1
    The human contribution in high technology systems   2
    The human contribution in low technology systems   5
    Ergonomics and other aspects of technology   7
    The philosophy of work   7
1.1.2 *The design of systems*   8
    The system concept   8
    The design of high technology systems   10
    The design of smaller systems   19
    The design of macro-systems   20

1.2   **Knowledge**   21

1.2.1 *Demographic data*   21
1.2.2 *Human resource utilisation*   29

1.3   **Principles, methods and procedures**   31

1.3.1 *Education, work and leisure*   31
1.3.2 *Socio-technical systems*   32
1.3.3 *Man–machine systems*   34
1.3.4 *Task analysis*   41
    Terminology   41
      Procedural task analysis   45
      Diagnositic task analysis   47
    Task analysis by observation   50
      Process charts   50
      Sequence charts   55

	Link design charts	56
	Flow charts	56
	Block diagrams	57
	Algorithm charts	59
	F.A.S.T. diagrams	61
	General functional diagrams	61
	Task analysis by discussion	61
	Responsibility charts	65
	Hierarchical analysis	66
	Protocol analysis	67
	M.C.I. Job–process analysis	67
	Conclusion	69
1.4	**Applications**	70
1.4.1	*Man-power planning*	70
1.4.2	*The design of procedures*	72
	Checklists	74
	Routines	75
	Knowledge texts	75
1.4.3	*The design of manuals*	76
2	**SKILL AND TRAINING**	80
2.1	**Concepts**	80
2.1.1	*Developmental aspects*	80
2.1.2	*Human skill*	81
2.1.3	*Acquisition of skills*	83
2.1.4	*Mental models*	85
2.2	**Knowledge**	88
2.2.1	*Individual differences*	88
	Capacities, abilities and aptitudes	88
	Intelligence and personality	89
	Age differences	90
	Sex differences	91
	Ethnic, cultural, climatic and economic differences	92
2.2.2	*Learning*	93
2.2.3	*Memory and thinking*	96
2.2.4	*Language*	99
2.2.5	*Learning and memory*	100

2.3	**Principles, methods and procedures**	102
2.3.1	*Interviewing*	102
2.3.2	*Psychological testing*	105
2.3.3	*Surveys*	106
2.3.4	*Task training*	108
2.3.5	*Skill training*	111
2.3.6	*Attitude training*	113
2.3.7	*Skills analysis*	113
2.4	**Applications**	115
2.4.1	*Selection and guidance*	115
2.4.2	*Placement*	120
2.4.3	*The design of training schemes*	121
2.4.4	*Programmed instruction*	123
2.4.5	*The use of simulators*	128
3	**NEEDS AND ORGANISATIONS**	135
3.1	**Concepts**	135
3.1.1	*Social factors*	135
	Activity involving others	135
	Conceptual approaches	136
3.1.2	*Human aspirations*	137
	The importance of context	137
	Terminology	138
3.2	**Knowledge**	139
3.2.1	*Small groups*	139
3.2.2	*Large groups*	141
3.2.3	*Leadership*	142
3.2.4	*Organisation theory*	143
3.2.5	*Motivation theory*	144
3.3	**Principles, methods and procedures**	146
3.3.1	*Group decision making (committees)*	146
3.3.2	*Role analysis*	147
3.3.3	*Job analysis*	148
3.3.4	*Depth interviews*	150
3.4	**Applications**	151
3.4.1	*Batch production*	151

3.4.2   *Construction*   153
3.4.3   *The management consultant*   154
3.4.4   *Ergonomics in developing countries*   155

4   **PERFORMANCE AND JOB DESIGN**   159

4.1   **Concepts**   159
4.1.1   *Fatigue*   160
4.1.2   *Arousal*   161
4.1.3   *Stress*   163
4.1.4   *Vigilance*   165
4.1.5   *Circadian rhythms*   167

4.2   **Knowledge**   168
4.2.1   *Human state*   168
4.2.2   *Mental load*   171

4.3   **Principles, methods and procedures**   176
4.3.1   *Experiments and trials*   176
4.3.2   *Job design*   180

4.4   **Applications**   183
4.4.1   *Design for operation*   183
        The general approach   183
        The specific approach   184
4.4.2   *Design for maintenance*   184
4.4.3   *Inspection tasks*   186
        Passive inspection   186
        Active inspection   187
4.4.4   *Shift systems*   187
4.4.5   *The use of VDUs*   188
        The casual user   189
        The continuous user   189

5   **INFORMATION PROCESSING**   194

5.1   **Concepts**   194
5.1.1   *Information acceptance*   194
        Sensation   194
        Perception   196
        Cognition   198

5.1.2   *Information transmission*   199
        Signal detection theory   199
        Information theory   201
        Transfer theory   202

5.2   **Knowledge**   205
5.2.1   *Data acquisition*   205
5.2.2   *Information transmission*   205
5.2.3   *Decision-making*   208

5.3   **Principles, methods and procedures**   208
5.3.1   *Displays*   208
5.3.2   *Controls*   217
5.3.3   *Interface design*   218
5.3.4   *Centralised control systems*   220
        System malfunctions and human errors   222
        Human limitations   223
5.3.5   *Alarm systems*   225
        Alarm interfaces   227
        The alarm recipient   229
5.3.6   *Computer support*   223
        The engineered mechanism   223
        The man–computer system   223
        The human–computer interface   235
        User requirements   235
        Robotics   237
        Conclusion   238

5.4   **Applications**   239
5.4.1   *Human-computer interface design*   239
        The U.K. organisational structure   239
        Input systems   240
        Display systems   241
        Conclusion   242
5.4.2   *Military control systems*   243
5.4.3   *Process control centres*   246
        A team work-space   247
        A plant interface   248
        A management centre   249
        An information centre   249

5.4.4	*Aviation psychology*	250
	The pilot	251
	The air traffic controller	253
5.4.5	*Checklists and standards*	254

6	**RISK AND RELIABILITY**	260
6.1	**Concepts**	260
6.1.1	*Risk*	260
6.1.2	*Safety*	262
6.1.3	*Accidents*	265
6.1.4	*Human error*	269
6.1.5	*Reliability*	271
6.1.6	*Disasters*	273
6.2	**Knowledge**	276
6.2.1	*Accident data sources*	276
6.2.2	*Accident data interpretation*	277
6.2.3	*Accident data*	277
6.3	**Principles, methods and procedures**	282
6.3.1	*Accident reduction*	284
	Design	285
	Procedures	286
	Training	287
	Management	288
6.3.2	*Hazard reduction*	290
6.3.3	*Error reduction*	290
6.3.4	*The safe system*	295
6.4	Applications	298
6.4.1	*Risk analysis*	298
6.4.2	*Reliablity analysis*	299
6.4.3	*Safety compliance*	300
6.4.4	*Accident research*	302

7	**THE CITIZEN AND THE ENVIRONMENT**	308
7.1	**Concepts**	308
7.1.1	*The technology-based society*	308
7.1.2	*The technology-based environment*	310

7.1.3   *Consumer ergonomics*   313
7.1.4   *Disabled individuals*   314

7.2   **Knowledge**   317
7.3   **Principles, methods and procedures**   319
7.3.1   *Control for ill-defined issues*   319
7.3.2   *User preference studies*   320
7.3.3   *The rehabilitation of the disabled*   321

7.4   **Applications**   324
7.4.1   *Office design*   324
7.4.2   *Car design*   328
        Design procedure   329
        Computer-aided design and manufacture   330
        The technological push   331
        Continuity and change   332
        The customer – designer loop   332
        Competition and fashion   333
        Continuing problems   333
7.4.3   *Ergonomics and disability*   334

        Author index   338
        Subject index   343

Key to symbols used in figures

Activity
Function
Analysis

Decision
Choice

Thing
Operator
Person
Object

Knowledge
Abstraction
Specification

1 Human resources and system design

1.1   Concepts
1.1.1   *The human contribution*
The human role as a system controller

The business of designing machines, processes and systems can be pursued more or less independently of the properties of people. Nevertheless people are always involved, the designer himself is a human being and his product will shape the behaviour of many workers and other users. More fundamentally, the design activity will be meaningless unless it is directed towards serving some human need. In spite of all this, the design process itself is often thought about and executed without any formal considerations about people. Inevitably the engineer, architect or other designer devotes most of his attention and expertise to devising mechanisms, buildings and so on which support some human activity more effectively than those currently available. The new machine or system must not be very different from the old one for a variety of reasons. The old one did its job, not perfectly but well enough to justify its existence. The new one is usually designed on the basis of copying the old one but removing as many as possible of the faults. There are other reasons such as commonality of components and, of course, shortage of imagination which lead to most design and development being a progressive iterative process. This happens to suit the human operators because most of their skills will transfer along the line of development of the machines and systems.

From the engineering point of view the hardware technology is central and the operators tag along supporting the activity of machines which are basically doing the work. In nineteenth century transport for example, the coach and horses was not a serious competitor for the steam-engined train, nor was the man with a spade as productive as the operator with a steam shovel. This was the earliest technology in which power was derived from sources other than animal muscles and the output was so obviously superior that men did not mind putting up with the inconvenience of machines which were uncomfortable or awkward to use. They even took pride in developing new skills which enabled them to use difficult machines which inexperienced people could not use. This attitude was reinforced by the second wave of technology which provided instrumentation, ways of sensing and recording data which gave more accurate and reliable data than that which can be detected directly by the human senses. At this stage the typical machine operator manipulated machine controls on the basis of data presented on instruments. The machine controls caused power to be applied and consequences to occur which resulted in changed readings on the instruments. The man was in the control loop (Hick and Bates, 1950). More recently, in the third wave of technology the man has been removed from the responsibility for continuous control (this is best done by computers working to a moderately flexible range of programs) but he remains as the monitor of the system performance and a selector of the appropriate program determined by the changing short-term objectives. He may keep the responsibility for setting-up and shutting-down the system or this also may be partially delegated to computers. This is the 'Supervisory Control' role (Sheridan and Johannsen, 1976). Information flow in these three phases of development of system control is shown in Fig. 1.1

Supervisory control is by no means universal, in fact it remains restricted to high technology systems such as aircraft, computer controlled machine tools, chemical plants and power stations. (Edwards and Lees, 1974). There are still many systems where the man is in the control loop, for example in vehicle driving and in most manufacturing production processes. There are many tasks where the operator is assisted only by hand-tools and simple powered machines, for example in craft-work and surgery. There are also plenty of tasks, although these are now perhaps more common in leisure than in paid work, where the man supplies the muscle power, for example the manual labourer and the active sportsman.

In general, the working man may function at any level from the senior partner in high technology operations to the provider of muscle power in physically demanding jobs. In all cases the ergonomic requirement is that the task as designed should make use of his abilities and be adaptive to his limitations.

The human contribution in high technology systems

All working systems, including those incorporating advanced technology of processes and process control, depend on skilled operators. There are social, economic and technical reasons for this.

Socially the public will not easily accept automatic systems. When seeking reassurance that a system is safe they study the people who are responsible for it. They have no means of assessing the reliability of automatic control systems but they can make some assessment of a skilled individual and without (*a*) Power supplemented human performance

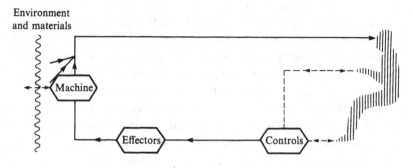

(*b*) Power and information supplemented human performance

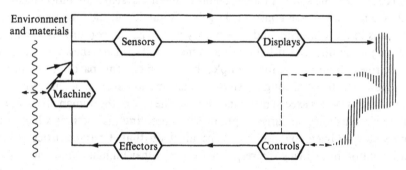

(*c*) Power, information and decision supplemented human performance

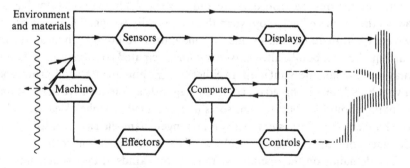

Fig. 1.1. The changing role of the human operator with technological development.

knowing very much about his working procedures they will trust his actions if he seems calm, competent and mature. The most direct example is the nervous airline passenger who is comforted by the belief that the middle-aged pilot he saw sitting on the flight deck is flying the aeroplane. Less directly but equally importantly, people living in the vicinity of a large plant would not take kindly to the idea that it was not under the control of human beings who are on the spot and are assumed to know exactly what is happening.

Economically it remains true that it is inordinately expensive to construct a system which must continue to be reliable without direct human intervention, for example under the sea or in space. Equally it is expensive to ensure that equipment will continue to function under rough handling conditions, for example the necessary 'ruggedising' of military equipment. A system can be designed much more economically if it can be assumed that skilled personnel are available to control and take care of it.

Technically the state of the art seems to be that systems are most efficient, reliable and safe when control is largely automatic but the human operator remains in a monitoring and supervisory role. That is, continuous dynamic dealing with minor perturbations is automatic and so also is the application of basic rules about safety; for example, the system or some part of it might be programmed to go through a step-change function such as a shut-down if certain parameters exceed prescribed limits. The role of the human operator in these circumstances is largely specified by operating instructions which are mandatory. Given this and this – he must do that. Characteristically his intervention in this way is a response to some other human requirement; for example, a maintenance man may wish to have a particular sub-system shut down for his attention or a user of the system product may wish to receive a different input to meet his purposes. Many of these interactions could be made automatic were it not for the basic need for a human presence for the social/economic reasons mentioned above and because the human operator has to act as the ultimate back-stop when things go badly wrong. Things go badly wrong when there has been some extreme untoward event such as a fire, an earthquake or a bomb, alternatively an unanticipated combination of faults may occur within the plant itself. In either case the human intervention must be a very high level one based on complex diagnosis and innovative design-type thinking about how best to cope so as to avoid a catastrophe. A catastrophe can happen when the system energy is no longer channelled as intended by the designers or because there is a release of toxic substances or both.

The demands on the operator stem from two kinds of task which are not compatible because they require very different levels of skill. On the one hand he must cope with routines where the demand is for precise obedience to established instructions and on the other hand he might suddenly be faced with a need to respond in a creative manner totally outside any instructions.

Superficially the solution would seem to be to have two kinds of operators, those who carry out the routines and others who are on call should unforeseen emergencies arise. There are two snags about this approach. Firstly there may not be time or it may not be physically possible to suddenly introduce a high level operator, for example we cannot put a different pilot on the flight deck when an aircraft gets into trouble. Secondly, the high level operator will not maintain his skill and familiarity with the system unless he operates regularly within it. His ability to intervene effectively must be a function of his 'hands on' experience supported of course by his conceptual knowledge of how the system functions.

This last proposition is based on experience of systems where the intervention requires complex manipulative activity, for example a surgeon dealing with an emergency during an operation or an aircraft pilot taking over manually. It is not so obviously true where the intervention takes the form essentially of a decision to initiate a single direct action such as closing a particular valve or starting up a stand-by pump. In these circumstances it is not clear whether or not the effectiveness of the intervention is quite so dependent on operating experience.

Taking for example the nuclear power plant control room, the question is whether the desk operators should be expected to cope with all emergencies which appear within the total information presentation or whether, for complex and dangerous situations, a more senior person such as the shift-charge engineer should be called upon to make the decisions. This policy issue must be cleared before the basic personnel decisions about selection and training of staff at the various levels can be made and before the information presentations can be designed.

The human contribution in low technology systems

The extreme case of man as a source of muscle power is dealt with in the previous book in this series – *The Body at Work*. Such working situations are now relatively rare in developed countries and the man is more usually employed in tasks where there is a considerable control element requiring extensive information processing. Such tasks range from the use of simple hand tools to tracking using complex powered machinery.

Human beings are needed for those tasks for a variety of reasons from their highly dexterous manipulative potential through to their ability to accept informal instructions. These reasons are given in detail in the discussion of man–machine function allocation (p. 35).

The demands on the human operator are difficult to quantify or even to describe because the process is essentially an interactive one. The skilled operator is working in harmony with his tools and machines. The concept of 'demand' is often not appropriate because it implies confrontation, the process is more aptly considered as one of cooperation and persuasion. The human operator is pursuing an objective, usually to make something or to go somewhere, and he achieves this with the assistance of the hardware at his disposal. This hardware, if it is well-designed, aids him in his progress toward his objective. There may be demands in the sense that there are always obstacles to be overcome but these stem from the nature and the variability of the situation he is in; that is, the materials he has to deal with or the environment he has to move through. The skilled operator will aim for efficient performance. Efficiency incorporates not only quantity and quality of achievement but also preservation of his own safety and health and that of others who might be involved as working partners, passengers or the general public in the neighbourhood.

Of course, if his tasks are badly designed they may well make unnecessary demands. These begin with bodily aspects of the operating posture required and the forces which must be exerted to operate controls. For a work-space which is used full-time very slight departures from the optimum may lead to problems in the long term, for example in strained ligaments, tendons and muscles. Posture is constrained not only by the physical dimensions of the work-space but also by the need to be in a position to see certain events and to feel others through control operations or machine movement. Other demands will arise if the information presented is inadequate in content, e.g. poor lighting may make it difficult to detect some relevant cues, or in structure, e.g. because of poor coding and presentation of information on dials, charts or screens. Correspondingly there may be output demands created by control operations which result in things happening too quickly or unexpectedly. The level of demand is to do not only with the tasks as they are done but also with the duration for which they must continue to be done. This applies particularly to routines and repetitive work where the main operator limitation is not capacity or skill but stamina.

In principle, repetitive work is best left to automatic machines but the flexibility of human performance is often needed because slight changes are required either to modify the product or to cope with different materials. Batch production work is often of this kind and in general it is by no means as unchanging or boring as it might appear to the casual visitor to the factory. In all the clothing trades for example there are continuous changes in sizes, materials, colours, styles and so on which provide the appropriate variety for the customers and incidentally for the producer. Work design must take account of the needs of the consumer as well as those of the worker.

Ergonomics and other aspects of technology

The technical specialist who represents the people point of view implicit in the approach just described is the ergonomist. In the previous book in this series the relationship of ergonomics to other aspects or kinds of technology was discussed in detail. The unique feature of ergomonics is its emphasis on the characteristics of human operators and their relevance to the design of work.

The role of the ergonomist is essentially an advisory one. In the case of high technology design he must provide a service for the engineers and scientists who carry the technical design responsibility. This service may simply be as a source of information or the ergonomist can have more power in that the design decisions involving people have to be approved by him. This is usually restricted to obvious cases of man–machine interaction such as the design of displays, controls and work-spaces. In the case of low technology design again he has an advisory role but with a general emphasis on awareness of the kinds and ranges of people who are being catered for. For systems which are already operating the ergonomist is likely to cooperate with occupational health and safety specialists and to play a part in the consideration of accidents and occupational diseases which might arise from unnecessarily stressful work situations (p. 294).

It will be appreciated that for most kinds of work and most working organisations it is not feasible to employ specialist ergonomists. In such cases those who have responsibilities for work design need to have some awareness of the principles of ergonomics.

The philosophy of work

Ergonomics is sometimes confused by questions such as, who is the ergonomist servicing – the employer or the worker? or, to whom is he ultimately responsible – the state, the employer, the producer or the consumer? Fortunately it is possible to dispose of these issues without taking up any particular political position. Ergonomics seems to flourish equally well in capitalist and socialist/communist systems, ergonomics activity can be sponsored with equal validity by employers organisations and by workers organisations.

This is because, as already mentioned, ergonomics is about efficient use of people. There can be no good reason to object to this when it is recognised that efficiency incorporates personal factors such as safety, health and quality of working life as well as system factors such as productivity and quality of work. There is rarely any conflict in that good ergonomics is in line with the objectives of the worker, the employer and the consumer or customer. There are sometimes larger issues of whether what the system does is acceptable or not, for example in weapon systems, and the ergonomist as a citizen will have his own opinion on these matters but the ergonomist as an ergonomist is confined to questions of efficiency.

There is an underlying necessary ethic which is best summarised as the social contract. An individual is a member of a community from which he obtains considerable benefits, in return he develops special skills which he applies for the benefit of the community. The application of special skills in this way is called work. The ergonomist has to believe that work is a good thing and that to conduct it efficiently is always better than to conduct it inefficiently.

1.1.2   The design of systems
The system concept

A system is a set of interacting parts which has meaning as a whole because it is possible to define a purpose – a reason why the parts are seen to be related to the whole and a justification for the concept of the whole (Singleton, 1974). Thus, systems theory is essentially teleological – explanations are in terms of consequences rather than causes. The parts may themselves be complex and may be conceived as having their own subsidiary purposes in confluence with the system purpose, these are sub-systems. The system in turn is part of a larger complex – the parent system. Thus, systems are hierarchical and at each level the unit is considered as a functional rather than a physical entity.

The systems approach is often a convenient way of looking at human behaviour either internally – this is man as a set of sub-systems or in terms of the man interacting with mechanisms – man–machine systems, or man interacting with organisations – socio-technical systems. The enormous flexibility of the systems approach has its penalties in potential confusion due to the highly variable relationship between functional and physical entities. Sometimes this relationship is fairly close; for example, in the nervous system, the endocrine system, the digestive system and so on, and sometimes it remains almost entirely unknown, for example, the perceptual system and the decision-making system. These last two are obviously each related to the nervous system and to the brain but not necessarily to a particular part of the brain and taken together they overlap in such obscure ways that they are best regarded as sub-systems in different domains, one can talk in terms of one or the other but not both simultaneously.

Systems theory is a useful way of identifying complex entities, particularly those which have a functional unity and of talking about relationships but it remains at some level of abstraction from reality. For example, to solve any design problem there has at some stage to be a switch from systems thinking to thinking in terms of physical entities because these are the things that can be created, precisely located and manipulated in the real world. Nevertheless, there are enormous dividends in being able to discuss functions independently of physical mechanisms and to explain relationships without being restricted to established and readily observable physical connections or separations.

For example, thinking of a power station as a way of translating energy from fuel into electric power enables the designer to consider various options. Should the fuel be of a fossil type such as coal or oil or should it be the radioactive elements in a nuclear reaction? When the heat has appeared how best should it be taken away – by pressurised water, by steam, by liquid sodium or by carbon dioxide? This heat has to be turned into mechanical energy, currently always by a steam turbine and the mechanical energy in a rotating shaft is then translated by a generator into electricity. The losses in this transfer of energy from one form to another can be calculated and the flow through the various sub-systems can be traced. The initial consideration of the power station as an energy processing system aids design discussions about the relative advantages and limitations of various mechanisms and their perform-ance in practice. As the system operates it has to be controlled. The control of the flow of energy is partly through automatic servomechanisms and partly through human operations. The design problem of which does what is also best thought about initially in system terms. Distinct from the flow of energy the designer is, at this stage, thinking about the flow of information. Energy and information are processed by systems and sub-systems. In these terms, the human operator is a particular sub-system. Mechanical devices and human operators are not comparable physically beyond the mundane level of size but they are comparable as different sub-systems whose performance can be described and assessed in terms of the common metrics of energy and informa-tion. Hence the importance of systems concepts to ergonomics. If the human operator is to control functions within other sub-systems he must receive information about the system state through a man–machine interface. This interface takes its physical form in the control room. The control room is part of the communications channel between the human operators and the mech-anisms and its design, as a man–machine interface, is one of the key ergonomics problems in power stations.

Office organisations also can be considered as systems. There will be certain physical mechanisms such as telephones, typewriters and computers but the flow of energy is trivial and the interest centres entirely on the flow of information. Consider, for example, a travel office. There is a vast amount of information available either in printed form or through computer networks.The objectives are to help members of the public to find their way through this information store and to transmit their orders for particular journeys or holidays to the providers of those services. The manager or designer of the office has to consider the various sub-systems he requires; one for dealing with enquiries, one for handling money, one for receiving new information, one for confirming orders and so on. The interface between the public and the information store is a counter manned by people. The counter assistants are parts of the interface. Information is exchanged verbally and through written documentation. In this kind of office the variety of requests for service is probably such that it would be necessary to provide a set of categories of the main kinds of activities or functions. It would then be possible to devise the appropriate system for presenting the required information. It is a very different situation from a power station control room but nevertheless the same principles of starting by the analysis of the required information apply.

The power station, the travel office and all other man-made systems have in common the employment of people so that sub-systems are required which are associated with personnel functions. It is necessary to attract and select staff, to train them, to provide them with various services and with potentiality for advancement as their skills increase with experience. The design of tasks is the common ground between personnel activities such as training and engineering activities such as workplace design.

Consideration of people in system terms provides the possibility of generalisations which apply across great varieties of physical and intellectual activities. The resulting knowledge is the content of ergonomics. Fig. 1.2 shows the outline of the systems design process in a way which emphasises the parallel roles of the engineer and the ergonomist concerned respectively with the design of the hardware and the personnel sub-systems and their common design problems of allocation of function and interface design.

The design of high technology systems

The insertion of an adequate Human Factors approach into a comprehensive design process is not easy, partly for the reason mentioned already that it has not habitually been regarded as necessary and partly because it cuts across all other decision-making. The Human Factors specialist can rightly be accused of wanting to have a finger in every pie because, as he sees it, behavioural considerations do affect every design decision. If ergonomics was confined to, say, the determination of the physical dimensions of the workspace then it would be more readily accepted by traditional designers, but the broad claim that ergonomics has a contribution to make to every design and operational aspect which involves the behaviour of people is a proposition which it is much more difficult for an engineer or other designer to digest (Fig. 1.3).

The questions begin with the formulation of the design objectives. What are

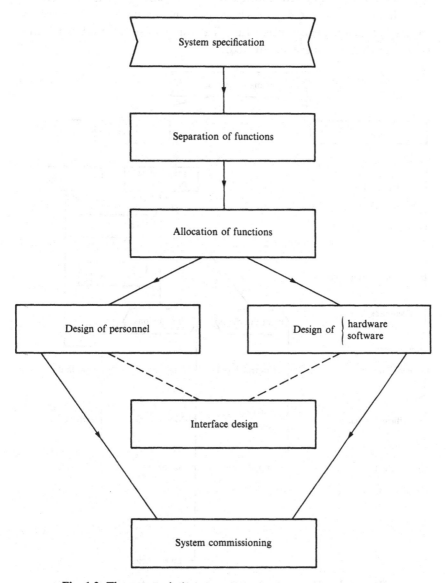

Fig. 1.2. The system design process.

the human requirements which the new product or process is intended to meet and how far are they not met by those already available? This would normally be regarded as a matter for economists and market-research specialists but behind the formidable array of evidence which they will generate are more fundamental questions of consumer preference, customer requirements and so on which are matters of human needs and prejudices. Competent market research should cover these aspects but the ergonomist can remind the policy-makers that such evidence is needed and that it should be acquired by studies of people which are properly conducted.

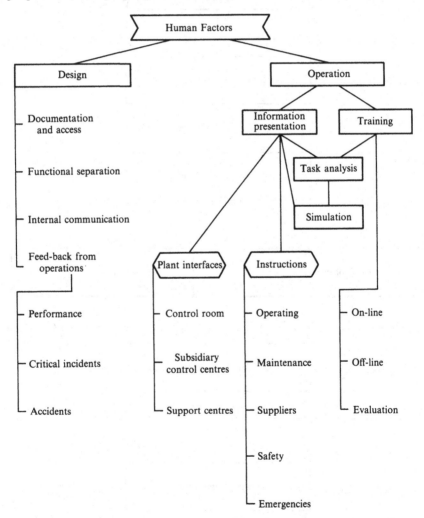

Fig. 1.3. The Human Factors contribution to system design.

If the evidence is favourable then the next step will be to set up a design team containing members covering the relevant range of expertise. How much design effort is needed in the different areas will not be clear at this stage but unless the system is very simple there are bound to be problems of overlap and of how far to arrange sub-teams by discipline, by function or by problem (Singleton, 1987). The usual compromise is that there should be problem-orientated sub-teams but with additional support available from discipline-orientated specialists. If these latter are part of the design team then already we have a matrix organisation but they may well be provided on a service basis from some other part of the parent organisation. Difficulties will emerge later unless considerable thought is given at this stage to the appropriate range of skills required and the consequent problems of interdisciplinary communication. The art of good sub-system design is to identify problem areas where work can proceed relatively independently of other areas so that the need for intercommunication is minimised. There will always be the need for some intercommunication and the appropriate interfaces should be provided. Nevertheless, if committees, working parties and task forces begin to proliferate within the design team, this is a sure indication that the basic allocation into sub-systems was not optimal. Communication should be mainly through the central command and control centre which may be no larger than the project leader and his small personal staff as may be a group of heads of sub-systems or both. These issues are discussed from another viewpoint in Chapter 3 (p. 140).

The analysis of required skills ought in principle to have an ergonomics input but in practice it is usually done on the basis of experience of similar system designs in the past. There can be a useful discussion between the project leader and an ergonomist where the former is invited to clarify how he sees these intercommunication problems being dealt with including such criteria as what is reported to him, what to the meeting of sub-heads and what occurs directly between sub-teams. Organisational rules of this kind can be very helpful in steering between the excessive information flow, e.g. memoranda copied to many people, and excessive unilateralism, e.g. refusing further discussion after the issue of formal documents. Having allocated the human and other resources needed for the overall design task it is then appropriate to develop a more detailed model of the system functions in terms of materials, energy and information flow. Most designers have an intuitive but unformalised picture in these terms but it is of great utility to produce these pictures in flow diagram form so that any differences of view are revealed and can be reconciled by discussions during the process of agreeing the diagrams.

When there are a number of individuals or groups from different disciplines and pursuing different objectives within some overall specification it is obviously crucial that all their activities should be in line with the common goal. To this end, it is necessary that there should be intercommunication not only about particular design decisions but also about underlying philosophies so that the ultimate system is conceptually as well as operationally coherent. Sometimes this is achieved by a dominant project leader who imposes his own philosophy and then makes many of the decisions leaving only detailing for team members. In recent times it is more usual to have some element of discussion, partly because of the increasingly democratic style of organisations and partly because the variety of relevant technology requires a correspondingly wide range of expertise. In any case there is a need for widespread intercommunication which may be mainly informal but requires some formality to ensure that clashes of attitude do not delay or distort decisions and to make sure also that finalised decisions are unambiguously recorded. If this intercommunication is not properly arranged there will be the familiar symptoms of frustrating reiteration, decisions being misunderstood or being constantly revised, political manoeuvring and even concealment of progress within one or more of the teams. As the overall design progresses the information storage system becomes increasingly important. If insufficient attention has been devoted to the design of this and also the related access procedures the symptoms are a plethora of documentation which no individual entirely understands, the temptation to do it again rather than waste time finding out how something has already been done and too much reliance on the human memory. The behavioural symptoms of inadequate organisation of design teams are summarised in Table 1.1.

As the system is made more definitive by the selection of particular physical mechanisms there should be parallel activity in the consideration of how these things are to be used and maintained by the human operator. Note that the philosophy here is that all the hardware is ultimately an extension of and a support for human functions. This is the concept of all systems as human beings with various kinds of engineering aids (Singleton, 1967a). Functions are delegated from the human operator rather than allocated to him. This extreme ergonomics stance serves as an antidote to the equally extreme engineering approach in which systems are regarded basically as hardware which for reasons of economic or technological limitations have to depend occasionally on some human performance. Even if there is no dependence on human performance in the on-line operational mode it is bound to exist in the maintenance mode.

In either case, there will eventually be a need for the consideration of the kinds of human operators required and how they are to be selected and trained. Traditionally these personnel functions were regarded as quite separate from

Table 1.1. *Behavioural symptoms of inadequate design team organisation*
(from Singleton, 1987)

---

1. Internal memoranda copied as a matter of routine to many colleagues.
2. The setting up of internal (and interminable) working parties, sub-committees and task forces.
3. Invitations to attend meetings not because of any potential direct contribution but in a representational or liaison role.
4. The setting up of committees which are allowed or even encouraged to write their own terms of reference.
5. Contention between individuals or sections particularly about demarcation.
6. Perpetual reconsideration of matters about which firm decisions have already been made, possibly because the previous decision is not accepted, more usually because there are inadequate records and insufficiently structured access to records of decisions.
7. Poor documentation and indexing of documents.
8. Excessive reliance on the human memory.
9. Secretiveness about progress to reduce the possibility of interference by others.
10. Inadequate leadership and communications so that there are insufficient consistencies in style of problem solving.

---

design functions and indeed they were often left until the hardware design and commissioning was virtually complete. The essence of the systems approach is that personnel decisions should proceed in parallel with engineering decisions, partly to economise on development time and partly to provide scope for trade-offs. One factor which has given renewed emphasis to this need for cooperation is the increased use of simulation (p. 128). Simulators were originally considered to be training devices but their use is now extending into other fields such as personnel assessment and as aids to the design of the information interfaces. It used to be considered that simulator specifications could only be proposed when the on-line system design had been completed but there are considerable advantages in developing the simulator before the on-line system so that it becomes a dynamic mock-up of the real situation. Detailed evaluations can be carried out on this mock-up before the real system is constructed.

All systems are constructed from bought-in components which may themselves be complex enough to warrant a human factors evaluation. For example, a motor/pump system may well have its own controls, there will be standard maintenance procedures and there will be an operation/maintenance manual. All of these can be assessed from the point of view of clarity of presentation and ease of use.

The system being constructed will require its own operating instructions, maintenance procedures and perhaps safety regulations. The design and preparation of this documentation has a Human Factors component. It is a matter of storage, access to and presentation of information. Even at the design stage it is useful also to recognise that all this material will require procedures for updating in the light of experience

Finally it must be accepted that technological and operational expertise is never complete. The operators of plant are bound to discover by experience aspects of the design which could be improved. There should be a mechanism for feeding this information back to the designers so that the succeeding system designs will avoid these problems. In particular, human performance within systems is impossible to predict with any precision and details of this performance as it occurs in practice or on simulators is the only basis for prediction on matters such as safety and system reliability either for the current system or for future systems. Potential human factors inputs to the large scale design process are summarised in Fig. 1.4.

In all behavioural matters and indeed in many technical matters also it is important to avoid the impression that when operations in practice contain undesirable features not predicted by designers then the designers have made mistakes. This may be true in a formal sense but allocation of blame is not usually a productive exercise particularly from a learning view-point. It is valuable to inculcate the attitude that everyone learns, that is, design and operating staff all improve on the basis of experience with feed-back. The exposure and remedy of facets of systems performance which are not entirely as predicted is in everyone's interest. One example of this is matters to do with safety: it is always useful to collect 'critical incident' data as well as accident data as one part of the feed-back about system performances. The setting up of routines for this communication is another aspect of ergonomics.

In summary, although the basic contribution of the ergonomist is to the design of information interfaces these interfaces extend far beyond the man–machine interface found in the control room. They include the documentation of the design itself, communication within the design team, between designers and suppliers and between designers and operators (Fig. 1.5). The operations staff include those who set it up, those who control it during operations, those who maintain it, and eventually those who have to dismantle it. To give one example of the size of the documentation problem it is not unusual for a large process plant to have two or three hundred volumes of instructions. These include the operating instructions, the maintenance instructions, the suppliers' instruction manuals, the safety regulations and instructions for particular emergencies.

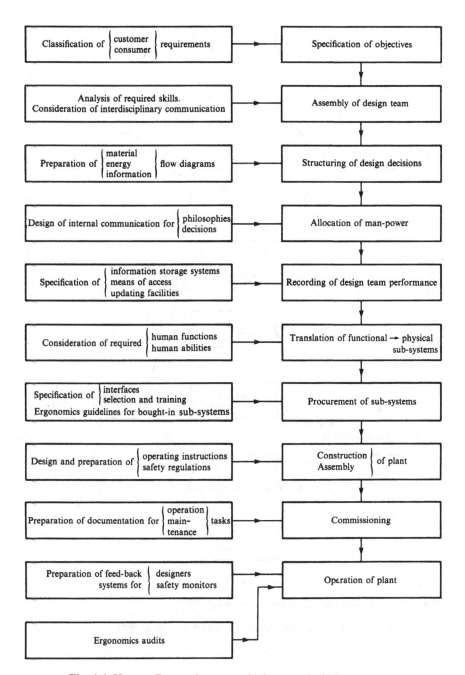

Fig. 1.4. Human Factors inputs to the large-scale design process.

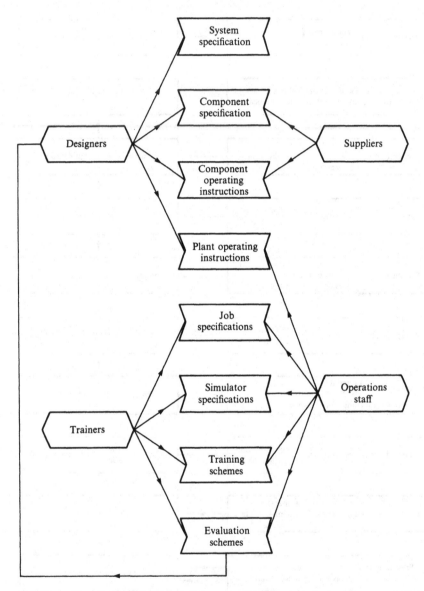

N.B. To avoid confusion only the main linkages are shown.

Fig. 1.5. Information sources in a complex system design.

The design of smaller systems

The design of a machine or device which is assigned as an aid for one person will not usually encounter the problems associated with elaborate design teams just described, but nevertheless some human factors sensitivity will help to provide a better product. This can be important not only from the point of view of efficiency in design and use but also in improving the sales appeal. It is increasingly common for advertisements to emphasise features such as 'man–machine harmony' or 'user friendliness'. The implication is that ergonomics has been properly applied.

There is a need for formal ergonomics in any design where the designer himself is not an experienced user. Some hand tools are beautifully designed to match the user, e.g. the two-handed scythe. In these cases it is clear that the design developed by constant trial in practice. There are others, however, where even after centuries of use this matching is not obviously satisfactory, for example violin playing would seem to be posturally a disaster, but there may be some subtle aids to very precise control of the sound generated in having the source of sound very close to the ear and perhaps some vibration transmission by the direct contact of this instrument and the jawbone.

Ergonomics is concerned with the transmission of information. For modest design enterprises information exchange is needed between the designer and the potential user, between the designer and the producer and between the designer/producer and the customer/actual user (Fig. 1.6).

The designer needs to know about the tasks which his new device is intended to aid and also about the kind of person who will use it. Clearly, designing for fit young men in the armed forces has different constraints from designing for middle-aged female workers in manufacturing. Some of the required informa-

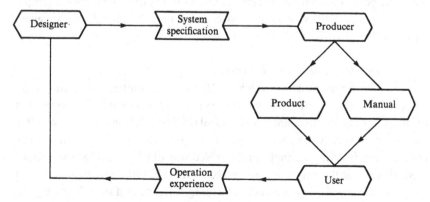

Fig. 1.6. Information interfaces in a simple design system.

tion may be susceptible to precise description in numerical terms such as body size and strength, but most of it will be of the 'awareness' kind when the designer recognises broadly that particular kinds of people have particular advantages and limitations. Similarly the range of tasks for which the device is required may not be known in the kind of detail which is available from comprehensive task descriptions but the designer will consider the extremes of what it is likely to be used for and the environment in which it will be used, for example designing a machine-tool for use in a factory has different requirements from designing a powered garden tool where the user could be wearing heavy gloves, will not be wearing safety-boots and will not receive any formal training.

Communication between the designer and the producer used to be done almost entirely by traditional engineering drawings but there is now a tendency to use sketches, schematic drawings, photographs and models including computer-based models, for example complicated shapes in three dimensions are difficult to represent as rectangular projections and are not easily interpreted.

Communication with the customer/user takes the form of operating instructions which are contained in an instruction book. The design of this book, booklet or even leaflet is a much neglected art and is frequently very badly executed – hence the common attitude reflected in the aphorism 'when all else fails try reading the instructions'. The most common failings are to rely too much on words rather than extensively labelled diagrams, to use technical terms and concepts which the user may not understand, to focus on what it is at the expense of what it does and to fail to separate the needs of the operator from the details which are needed to set up the device, to locate faults, to provide remedies and to provide routine maintenance. An extended booklet should have a very good index or other access system to the information. The designer is not the person to evaluate the clarity and usability of instructions, a sample of actual users will provide a much better assessment. Further details are given on p. 76.

The design of macro-systems

The larger systems which make up communities and nations are currently in a state of flux because of the impact of technology. The provision of such a variety of telecommunication and travel facilities makes it impossible for any community however large or small to develop in isolation. The consequence is an increasingly standardised way of life or at least aspirations towards a particular way of life across the world. The differences which remain are enforced mainly by differences in average income and in style of government. Technology continues to change jobs with consequent changes in ways of life and it also changes life-expectation which has profound effects on all communities.

However, just as hardware systems are dominated by engineering thinking, macro-systems are dominated by economic thinking. There is excessive reliance on the adaptability of people who are required to adjust to whatever is dictated by economic and technological policies. Politicians in all countries would accept the proposition that the system should be designed to serve the people but whatever the political philosophy behind the system, the people always seem to be more its servants than its masters. Economic issues are real enough and it is often pointed out that politics is about priorities. The priorities are assessed on the basis of evidence and unfortunately evidence about people is not so readily quantified as evidence about financial and physical resources. The result is that systems at every level from the state to the small company are evaluated and policies are developed which are not sufficiently orientated to the needs and aspirations of the people within the system. This is a very large issue mostly beyond the scope of this book except to note that ergonomics is an exemplar of a style of thinking which is based on characteristics of people. Ergonomics can be defined as systems design with the attributes of people as the frame of reference.

Although the human operator is for many purposes within ergonomics appropriately considered as a mere information processing device, any design issue must be considered in the context that these human operators are individuals and citizens within communities. What they believe, what they want, what they like, what they dislike and whether they work efficiently or not are determined by the societal context as well as by the physical environment. It is therefore appropriate to bear in mind the position and trends in human resources in the community of which the workers are members.

For such macro-systems, the principle that the designer produces what he thinks the users need is being replaced by the principle that the users themselves decide what they want and the professionals assist them in designing as specified by the users. This approach generates another duty for designers and ergonomists, to present to the users an array of possible options which will aid their discussions and choices.

1.2　Knowledge

1.2.1　Demographic data

Currently there are about 4.5 billion people in the world, 1 billion in the developed world and 3.5 billion in the developing world (Table 1.2). This puts a correct perspective on the contents of this book which are mainly concerned with technologically-based societies although there is a section in

Table 1.2. *World population 1983*

(U.N. demographic year book)

		Population (millions)	Proportion of total
Oceania		24	0.5%
North America		259	5.5%
U.S.S.R.		273	5.8%
Europe		489	10.4%
	Sub-total	1045	22.3%
South America		388	8.2%
Africa		521	11.1%
Asia		2731	58.3%
	Sub-total	3640	77.7%
	Total	4685	100.0%

Table 1.3. *Age distribution of populations*

(*The Economist*, 1981)

	Age Group %			Life Expectation (years at birth)	
	<15	15–64	65+	Male	Female
U.S.A.	24	65	11	69	77
U.K.	22	63	15	70	76
Australia	27	64	9	68	74
India	41	56	3	42	41
Ethiopia	43	54	3	37	40
Guatemala	45	52	3	48	50

Chapter 3 on ergonomics in developing countries. Most of the evidence and experience reported here has been derived from the 16% of the world population living in Europe and North America.

The two worlds differ markedly in the distribution of populations, developed countries have about 65% of the population in the economically active age range from 15–64 years, about 25% under 15 and the remaining 10% in retirement. This last group is still increasing quite rapidly. The retired group is much smaller in developing countries where about 55% are in the economically active age range and more than 40% are under 15. Life expectation at birth is about 45 years in developing countries and more than 70 years in developed countries. The longer life expectation of females is more marked in the developed countries (Table 1.3).

The age distribution of the working population for two countries, one developed and one developing, which happen to have the same sized labour force is shown in Fig. 1.7. West Germany has a greater proportion of people economically active but they start work later and retire earlier than do workers in Pakistan.

There are about 4 million research and development scientists and engineers in the world, 3.5 million in developed countries and 0.5 million in developing countries, almost all this latter 0.5 million are in Asia, the numbers in Latin America and Africa are very small (UNESCO statistical year book).

The differences in various amenities are shown in Table 1.4. The energy consumption is about 100 units (kg of coal equivalent per person) in a developing country and about 10 000 units in Europe and the U.S.A. This is affected by the fact that developing countries mostly have tropical or sub-tropical climates while developed countries are in the temperate zone, but there is a similar difference of about 100 : 1 in income per head between the rich countries and the poor countries (*The Economist* – the world in figures).

Within any country the Human Resource situation can be approached by this basic division into the 'economically active' and others who, for one reason or another, are supported by the workers. Those supported include young children, students, retired persons, seriously disabled persons, people living on independent means and, somewhat unfairly, women doing domestic work. The numbers and proportions of those economically active in a sample of developed countries are shown in Table 1.5. It will be seen that in each country this economically active group is about half the total population. For males the proportion is usually about 55% and for females about 45%. A very large economy such as the U.S.A. has more than 100 million workers, the large European countries have about 25 million workers. Japan is about half-way between with about 60 million workers. The smaller European countries have less than 5 million workers. Workers in this sense are a country's Human Resource which is deployed for the benefit of the community generally.

The primary need of any person or population is water and food and in primitive societies the supply of these commodities will absorb the effort of almost all the workforce. As food supplies improve it is possible to move some of the Human Resource into construction and manufacturing. In the U.K. the concentration on manufacturing in the nineteenth century was balanced by the importing of food. France, by contrast, had a smaller manufacturing base but remained self-sufficient in food so that the dramatic fall of proportion of

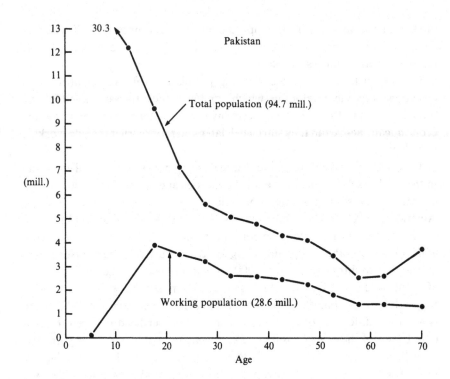

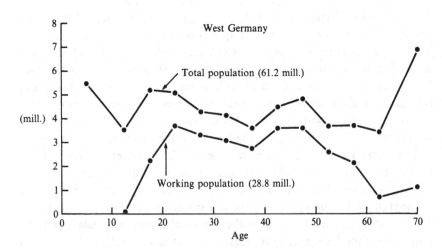

Fig. 1.7. Age distributions of populations and labour forces (I.L.O. data).

Table 1.4. *Available amenities (1978/1979)*

(*The Economist*, 1981)

	Electricity billion kwh	Cars per 1000 pers.	Telephones per 1000 pers.
U.S.A.	2340	531	769
U.K.	300	267	442
India	106	1.3	4
Nigeria	5	5.5	2

Table 1.5. *The 'human resource' of a sample of countries*

(I.L.O. data)

	Economically active (in millions)			Population Total
	Males	Females	Total	
U.S.A.	63.8 (56%)	49.7 (41%)	113.5 (48%)	236
Japan	35.8 (61%)	23.5 (39%)	59.3 (49%)	120
France	14.0 (53%)	9.6 (35%)	23.5 (43%)	54
U.K.	16.0 (59%)	10.3 (36%)	26.3 (47%)	56
West Germany	18.0 (60%)	11.3 (35%)	28.8 (47%)	61
Switzerland	2.0 (63%)	1.0 (34%)	3.1 (49%)	6
Sweden	2.2 (54%)	1.8 (43%)	4.0 (48%)	8
Netherlands	3.8 (54%)	1.9 (26%)	5.7 (40%)	14

The percentages are of the total male, female and grand total populations respectively.

workers in primary industries did not occur until after World War II (Fig. 1.8). In the U.S.A. even at the time of President Lincoln about 1860 there was serious debate as to whether the economy should remain agricultural or whether there should be a positive attempt to develop manufacturing. In India the total population is currently about 665 million of which 244 million (37%) are economically active. 153 million are engaged in agriculture and fishing, that is 63% of the working population (I.L.O. data). In the U.K. less than 3% of the working population are now employed in agriculture, in most advanced countries this figure is now well below 10%, as illustrated in Fig. 1.9. This also shows that the predominant way of earning a living in a developed country

Primary – agriculture, fishing, forestry
Secondary – manufacturing
Tertiary – commerce, transport, services

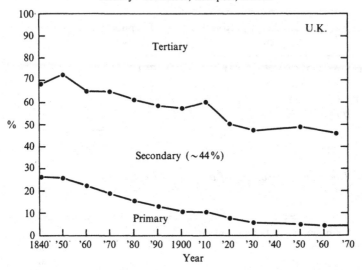

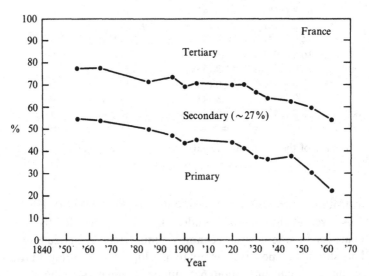

Fig. 1.8. Distributions of labour forces and changes over a century (I.L.O. data).

now is in the service industries. Fig. 1.10 shows the current distribution of U.K. Human Resources. The former basic industries – mining, agriculture, construction and manufacturing – now employ about a third of the total workforce. In manufacturing between 1980 and 1985 output measured per person-hour or per person employed increased by about 25% but the total

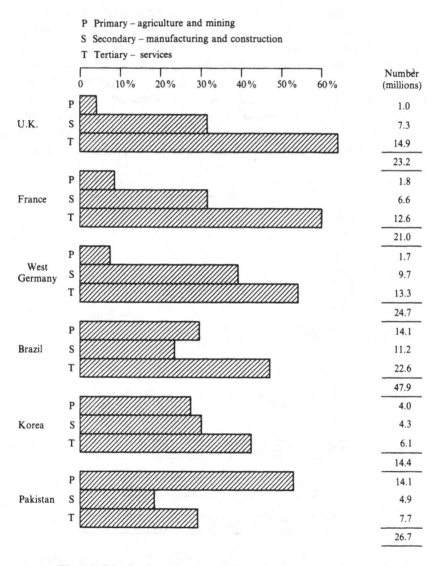

Fig. 1.9. Distribution of economically active population between industries (I.L.O. data 1984).

output remained roughly constant, that is the manufacturing labour force is still falling rapidly (*Economic Trends* 1985). Some consequences of these trends are discussed in more detail in Singleton and Crawley (1980).

From the end of World War II to the early 1970s there was virtually full employment in developed countries, but in the last ten years the position has changed considerably as shown in Fig. 1.11. Apart from Ireland it would seem that the smaller European countries have contained the situation better than have the larger ones, but this is an artefact since other small countries such as Belgium, Netherlands and Denmark follow the same trend as the larger countries. It should be noted that the trend of an increase in unemployment from about 5% to about 10% over ten years is sufficiently general to indicate that it is not a function of the style of government. These data for countries do not reveal considerable underlying differences within countries. In England for example, unemployment in the North is twice that in the South-East, and in most European countries there are lesser employment opportunities in rural

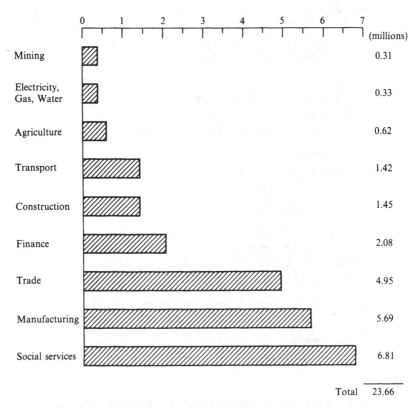

Fig. 1.10. Distribution of U.K. labour force (I.L.O. data).

areas as opposed to urban areas resulting in depopulation of the countryside and an increase in the size of cities. This trend is even more marked in developing countries.

1.2.2 Human resource utilisation

This brief excursion into the complex field of labour statistics is intended to illustrate the following points which are relevant to the theory and practice of ergonomics.

1.   Since the beginnings of technology, now about 200 years ago in the case of the U.K., the labour market has been in a continuous state of flux.
2.   The overall shift has not been so much from agriculture to manufacturing but rather a steady rise in the service industries, and a fall in primary industries.
3.   The manufacturing labour force in developed countries is now in

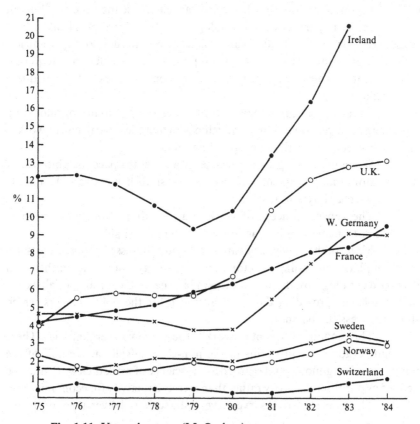

Fig. 1.11. Unemployment (I.L.O. data).

accelerating decline as productivity and the investment per worker increases, this is resulting in a further increase in service industries and an increase in unemployment.

4.   There are considerable differences between the problems of so-called developed and developing countries. This dichotomy is useful but is an oversimplification; degree of development as measured for example by income per head or technology utilisation is best described by a continuous scale. A particular country is at one point on that scale at one time by one measure.

5.   Accelerating technological development has pushed the government of every country off-balance in the past decade. This is illustrated in developed countries by the increase in unemployment which is fundamentally a failure to properly utilise the total Human Resource. In developing countries there are many contrasts in that high technology (airlines, nuclear power, information systems, etc.) exists in small pockets alongside the still unresolved traditional problems of inadequate nutrition and health.

6.   Ergonomics also is pushed off-balance because the variety of human work increases in parallel with technology. The traditional problems of heat stress and physical work-load remain, particularly in the developing countries, while new problems appear as more complex systems are designed requiring new operator roles and more serious consequences of inadequate performance.

7.   Nevertheless technology now provides the possibility of allocating high energy and repetitive work to machines so that the typical man at work is in a supervising rather than an operating mode.

8.   When machines provide the energy and set the pace the objective of the operator (and consequently of ergonomics) shifts from rates and amounts to quality, reliability and safety.

9.   The general concept of work is also shifting from man–machine interaction to man–man interaction with machines as aids.

10.   Many of the policy issues are mistakenly addressed in that there is too much emphasis on finding uses for what technology can provide rather than driving technology by the needs of people. The behavioural specialists are responsible for providing data and attitudes for the policy-makers which should redress the balance.

11.   The economic concept of work is too narrow for ergonomics. There are many ergonomics problems in the non-economically active half of the population. If ergonomics is regarded as the science of work then work must be defined as purposeful activity rather than merely as activity for economic gain.

12.   This brief statistical survey reveals the scale and diversity of problems

associated with the mind at work. This is daunting but it is also challenging and stimulating.

1.3   Principles, methods and procedures
1.3.1   Education, work and leisure

Virtually all human societies have developed the principle that the pattern of personal activity should change with age. In the early years there is extensive leisure devoted to play in which the basic manipulative and social skills are developed. There is also more formalised learning through an educational system which concentrates mainly on information processing: reading, writing and arithmetic and more elaborate symbolic and organisational skills. When the individual has matured he usually accepts responsibilities for child-rearing and for work. In his declining years the proportion of leisure increases again, sometimes suddenly when he 'retires' but preferably gradually as his energies diminish.

Thus we can normally expect a mature mind in a person at work and although developmental processes of growth and senescence are of some interest, studies of the person working usually assume that we are dealing with a mind which is equipped with the basic skills derived from play and education but one which has not been subject to any serious diminution of capacity. This is not to suggest that the age variable can be ignored. It is accepted that ageing is a continuous process from birth to death and there are considerable differences between the average worker in the 25–45 age group and the apparent equivalent in the 46–65 age group. The age distribution of a particular workforce can materially affect the problems of work design and training.

Correspondingly it must be recognised that an individual has entered work with a particular educational standard. During his working years he has considerable leisure which is bound to have some interactions with work. For approximate computational purposes it is normally assumed in the western world that a full working year is no more than 200 man-days. The remaining 165 days disappear in week-ends, holidays and absence for training, sickness and so on. There is also a widespread convention that the working day should be 7–8 hours, that is about a third of the total day. Thus the full-time worker is in fact working for less than 20% of the total time.

The distinction between work and leisure and between work and education is an arbitrary one from the point of view of stress on the person. For example, many city office workers regard the main stress of the day as the difficulties in getting from home to work and back again with work as a relatively relaxed period between. Even more strikingly, some working mothers regard a period at work, particularly if it is part-time, as a welcome respite from the great variety of stresses arising in looking after a home and children. Some of the most exacting university degrees, such as those in the biological and physical sciences demand a level of work load from the conscientious student which is greater than that expected in most occupations.

One would expect self-selected leisure activities to be different from and complementary to those at work. For example, the manual labourer is unlikely to take up an energetic hobby such as cycling and he is likely to spend his holidays relaxing at the seaside rather than walking in the mountains. The young office worker in a safe sedentary job may well take up rock-climbing as a dangerous, physically exacting antidote for the dull occupational part of his life.

Although it would be convenient scientifically and sometimes personally to regard work as a separable part of a human life this separation is never entirely valid and can be misleading. The mind at work is part of the person at work and that same person has many other activities in the past and the future and in parallel which have their interactions with the work.

In system jargon, the working world is one sub-system within a complete set of sub-systems which make up the total environment or life space of the individual. To study one sub-system in detail without regard to interactions with the others is usually inadequate, but on the other hand, to try to examine simultaneously the whole complex of sub-systems is to invite disorientation. The remedy is a compromise in which activity in one sub-system such as that which incorporates work is studied but in the context of sensitivity to external influences.

Systems theory can be applied in many ways to behaviour at work. The two main theories emphasise respectively interactions with other people; *socio-technical systems* and interactions with machines; *man–machine systems*.

1.3.2 Socio-technical systems

In the period of technological innovation following the second world war a group of human relations specialists, working from the Tavistock Institute in London, noted that the social behaviour of workers and their organisational structure in groups and teams was influenced by the technical systems associated with that work.

The first studies were in coal mines where there were different degrees of mechanisation associated with the same type of working group and it was also possible to distinguish different social organisations working in similar technical environments (Trist and Murray, 1948). Some groups were organised so that each worker carried out an independent part-task with little reference to the total task, whereas in other cases each worker had a commitment to the total task and carried out various sub-tasks in this context. This latter, labelled a 'composite' group as distinct from a conventional group, had greater productive achievement and lower absenteeism.

More generally, the effectiveness of the production system depends on the way the social system is adjusted to the technical requirements (Emery and Trist, 1960). Technological decisions necessarily dominate the design of the system in the sense of how the collective task of transforming inputs into outputs is achieved. Nevertheless, the social system which integrates the activities of the workers and provides the flexibility for relating separate tasks to the needs of the production system as a whole must be considered. Hence the concept of the socio-technical system where technical and social requirements are harmonised into one effective organisation.

The organisation, like a living organism, maintains a dynamic equilibrium with the environment. Thus it is an open system rather than a closed one and its behaviour cannot be understood by simply looking at the relationship between inputs and outputs. The adaptability of the enterprise may lie in providing appropriate outputs to match the changes of the market from relatively stable physical inputs or may lie in providing a fixed output with changing sources of inputs. In either case there is no fixed relationship between physical inputs and outputs, the system responds to the environment. It follows that one of the main tasks of management is to control the interaction with the environment. The implication also is that, if management has got the technology right within the system design, it should then attend to the environment and should allow, within the internal activities, scope for self-organising into autonomous groups. If, on the contrary, there is a rigid internal separation between the roles of setting standards and meeting standards then conflict has been built into the system (Klein, 1979).

This approach can legitimately be regarded as the parent of organisation theory (p. 143), and of the 'quality of working life' (QWOL), sometimes also called the 'job design' movement (Davis and Cherns 1975, Davis and Taylor 1972). It provides considerable insight into the eventual difficulties of the early twentieth century mass production methods as exemplified by the moving belt type assembly line. On the other hand it does not provide remedies for production problems which can be applied as standard recipes or procedures. Again, because of the elusive if all-pervading nature of the theme, it is difficult to formalise into legislation on humanising work as several European countries have discovered by experience.

It has emerged in many countries that, as the standard of living rises, it is more and more difficult to run an autocratic production system using the indigenous labour force. The first management remedy is to import a more docile labour force from another country or from a less developed part of the same country. This is only a temporary solution and there have been many attempts to organise more humane working systems. The danger here is that, although things may be pleasant for the workers, the incentive to work very hard is not so direct and it may not be possible to maintain a competitive position in comparison with the same industry in a developing country. Hence a further development of research on work motivation (p. 144).

Taking a more global view, one opinion is that the manufacturing industries should indeed move to developing countries whilst the advanced industries orientate their labour forces toward information and other service industries. There is a trend in this direction (Singleton and Crawley, 1980), but, of course, it is not the complete answer. There are other complications. Robots, for example, are best suited for the highly repetitive manufacturing tasks which are the ones least suited to human efforts so that robotisation can cure some of the ills of mass production. Looking at the environment, as market demands become more sophisticated so there is a need for operator flexibility in production system outputs, which has its counterpart in greater variety of work within the production system (Lupton and Tanner, 1980).

Socio-technical system theory has been highly fruitful in generating other academic lines of development: organisation theory, quality of working life concepts and work motivation, in stimulating many innovations in production organisation and in provoking governments to consider legislation in matters such as humanisation of work (Germany) and co-determination at work (Sweden). Paradoxically it has not developed a formalised set of principles or immutable knowledge which could, for example, be structured into an academic text-book about socio-technical systems. The problem seems to be that it is fundamentally about attitudes to work and such attitudes are subject to an inextricable and non-monotonic range of influences not only from work itself, with all the pressures of technological change, but also from prevailing economic, social and cultural changes in the community generally.

1.3.3 Man–machine systems

Work is very rarely performed by a man without the aid of some machinery and correspondingly machines rarely function for very long without human intervention. Man and machine can be regarded as sub-systems each making a distinctive contribution towards the achievement of the purposes of the working system. The system itself can be described as a set of functions necessary for the overall purpose. The emphasis on defining the system in terms of its purposes or objectives and analysing it in terms of its functions are the characteristics of the systems approach.

It follows that at some stage in the design process it should be useful to consider how the various functions are most effectively allocated – to man or to machine. Fig. 1.2 shows the essentials of the system design process but since feed-back paths are omitted this figure does not indicate either the repetition and iteration which goes on in operational design or the different possible priorities and variability in the order of decision-making. The engineering emphasis will be on the search for mechanisms which can most effectively perform the required functions with the human operator in a support role undertaking functions which are not readily mechanised. The ergonomics emphasis will be on the human operator as the navigator moving towards the system objectives supported by various mechanisms. One neutral viewpoint is to consider formally the relative advantages and limitations of men and machines. These can be listed (Table 1.6) on what is called a 'Fitts List' after Paul Fitts who originally proposed this approach (Fitts, 1951). At the time it was hoped that eventually it would be possible to refine the quantitative distinctions between the performance of men and machines so that allocation of function decisions would be unambiguous (Wulfeck and Zeitlin, 1962), but this has not happened. The reason seems to be that men and machines are fundamentally complementary rather than comparable, this point was originally made by Jordan (1963). If a required function can be specified precisely then a mechanism can be designed to perform it. The reasons for incorporating men in systems are to do with properties such as flexibility and adaptability which by their nature are not specifiable in numerical terms.

Incidentally this clarifies why the man–machine system is such a potent combination. Each provides attributes which are not easily available from the other. A man without the support of machinery is physically weak and informationally slow. A machine without human guidance is inflexible and highly limited in recognition and learning facilities. Nevertheless it is not common practice to consider the man–machine allocation of function as an isolated design decision. More usually the allocation emerges from a pattern of related decisions including what can be reliably and economically achieved by hardware and software, what the allocated tasks look like as integrated jobs for the human operators, the skills and traditions of the available work-force, the importance of safety and reliability and so on (Table 1.7). As potential functional weaknesses emerge during the design appraisal further consideration is given to what functions might be allocated to the man or machine to provide greater mutual support. The result of selective competent design along these lines should be a system with optimal man–machine allocation given the technological state of the art and a comprehensive sensitivity to the feasibility of the human tasks. A detailed discussion of the historical development of the allocation of function concept is given in Singleton (1974).

Table 1.6. *Relative advantages of man and machines (Fitts' List)*

Attribute	Machine	Man
Speed	Much superior	Comparatively slow, measured in seconds
Power output	Much superior in level and consistency	Comparatively weak, can spurt to about 1500 watts, less than 150 watts over a working day
Consistency	Ideal for consistent repetitive activity	Not reliable, always subject to learning and fatigue
Informational capacity	Can be multichannel. Information transmission in megabits/s	Mainly single channel. Low information transmission rate – usually less than 10 bits/s
Memory	Ideal for literal reproduction, access restricted and formal	Better for principles and strategies, access versatile and innovative
Reasoning	Good deductive	Good inductive
Computation	Tedious to programme. Fast. Accurate. Poor at error correction.	Easy to reprogramme. Slow. Inaccurate. Good at error correction
Sensing	Specialised and relatively narrow in range	Wide energy ranges, some multifunction
	Good at quantitative assessment. Poor at pattern assessment	Poor at quantitative assessment. Good at pattern detection and interpretation
Perceiving	Poor at coping with variation in written and spoken material. Poor at detecting messages in noise	Good at coping with variation in written and spoken material
		Good at detecting messages in noise

This approach contravenes currently fashionable Human Factors methodology that there should be a formal attempt to carry out man–machine allocation. Operational experience of real systems design reinforces doubts about the allocation of function concept as a basis for a unitary systematic procedure. The paradigm illustrated in Fig. 1.12 has the virtue of simplicity. Like many block diagrams this conceals the practical problems. From such a simple diagram it is easy to assume that all the thinking is done in terms of functions. This cannot be sustained because the only way to validate task analysis is to switch from functional concepts to behavioural concepts and the only way to validate hardware concepts is to switch to thinking in terms of

Table 1.7. *'Allocation of function' design decision-making*

1. How has technology advanced since the previously designed system? Can new substitutions be made for human tasks? Can new aids for human tasks be provided?
2. Is there any evidence of excessive stress on human operators in earlier systems? e.g. accident data, illness and absence data, data on systems failures due to human error?
3. Did jobs in earlier systems function well as integrated sets of tasks? Do managers report any problems of obtaining, training, supervising or keeping good operators?
4. Have there been relevant labour market changes? e.g. costs, attitude changes, availability.
5. Is there any case for upgrading or downgrading required levels of operator skills? Is there any case for increasing or decreasing staff numbers?
6. Are there any changes in problems of safety and reliability either externally, e.g. new legal requirements or internally, e.g. more dangerous technical processes?
7. Does the external or internal industry image need to be changed or reinforced?

specific mechanisms. Thus, allocation of function requires a continuous juggling of functional, mechanistic and behavioural approaches.

In addition to the separate criteria related to men and mechanisms there are others to do with information acquisition, storage and presentation focussing on the interface design which has its own design criteria. Note that a real problem usually involves men rather than one man and thus there are extensive man–man communication issues where few of the functions could conceivably be allocated to non-human mechanisms. In a military command and control situation these will typically be sub-system operators, supervisors and customers using the output (p. 243). Even when design attention can be focussed on the interaction within a single man–machine sub-system it emerges that the man may have very different roles in setting-up, operation and maintenance of his particular machine and each role may require separate man–machine allocation considerations.

A designer is often restricted by various mandatory requirements based for example on imagined safeguards against accidents. There are also unspecifiable but none the less potent political restrictions, some from within the organisation, some from outside it. For example the use of nuclear power in either the military or the civil sense is regarded as qualitatively different from non-nuclear power in its safety, control and management requirements.

Design is never an isolated logical process. There is a legacy of experience from earlier designs which inevitably guide and inhibit a new design. The shifts of allocation of function from this point of view are illustrated in Fig. 1.13.

Swain and Wohl (1961) argue that the man–machine concept is oversimplified, it should be man–machine procedures allocation and also that prime equipment should be separated from check-out equipment (Fig. 1.14).

In equipment involving advanced technology the allocation of the control function is between the on-line operator and the designer. The latter builds decisions into the hardware and software based on his knowledge of the limitations of the mechanisms. High technology can also be used to provide the operator with flexibility in the allocation of functions, he can make his own

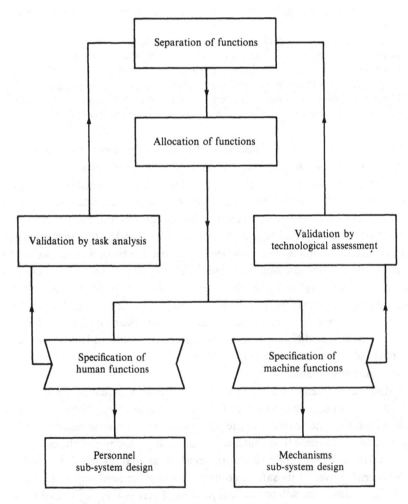

Fig. 1.12. The 'Allocation of Function' concept.

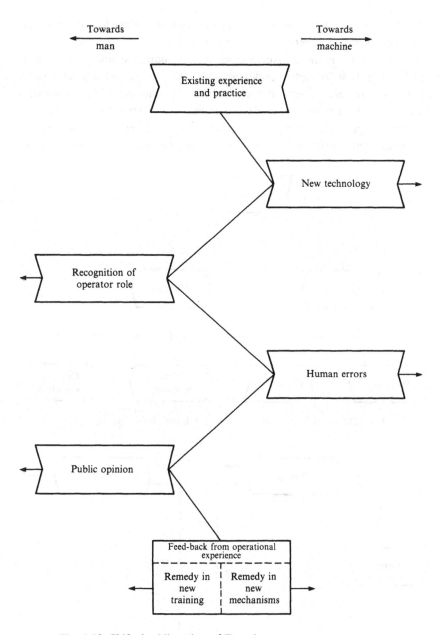

Fig. 1.13. Shifts in Allocation of Function.

decision about when to control manually and when to leave it to the mechanisms. This is called supervisory control (Fig. 1.15)

It emerges from the above discussion that man–machine allocation of function is at best an oversimplification and it may lead to the neglect of some key features of human performance. Only the human operator can cope with the concept of purposes and goals and more particularly with their modification in the light of changing circumstances. Knowledge of circumstances is communicated partly by information exchange across man–machine inter-

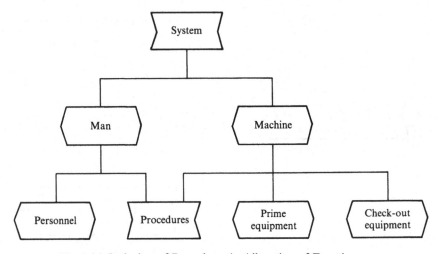

Fig. 1.14. Inclusion of Procedures in Allocation of Function.

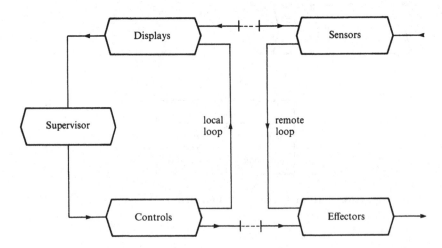

Fig. 1.15. Supervisory Control (after Sheridan and Johannsen, 1976).

faces but also by verbal exchanges between people. These verbal exchanges can be factual but can also be diffuse in the sharing of attitudes, beliefs, urgencies, doubts and so on. These features are just as important to efficient performance as are data about plant functions but they cannot be incorporated in a man–machine allocation process.

Implicit in the attempt to complete a systematic man–machine function allocation is the principle that some trade-off is possible. More attention to the hardware and information presentation will yield improved operator support whereas more attention to operator training will minimise the difficulties of interpreting information presentations and thereby making full use of machines (Singleton, 1967b). These alternative procedures are summarised by the expressions 'fitting the man to the job' or 'fitting the job to the man'. The systems approach indicates that the two should be balanced on technical, economic and behavioural criteria (Table 1.8.). To proceed systematically, both require that there should be the greatest possible understanding of what the man is required to do. The design of the man–machine interface must develop from an understanding of how the man is expected to interact with the machine and correspondingly the design of selection, allocation and training schemes depends on knowing what is required of the operator. The study of demands on the operator requires task analysis. In this context the term 'machine' is used as shorthand for the total hardware and software system or, in other terminology, the plant.

For information systems the allocation of function and interface design issues merge into the procedure for considering the required points of human intervention in the total information network. From this point of view the allocation of function and interface design are one core design activity based on the man–machine concept.

1.3.4 Task analysis
Terminology

In the context of systems design, task analysis has become the generic term applicable to the field study of human performance. This is somewhat confusing because the centre of interest may be jobs or skills rather than tasks, and strictly the procedure is often more accurately described as one of synthesis rather than analysis. For example, a designer may build up a sequence of actions which an operator must follow in order to cause his product to function properly – he has synthesised the task from a knowledge of how the machine or other product was designed to function. Nevertheless, such activity comes under the heading of task analysis (Fig. 1.16).

Tasks represent the human contribution to system performance but for

Table 1.8. *Trade-offs in 'allocation of function'*

Economic Criteria

1. Manning costs are particularly high if there is a requirement for a twenty-four hour presence. Five or six teams are needed to work a full shift system (p. 187). Considerable investment in automatic equipment is justified to remove the need for one such operator

2. Broadly the human operator is not directly expensive in initial cost but requires very high continuous expenditure. Thus using human operators can reduce capital cost at the expense of greater running costs

3. Full overheads are usually more than 100%, that is the total cost of operator is more than twice the wages cost but on the other hand equipment overheads (maintenance and spares) are of the same order

Technical Criteria

4. The technical support per operator is so extensive in high technology as to warrant the highest quality operators

5. Increased technical support for maintenance operations is still best developed as human aids rather than as independent automatic devices

6. Automatic systems are particularly efficient if they can function for a matter of days without any human intervention, e.g. if they can be left working overnight and over weekends

7. Increased automation is usually at the expense of flexibility and adaptability unless the technical support directly aids human performance, e.g. in computer-aided decision-making

Social Criteria

8. Tasks may be allocated to human operators for secondary reasons. For example, to round off a job which otherwise is not integral, to provide slots for operators who are employed but not otherwise needed, and to maintain arousal level by insertion of regular checking and recording tasks

9. Tasks are often allocated to human operators because of the trends and traditions in particular industries rather than because of an unavoidable technical demand

10. Tasks may be allocated to human operators to avoid redundancies which have considerable social and economic costs

---

purposes of personnel selection, training and allocation, it is necessary for tasks to be separated or combined into jobs. For systems which have evolved on the basis of operational experience rather than those which have been created by a formal design process, job analysis rather than task analysis may be the starting point of human factors studies. The ergonomist will begin his investigation by the consideration of what the personnel actually do in their jobs which have emerged and been refined by practice and personal preference rather than design.

A *task* is usually considered to be an integrated sub-activity with a particular purpose as distinct from a *job* which is a particular kind of work carried out by an individual in a system context. Jobs are collections of tasks or parts of tasks. *Occupation* is the wider term which covers a range of jobs and the career of an individual in a community context. For example, management is an occupation, a production manager is a job, and work scheduling is a task. These distinctions are demonstrated in Fig. 1.17. Another source of ambiguity is that task analysis is often used as a generic term covering any study and description relating to people at work. Sometimes this is no more than a description of what has to be done but sometimes it incorporates how the operator does it or should do it. Strictly, this latter should be called a *skill description* rather than a task description. In principle a task description is not necessarily an activity of

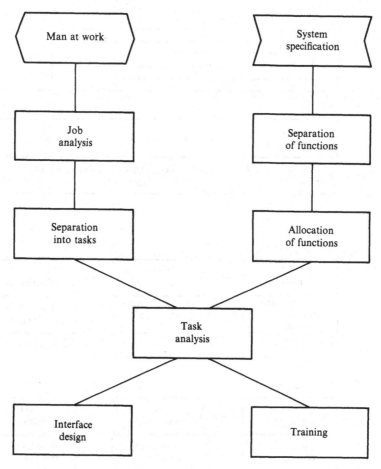

Fig. 1.16. The central role of task analysis.

a person, the task might possibly be completed automatically. There is no such ambiguity about a *skills analysis* which is always person-orientated and not just system-orientated. This confusion of terms obscures even further the difficult technical problems of moving from a task description to a skill description. The task description should emerge logically from the system design and more particularly from the allocation of functions. There is no such deductive way of getting at the skill description. This can only be done by studying operators.

There are two problems in analysing tasks: one is to acquire the evidence on which to base the task description, the other is to record what has been found out in a way such that other people, notably the interface designers and the personnel specialists, can use it effectively to assist in their work. It aids clarity

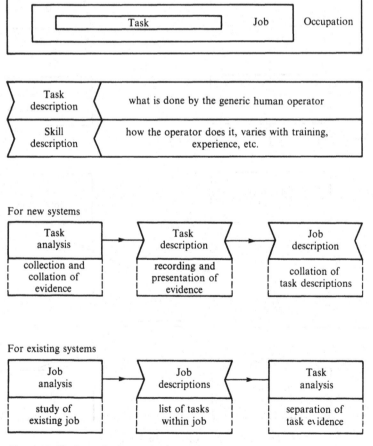

Fig. 1.17. Task analysis terminology.

to reserve the term *analysis* to mean the acquisition of evidence and *description* to mean the presentation of the evidence.

The test of a task description is: does it indicate a necessary function within the system performance? The test of a skill description is: does it indicate how an individual goes about a task, does it allow for individual differences such as those between a highly skilled operator and a mediocre one? For routine low-level tasks there may be no great distinction between a task description and skill description but for high-level tasks there will be a considerable difference. Skills analysis is an attempt to get at what is going on in the operator's mind. For a repetitive task there may be comparatively little going on in the mind which emerges at the level of consciousness. For example, the assembly of a set of components will be carried out by an experienced operator without thinking about it. He may be surprised when the analyst reveals the complexities of his hand movements and finger manipulations. The only way he can recall what he does is by doing it, literally 'going through the motions'. On the other hand, for a task such as fault diagnosis he will be thinking about it in various structured ways which he can reveal by talking about it and exploring verbally why he looks at particular indications or takes particular actions.

Human tasks and the purposes of task analysis are too varied for there to be one standard procedure for either analysis or description. Analysing a task where the main requirement is speed of response is different from analysing a task in which problem solving is required. A task analysis in the context of 'fitting the man to the job' can be very different from one designed to assist in 'fitting the job to the man'. As mentioned above the two extremes of human tasks are the procedure and the diagnosis.

Procedural task analysis is usually initiated on the basis of technology and logic by the designer. A task has been allocated to the human operator and what he must do is a function of the needs of the hardware. Such tasks may be in operation or maintenance. In either case the designer writes down the sequence of actions which must be taken coupled with informational indications of what should be happening. For example, in starting up a machine or system (Table 1.9). Effectively the operating instructions are the task description. It is, of course, desirable to check that nothing has been forgotten and to this end it is usual to ask an operator to go through the designed procedure while observing what he does and also observing that the system performs as expected. This may be done on the machine if it is available, or on a simulator or on some kind of mock-up of what the system will be like. This is known as the *talk through* or *walk through* method of task analysis. The difference is only in the kind of task and size of hardware. For example, in the case of starting up a machine at a control panel the operator will be given the instructions and

Table 1.9. *Start-up procedure for a machine tool*

Purpose	Action	Indication
1. Check that no tools, components or other materials have been left in positions where there might be interference with machine running	General inspection and walk around	nothing out of place
2. Check that all tools and controls are in neutral or off positions	General inspection and walk around	positions of tools and controls
3. Provide power supply	Operate isolator lever	lever position noise and feel
4. Switch on	Press labelled button	red light and noise
5. Switch on lubricant motor/ pump	Press labelled button	red light and lubricant flow
6. Switch on main motor	Press labelled button	red light and noise
7. Switch on auxiliary motors	Press labelled buttons	red light and noise changes

asked to provide a verbal commentary as he actuates the various controls and checks the various indications, this is a 'talk through'. On the other hand, a maintenance check of a series of related machines may involve moving to and fro between them while activating this and that, this is a 'walk through'.

The operating instructions/task description can be modified if the analysis reveals any problems from the operator's point of view; anything which the designer may have omitted or any difficulties the operator has in moving around, manipulating controls or checking information presentations. Ultimately, the machine layout or interface design may be modified to make the operating instructions easier to follow.

For complex processes the procedures can include stages of diagnosis (see below) because the operator has to monitor and interpret what is happening in the plant. In particular he is aware of various conditional constraints which form a multidimensional envelope, and whatever happens he must keep the plant state within this envelope. Thus he must have extensive knowledge of the parameters and their relationship, e.g. pressure/temperature curves, together with the safety limits of each parameter. Sometimes the safety limits are fixed, sometimes they are conditional on the state of other variables or plant, sometimes they are merely probabilistic. This is an extremely difficult task, and

Table 1.10. *Increasing order of diagnostic task difficulties for a control room operator*

Fault	Indication	Likely cause
1. Single component	Changes in pressures/ voltages	Routine malfunction
2. Failure of an instrument	Inconsistencies in readings and displays	Routine malfunction
3. Simultaneous failures of components	Confused pattern of display changes	Series of failures: one component has overstressed others causing them also to fail
4. Simultaneous failures of instruments	False indications which may be difficult to reconcile	Common mode failure
5. Simultaneous failures of some components and instrument readings	Mixture of true and false indications	Accident in plant such as fire or collision
6. Widespread failure of components and instruments	Extensive display discrepancies	Accidental or malicious but unstructured damage
7. Strange pattern of failures	Indications which suggest that the plant is fighting the operator	Deliberate expert damage

the operator requires various aids such as alarm systems and automatic cut-out devices which are also effectively monitoring the parameters approaching limits (see alarm systems p. 225).

    Diagnostic task analysis is even more complex and may indeed be virtually impossible to complete. It depends on the complexity of the task faced by the operator. The range of diagnostic task difficulties for a control centre is shown in Table 1.10. The operator is assumed to be reacting to a situation in a control room, containing a great variety of dials, charts, and computer driven displays together with the controls needed to take action in any part of the system. The simplest thing that can go wrong is the failure of one mechanism such as a pump, valve or thermostat. This will be indicated in the control room by changes in pressures and temperatures which the skilled operator will trace readily to the particular failure. Usually there will be some redundancy in the system so that other mechanisms can take over. If the hiatus is serious he may have to shut down all or part of the system or it may trip automatically and the operator's task is to observe/control the shut-down to a quiescent state.

The worst possible condition that can be envisaged is one in which there is an expert in the plant aiming to do the maximum possible damage and aware of the indications of his actions which are transmitted to the operator – this is not quite science-fiction, it could happen as a form of sabotage. A much less demanding condition is one in which the saboteur is attempting to damage a plant about which he has little or no technical knowledge.

However, the difficult condition which requires the most consideration because it is not that unlikely is one in which the operator is faced with a situation where various things have gone wrong naturally or by inadvertent human interference in the plant or instrumentation. His diagnostic task is somehow to differentiate between the information he is receiving which is false and that which is valid and follow this by the selection of a remedial strategy. There are further complications in that, because of the plant failures, not all the standard range of remedial actions will be available. Some automatic reactions may be taking place which might help or hinder, and he must also stay within the mandatory operating instructions. Unfortunately, because such situations are created by combinations of events the number of possibilities is very large and it would be prohibitively tedious to enumerate all of them. A complete task description is impossible and the appropriate preparation for the operator is not in direct training but rather in education/understanding of the system and the way it operates. He must attempt his diagnosis by returning to the relevant scientific and technological principles. How he does this in general terms is illustrated in Fig. 1.18. The task analysis will take the form of a consideration of the most likely or most dangerous failure and combinations of failures and the ways in which these will appear as indications in the control room. This should occur not only at the design stage but also as experience develops in operating the plant and data on actual failures and failure rates become available. Such task analysis can only be carried out to some cost-effective limit beyond which the skilled operator must be trusted to get things right by applying his broad expertise. This is not as much of a gamble as it may appear at first sight, there are general principles of how to cope with the system, some of which can be built into automatic safeguards and some of which can be conveyed to the operator as knowledge and instructions. In serious cases the aim is to shut down the system safely. In less serious cases the operator may for a while maintain certain parameters at appropriate levels without diverting his attention to detailed diagnosis, this is called *function control*.

In dealing with lower technology or less formal system design, there is a range of relatively standard ways of finding out about operator performance

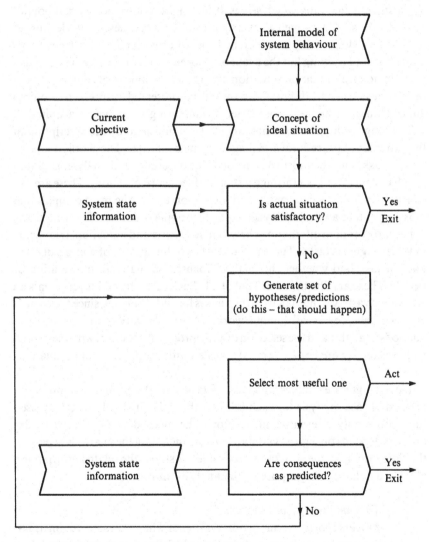

Fig. 1.18. Generic diagnostic procedure.

by studying it directly. Task analysis, in common with every other perceptual process, is a matter of setting up mechanisms for categorisation and filtering. The analyst is faced with an activity which is continuous, homogeneous and full of detail, some of which is significant and relevant and some of which is of no consequence. For example, the worker may pause at one point and scratch his nose, this may indicate that a critical decision is being made or it may indicate simply that his nose was itching. The art of task analysis always is to select what does matter, reject what does not matter and separate into categories or stages something which seems at first sight to have no internal boundaries. As already mentioned what is significant for a task description leading to an interface design may be different from what is significant for personnel allocation and training but the available procedures are the same. The acquisition of evidence and the presentation of evidence are linked, of course, in that it may be necessary to decide what should be presented before it is acquired although more usually it is a matter of presenting what can be acquired.

The range of human tasks has already been indicated by the description of the extremes of procedural and diagnostic task analysis. The simplest kind of human task, and the most straightforward to observe and analyse, is that in which the operator goes through a standard sequence of actions. These are still common in industrial assembly and inspection tasks. The most complex and most difficult to analyse are tasks requiring original thinking often with many apparently random alternations between deduction and induction, this occurs in fault diagnosis tasks. There are at least two dimensions of complexity: the kind of task and whether the analysis focuses on material, information or people. These are illustrated in Table 1.11. Each cell in this table represents an enormous variety of human work but this is hardly surprising since the total of eighteen cells covers all human work. There is a variety of task analysis methods available and the selection of an appropriate set varies with the kind of work (as represented by these cells) and also with the purposes of the analysis.

Table 1.12 gives examples of kinds of task and the probably appropriate method of task analysis for each cell in Table 1.11. It should be emphasised that this is only a tentative illustration. The method used for a particular analysis depends on a great variety of factors including the analyst's expertise, the time available, the situations accessible for study, the related information already available, the purpose of the analysis and so on.

Task analysis by observation
Process charts. Accurate observation of what a person is doing is not easy. The observer needs some discipline which ensures that he really does

Table 1.11. *Kinds of task requiring different methods of task analysis*

Focus of analysis Kind of task	A. Material	B. Information	C. People
1. Sequential	Assembly	Data entry	Data collection
2. Purpose-centred	Craft	Clerical	Serving
3. Dynamic interaction	Tracking	Process control	Negotiating
4. Resource allocation	Feeding	Supervisory control	Managing
5. Intellectual analysis	Fault finding	Data analysis	Consulting
6. Intellectual synthesis	Hardware design	System design	Work design

focus on the detail and separates the action into a coherent sequence. The required discipline is provided by the attempt to complete a chart such as a flow process chart using the A.S.M.E. symbols. These were originally standardised by the American Society of Mechanical Engineers. The symbols and an illustration of a flow process chart are shown in Fig. 1.19. It is assumed that whatever an operator is doing can be classified into one of five categories: operation, inspection, transport, delay and storage. Delay occurs when the operator is doing nothing – usually waiting for a machine to complete a sub-task – it differs from storage where there has been a particular decision to put something aside. For example, storage for a hand implies some static work – the operator is holding something or exerting a force of some kind although there is no resulting movement.

Process charts may concentrate on material, operator actions or the events in the process. These are known respectively as material-type, man-type or process-type charts. More details of these charts and how to complete them are given in ILO (1979).

The same symbols are used for a two-handed process chart in which a detailed description of what each hand is doing separately is provided (Fig.

Table 1.12. *Examples of tasks and task analysis*

Ref. Table 1.11	Kind of task	Example	Analysis
1A	Assembly	Switch assembly	Two-handed process chart
1B	Data entry	Computerised data updating	Input/output errors and timing
1C	Data Collection	Accumulating biographical data	Time-lapse film
2A	Craft	Carpentry	Sequence listing and posture
2B	Clerical	Transposing data	Data tracking
2C	Serving	Secretarial work	Discussion to identify key features
3A	Tracking	Car driving	Protocol analysis
3B	Process control	Chemical plant operating	Progressive redescription
3C	Negotiating	Employer/union representative discussion	Recording and identification of key features
4A	Feeding	Mixing animal feed stuff	Protocol analysis
4B	Supervisory control	Nuclear power-plant control	Critical incident analysis
4C	Managing	Production control	Discussion to identify key features
5A	Fault finding	Car failure	Protocol analysis
5B	Data analysis	Statistical studies	
5C	Consulting	Medical diagnosis	Construction of functional diagrams
6A	Hardware design	Engine design	
6B	System Design	Aircraft design	
6C	Work design	Training course design	

1.20). The meaning of the symbols changes somewhat because the separation of events is much more detailed. The same symbols can also be made to follow the concurrent behaviour of members of a team (Chapanis, 1959).

Note that, apart from the inspection category, the emphasis is entirely on what the operator does. Little attention is paid to the input side as distinct from the output side, the sensory information and feed-back which the operator is using to control what he is doing is neglected. This is appropriate enough for highly repetitive routine tasks because, as mentioned earlier, the operator is probably proceeding with little conscious attention and the limitation on performance is in the speed of the action rather than in the informational control.

To broaden the emphasis on a two-handed process chart it is possible to add

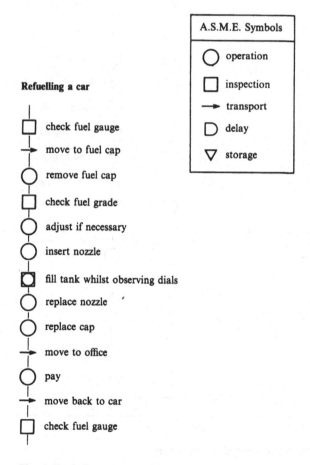

Fig. 1.19. A flow process chart.

Filling a car fuel tank

Left hand	Symbols	Right hand
check fuel grade	D □ ▽	hold key
adjust grade selector	○ □ ▽	hold key
lift cap cover	○ →	move key to cap
hold cap cover open	▽ ○	unlock cap
	▽ ○	remove cap and key
look for somewhere to put cap, release cover	○ □ ▽	hold cap and key
	D →	move cap and key
	D ○	place in safe location
	D →	move to nozzle
	D ○	pick up nozzle
reopen cap cover	○ →	move to filling tube
hold cap cover open	▽ ○	insert nozzle
replace cap cover	○ ○	press trigger
check fuel flow	D □ ▽	hold trigger on
	D ○	release trigger
open cap cover	○ ○	remove nozzle
release cap cover	○ →	move nozzle to pump
	D ○	release nozzle
	D →	move to cap and key
	D ○	pick up cap and key
open cap cover	○ →	move to filling tube
hold cover open	▽ ○	replace and lock cap
release cover	○ →	remove key
check pump dials	D □ ▽	hold key

N.B. This particular car has a spring loaded cap cover

Fig. 1.20. A two-handed process chart.

Table 1.13. *A sequence chart – starting a car*

Action	Indication
1. Adjust seating posture by manipulating height, back rest and distance controls if necessary	Feels comfortable, controls reachable, surroundings visible
2. Fit seat belt	Feels comfortable
3. Adjust interior and exterior mirrors	Rear vision satisfactory
4. Check that gears are disengaged by wiggling lever	Feels and looks satisfactory
5. Adjust choke control if not automatic	Feels and looks satisfactory Amber light appears
6. Switch on ignition	Warning lights appear
7. Engage starter motor	Characteristic noise
8. Check that engine is running	Red light disappears, characteristic noise and vibration if accelerator is pressed
9. Prepare to move and switch on direction indicator	Road clear front and rear, winking green light
10. Engage gear	Slight car movement
11. Press accelerator and release clutch if not automatic	Car moves

another column labelled 'attention' or 'sensory activity' and to try to describe human activity in these areas at particular points in the sequence. This goes beyond direct observations and requires some inference or speculation on the part of the observer.

Finer analysis of hand movements is possible using classifications such as Therbligs (Shaw, 1952), or Methods-Time-Measurement symbols (Maynard *et al.*, 1956). Analysis at this level of detail is not usually attempted by direct observation but rather by film or video analysis.

Sequence charts. These are similar to flow process charts except that no standard symbols are used, the chart is simply a list of the actions the operator takes but there may well be additional columns referring to the events which occur and the consequent information which appears. A sequence chart is more appropriate for a routine interaction with a machine rather than a physical manipulation of objects. An example is given in Table 1.13. Sequence charts are particularly useful for the study and description of starting up and shutting down procedures. They form the basis for procedural training.

Table 1.14. *A link design chart: Starting up a micro-computer*

Purpose	Trigger	Action	Check	
Provide power	Wish to start	Press wall-switch	Red light	A
Check no discs in place	None	Open drive doors	No discs visible	B
Switch processor on	B complete	Press switch	Fan motor noise	C
Switch printer on	C complete	Press switch	Print head zeros	D
Insert discs	D complete	Insert discs close doors	Display illuminates	E
Load discs	E complete	Press keys	Loading noise. Display indicates loading	F

Link design charts. This is a detailed sequence chart orientated more towards operator choice of actions and correspondingly relevant to the study of interface design rather than training (Singleton, 1964).

It is assumed that for every action the operator has a purpose, the choice of the particular action at the particular time or point in the sequence is triggered by some other event, usually the successful completion of an action is indicated by a particular information presentation which also is noted on the chart. The chart is particularly useful for detecting when information about action completion is not available and when an action is required which is not triggered by information from the situation. That is, the operator has to depend on his memory (which is unreliable). An example is given in Table 1.14.

Flow charts. These are more graphical presentations as distinct from verbal listings. They are used to indicate the spatial location and separation of events which are integral parts of the same process. An illustration of a flow chart is given in Fig. 1.21.

It is possible to obtain a kind of flow chart automatically as it were by using successive photographs of operator positions on the same photographic plate. More usually, this is done by attaching lights to the wrists or to other parts of the body, if the light is flashing at a known frequency the relative time of particular positions as well as the sequence can be measured. This is called a *chronocyclograph*. Flow charts are a useful record of a process but are not particularly suited as a basis for analysis which might lead to improved job design or training. On the other hand, they can clearly indicate differences in ways of doing something.

Block diagrams. These are particularly useful to describe situations where events occur in parallel or in patterns rather than in a single series. The block diagram is highly versatile as a spatial representation of any process at any level, that is the same process can be represented by one block or by very many blocks which provide more detail. The art of useful block diagram production is to select the appropriate level of detail. Most people find such diagrams much easier to understand than paragraphs of explanatory prose but the flexibility itself can lead to the difficulties illustrated in Fig. 1.22.

Taking a car out of a garage with a pull-up door

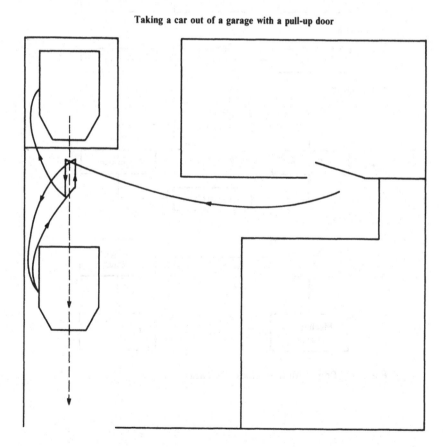

Fig. 1.21. A flow chart.

1. Avoid mixed levels of complexity

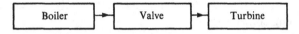

2. Avoid mixed categories in blocks

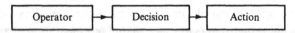

3. Avoid mixed categories in lines/arrows

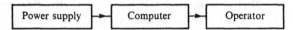

4. Do not confuse diagrams and inverse diagrams

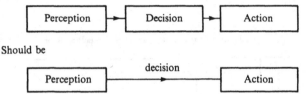

5. A block/line diagram

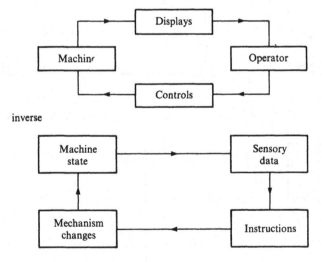

Fig. 1.22. Preparation of block diagrams.

It is important that blocks are at about the same level of complexity within one diagram. Blocks may represent physical entities, topics, concepts, decisions, actions or processes. If these are mixed in the same diagram the distinctions between categories should be indicated by using differently shaped blocks. Many of the figures in this chapter illustrate this convention.

Homogeneity is also desirable in the meaning of lines and arrows. A line may indicate a causal link but simple cause–effect relationships are destroyed if there are feed-back lines. Usually the line represents the flow of something but that something might be material, energy, information or time but again these should not be mixed on the same diagram unless differently coded lines are used.

It is usually possible to invert a diagram so that blocks and lines are interchanged. One of the more subtle failures is to confuse a block diagram with its inverse. An inverted block diagram can be a path–node diagram. The advantage of these is that the length of the path can be used to indicate time taken. This is the basis of 'critical-path analysis' where such a network can be analysed. The shortest path through a network is the minimum time in which the whole process represented could be completed. The longest sequence of required activities is the time it will take if no adjustments are made. An optimum path can be selected and other activities adjusted to phase in with those on this 'critical path'. There are formal techniques of network analysis which occasionally prove useful; for example, in identifying equivalent diagrams or ways of simplifying diagrams (Battersby, 1970).

Algorithm charts. These are a particular form of block diagram where the emphasis is on binary choices. Again there can be concentration on events or on operator decisions. In the latter case these are usually an oversimplification because there is an underlying assumption that decisions are being made in a simple logical sequence. In practice, the operator jumps forwards and backwards within the pattern indicated on the chart rechecking some decisions and anticipating others.

Nevertheless, by relating required information to decision points any lack of information can be revealed. It invariably turns out that an operator makes a series of decisions partly on the basis of what is currently displayed (*on-line information*) and partly on the basis of other material obtained from his knowledge of the system performance, his briefing and his operating instructions (*off-line information*). Adequate on-line and off-line information is essential for apposite decision-making. Fig. 1.23 shows such a chart.

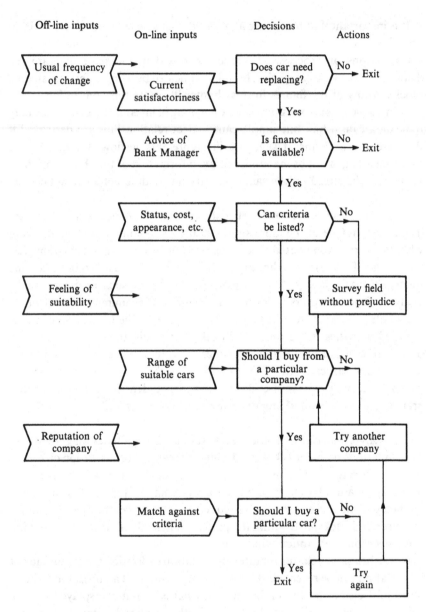

Fig. 1.23. Algorithm for car replacement.

F.A.S.T. diagram. Function Analysis System Technique was developed by Bytheway (1977) within value engineering. It imposes useful discipline on the production of a functional diagram in two ways. Within each block the function should be described by a verb and a noun. The functions are arranged in a sequence such that an arrow to the right on any line indicates HOW? and an arrow to the left indicates WHY? If these criteria cannot be met then either the functions are in the wrong order or some are missing. The diagram should be produced by writing each function on a card, the cards are then arranged to meet the criteria. Unfortunately the resulting diagram is not so easy to interpret as are some of the other forms of chart. In particular there is no obvious starting or ending point and the lines do not indicate a sequence. Fig. 1.24 shows an example.

General functional diagrams. As a Task Description, a block diagram is intended to illustrate the dynamic behaviour of the system with emphasis on human interactions within the system. For some purposes it is appropriate to use blocks and lines to indicate the flow of energy or material and to indicate all the ways in which the human operator can affect this flow. This is not a performance diagram but a potential performance diagram (Fig. 1.25). For other purposes it is appropriate to concentrate on a specific sequential task and illustrate the order of events involving human actions (e.g. Figs. 1.19 and 1.20). If a particular dimension (usually left to right or up to down) indicates a time scale as well as sequence this is called a *time-line diagram*. The blocks may even be omitted to further emphasise the relative timing of events. (Fig. 1.26).

Alternatively if the process is highly complex the emphasis may be on the pattern of events as indicated by a network of blocks with a specialist symbol indicating the many points within the system for which information for the operator might appear and another symbol for points where he can interfere in the system dynamics (Fig. 1.27).

Task analysis by discussion

Observation of operator performance within many high technology systems reveals nothing more than a person sitting at a desk scanning various kinds of displays at intervals and just occasionally picking up a telephone, making a note in a log-book or manipulating a control. In such situations, the task analysis requires extensive discussion rather than observation. Such discussions will centre on the operators themselves but may also involve others such as the management, the training officers, the safety specialists and the system designers. There will often be complications in that there can be two or more operators working simultaneously with overlapping tasks. The supervisor may also monitor the same information or may have his own separate displays or both. In such a team operation there will normally be a clear standard mandatory difference of responsibility but in practice what they actually do can overlap and overlap differently for different teams. Inevitably, discussion with different individuals about a particular task will yield very

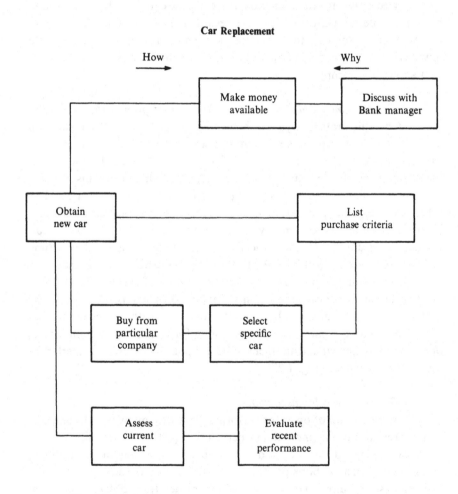

Fig. 1.24. F.A.S.T. chart.

different versions of what is being done or should be done. If there is a written version of what ought to be being done this is a useful basic document. However the supervisor will point out that things have changed since that was produced and he will have his own view of the essentials of the task. The operators themselves will again have a different version. The differences will be

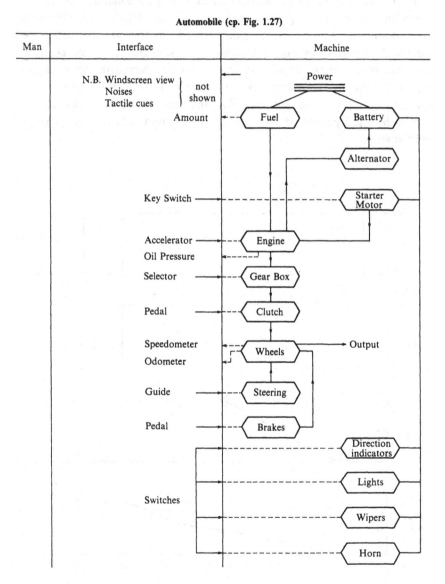

Fig. 1.25. M.M.I. chart.

mainly in emphasis on what is important central activity and what is peripheral. Even between operators carrying out what is ostensibly the same task there will be discrepancies, particularly if the discussion extends from what is required to the way these requirements are met. Similarly the specialists, the training officers, task designers and safety officers will have their own version structured in terms of the particular difficulties they have had in their specific contributions to the task performance. Finally, task descriptions differ with the personal biases of analysts and the reasons why they are conducting the analysis. However, in spite of all these sources of ambiguity the comprehensive task description is the essential starting point for most human factors work. An approach structured by a particular procedure is of considerable assistance in reducing ambiguity and ensuring that the result is comprehensive. The approach might consist of any one or any combination of the following techniques.

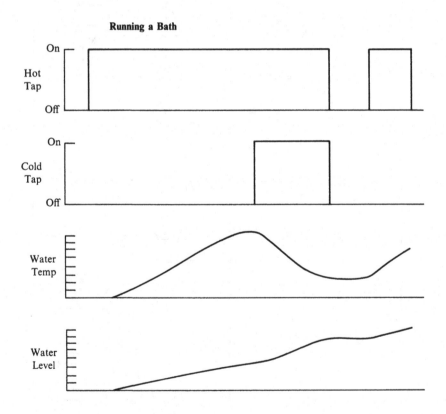

Fig. 1.26. Time-line diagram.

Responsibility charts. A useful starting point for the study of any system is a responsibility chart. This can indicate not only the hierarchy but also the different levels of modelling the system. Normally, the operators closest to the plant will have the most detailed information and this gets condensed or reduced as one moves up the hierarchy. For example in a power station the desk operator will monitor the detail of the plant performance, the supervisor will have more summarised information and greater contact with the national grid, while the station manager's on-line information about the plant is presented on one or at the most two dials in his office which indicate station output. A responsibility chart can indicate not only decisions and duties but also the information needed to discharge these duties (Table 1.15).

Although it is usual to model responsibilities in terms of a hierarchical tree there are bound to be overlaps between what appear to be different levels of the hierarchy. These shared or duplicated responsibilities are unavoidable and often in fact are desirable because the process is one of mutual monitoring which usually improves reliability. Occasionally overlap may have the opposite effect due to the 'falling between two stools' phenomenon, two operators at the same level or at different levels may each assume that the other has taken a particular action which they both know is required. The remedy is adequate information feed-back and continuous checking but the need for this may not

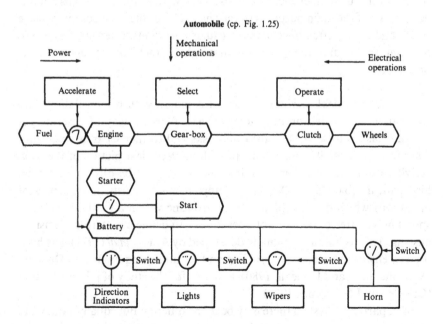

Fig. 1.27. Interface-Network diagram.

Table 1.15. *Responsibility chart*

Hierarchy	Responsibilities	Information needed
Production director	Liaison with Sales / Marketing	Sales achieved Marketing objectives Production performance
Production manager	Meeting production targets Provision of resources Costs	Production schedule Details of people, machines, materials, power, costs, etc.
Foremen	Quality / Quantity of products at a particular stage	Current functioning of people, machines, production
Production planner	Flow of work Availability of materials	Production schedule Production flow Materials position
Operatives	Quantity / Quality of products for each batch	Work available / completed Standards achieved

be obvious from the chart because the areas of overlap are difficult to illustrate. It makes for much neater charting to assume that there are no overlaps but this defeats one of the main purposes of the chart. Hence the most comprehensive and useful charts often have many irregular comments, asterisks, footnotes, directing arrows and so on, which at first sight detract from the clarity of the presentation.

Hierarchical Analysis. Tasks, in common with responsibilities, are susceptible to subdivision at different levels. A useful way of describing a complex task is to separate it into sub-tasks and further separate these sub-tasks into even smaller units. This provides a very clear picture of the total activity although the order of doing things may not be obvious. Such an hierarchical table (Fig. 1.28) can be supplemented by lists or sequences of operations which define a plan or a sub-routine within a total task. Correspondingly, a tree or network of operations can define a pattern of decision-making. This technique, originally developed by Annett *et al* (1971), has been used extensively as a basis for training and retraining requirements (Duncan, 1975, Shepherd and Duncan, 1980), and also for the study of job satisfaction (Crawley and Spurgeon, 1979).

For a particular system there may be many different but equally valid ways of separating tasks into sub-tasks depending on the relative emphasis on training, interface design and other system design aspects. Sometimes a 'bottom-up' approach may be better than a 'top-down' one.

Protocol analysis. An operator carrying out a task can be asked to talk about what he is doing as he does it. Clearly this is useful for tasks which involve extensive scanning of information sources and deliberations about what action to take. The visible action may apparently be trivial – adjusting one or two of very many available controls – or may even be non-existent. This sort of task is very common in process control situations where the operator often makes a preliminary three-way decision corresponding to the world-wide system of red, amber and green traffic lights. That is, he does nothing, he does nothing at the moment but prepares for action, or he takes action. Because so much of the activity is in searching for information and processing it leading to a decision, the observed output is obviously a poor indicator of total activity and his verbal commentary is a much better guide to his task performance. Such a commentary can be recorded or notes can be taken directly by the analyst. The snag about recording is that an enormous amount of material is produced which is very tedious to analyse. The presentation of the result may use any of the charting methods described in this chapter, or may take the form of a descriptive narrative.

M.C.I. Job–process analysis. Man–Computer Interaction has further complicated the relationship between human operators and other parts of a system but the computer can help to analyse these interactions. Tainsh (1985) has developed a technique in which a computer-based simulation of a generic information handling task is used to assist in analysing the behaviour of an operator or a team of operators. There are two V.D.U.s, one displaying alpha-numeric data, the other graphical data. A group of operators (note, these are people with extensive experience of the same or similar tasks, not the unskilled

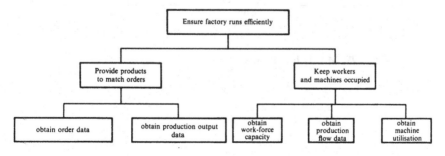

Fig. 1.28. Hierarchical task analysis – production controller.

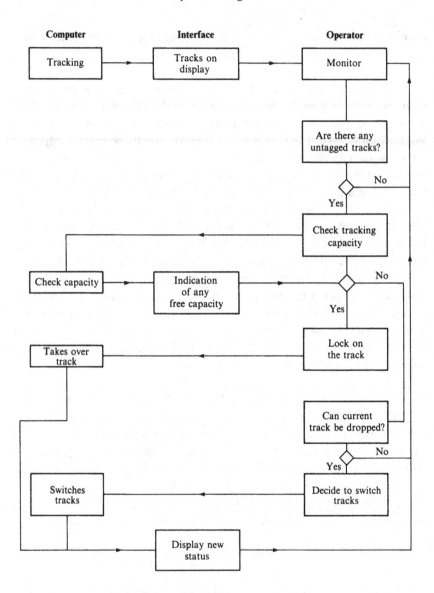

Fig. 1.29. M.C.I. Job–Process chart.

performer normally used in human performance experiments) run through a task using this equipment. Their behaviour and achievements are observed and discussed amongst themselves and with the analyst (Fig. 1.29).

Conclusion

Task analysis has not and cannot be reduced to a set of standardised procedures which the aspiring analyst could acquire in a formal training course. The techniques just described are no more than guidelines in what remains the creative art of studying and describing what an experienced worker is doing or will be required to do. The danger in being too rigid is that justice will not be done to the flexibility and complexity of human perform-ance. The danger of being too flexible is that the ergonomists will have an inadequate basis from which to design interfaces, training courses and other operator aids. If a comprehensive task description can be completed then it is legitimate to enquire why the task cannot be allocated to a technical device rather than a human being. Yet without a reasonably comprehensive task description the total system performance may be unreliable or unpredictable. There is a necessary compromise which can only be arrived at in the context of a particular system.

As mentioned earlier there are always the twin problems of how to get the information and how to present it. It is sometimes easier to proceed on the basis of: 'If I were doing the job this is how I would do it', but this can be delusory even for analysts who have past experience as operators. For analysts who are designers creating a new task there may be no alternative, but any task description arrived at by this method should be checked against the behaviour of real operators as they gain experience. A particular difficulty about task synthesis is that there is no easy way of confirming completeness.

A task description which is part of a design process should be fully documented in terms of the origins of information, the assumptions made and the methods used.

The standard method of producing task descriptions is to write all the separate sub-tasks at various levels on cards and then assemble the cards in a network. There is a temptation to make these final diagrams very large, but often it is more useful to separate into small units with cross-referencing. The optimum size seems to be A3, this is easily copied and circulated but is large enough to contain considerable detail. The procedure can be computerised, there are programmes available for the easy production, manipulation and storage of block diagrams with useful cross-referencing facilities.

There is an inherent difficulty in that often the main dividend from a task analysis is from the act of obtaining it. Those not involved find it difficult to gain very much from a presentation of a task description. Like reference books, they have to be used rather than read.

Task analysis can be very expensive in skilled manpower, but in looking at cost/value it is important to include in value the increase in mutual understanding which occurs when a multi-disciplinary team conducts the analysis. If such a team is used the required man-hours can be optimised by using the Delphi method rather than a long series of group meetings.

Political, economic and social issues which arise in conducting Task Analyses are discussed in the context of Job Analysis (p. 148).

1.4 Applications
1.4.1 Man-power planning

The 'Human Resource' concept of man-power as the central profit-generating asset of any organisation has made some progress over the past twenty years. There was particular interest around 1970 when companies were prosperous, stable and innovative (IPM, 1972, Patten, 1971). The objective is to revise and almost reverse the traditional accountancy concept of man-power as a resource consuming factor requiring regular payments, overheads in the form of heated, lighted, equipped workspaces and so on. From the narrow accountancy viewpoint, people are a cost and it is desirable to keep this cost as low as possible. In these terms it is very difficult to justify, for example, sending a member of staff on a training course. The training requires expenditure and so also does the replacement for the person away. Where is the return? The return is actually in the improved human resource but this is not readily measurable in terms which accountants use.

There have been two attempts to reduce human resources to this form of measurement (Giles and Robinson, 1972). One is to acquire a human asset multiplier for each level of staff. The multiplier for manual staff might be unity but it increases with staff level and becomes three or more for management. The other is to add together all the personnel costs for each kind of worker from the original job advertisement through to the retirement or redundancy payments. The first does attempt to obtain a value, the second remains essentially a cost and not a value. It would be unduly optimistic to assume that management skills have risen to a level such that costs undertaken can be assumed to be equivalent to value. A less direct measure which is applicable only to the most senior management is to observe the fall or rise of the share price when a particular executive leaves or joins a company. This can be very high, for a large company a change in market value of millions of pounds is not unusual.

The most serious consequence of the accountancy view of man-power is that high level policy decision-making does not give this factor sufficient weight. For example, the main board of a company will have complete details of cost and values of physical resources such as buildings and equipment but relatively scanty data about the man-power which is their most important asset. Indeed it will be described almost entirely as a liability because the costs will be known. Similarly, broad factors such as the state of morale will again only be described by negative features such as absenteeism, stoppages, strikes, low quality output and so on. It is obvious that company output and projects must reflect the man-power and its performance level, but, if this is acknowledged at all, it is only in brief verbal terms within, for example, the chairman's annual report.

The obsession, of current management, with measurement and the reduction of every variable to numbers for ease of computer manipulation has worsened the situation. Unfortunately there is no easy remedy. Human resources are too complex a variable to be easily susceptible to measurement beyond the level of counting heads and trades. Key variables such as the quality of staff at any level and the current morale are only expressible in general verbal descriptive terms.

It is generally accepted (p. 145) that 'hygiene' type variables such as pay and working conditions can, if they are inappropriately specified, depress morale and motivation but they will not in themselves result in very high levels of these parameters. Morale and motivation are influenced more by conditions of work in the sense of work variety opportunities and attitudes of management. These factors are worthy of emphasis because in practice they are still dealt with very badly in many organisations and yet it takes little trouble or expertise to make an enormous difference. For example, very few senior managements take the trouble to keep workers fully informed about policies and likely changes. The result is excessive reliance on rumour and continuous speculation which is not only time-consuming but is also highly deleterious in morale terms.

The two human factors which can be unambiguously measured are age and sex. The age distribution of a work force is always an interesting and important source of information. For most purposes a rectangular distribution is the most desirable because it provides the appropriate mix of youthful enthusiasm and ageing experience. It also makes for regular changes as staff retire and are replaced. Many distributions show a peak in a particular age group mainly associated with taking on a large number of young people when the organisation was started or reorganised, this is not desirable because it leads to excessive competition for promotion at particular stages. These comments are obviously most relevant for work forces where there is little tendency to move out, this is characteristic of a surprisingly large number of organisations in European countries and in Japan but much less so in the U.S.A.

Stable work forces have their advantages in terms of familiarity with the enterprise and its peculiar needs but they do result in problems if the market for the products is erratic or otherwise unpredictable. This is particularly so in high technology e.g. design and construction of ships, aircraft, power stations and chemical plant, where the product unit is large and expensive and the variety of required expertise is extensive. Some peaks of demand can be dealt with by using consultants, but they tend to be expensive and do not always fit well with ill-defined but important factors such as the favoured style of the organisation. In well ordered systems it may be possible to calculate the length of in-house experience required to achieve the required level of expertise in particular topics and compare this with the lead time for particular product requirements. Given time available to train new staff it is not necessary to keep more than a nucleus in that particular expertise. On the other hand, if there is usually insufficient notice of need it may be necessary to keep staff who have periods with little to do between projects. It is also desirable to have the possibility of shifting staff between design and operational duties. This not only provides flexibility in the use of man-power, it also improves communication. These real difficulties of man-power utilisation are such as to force many organisations to become larger and larger if they are to remain economic. Size provides a cushion to the vicissitudes of markets but it creates other problems. For example, difficulties of communications and in particular, how to inculcate the feeling within each individual that he and his performance are important to the organisation. This is considered in more detail in Chapter 3.

Human resources should be fundamental to subjects such as ergonomics which are essentially people-centred but the concept remains procedurally undeveloped at any level from a continent through countries, regions and companies down to particular working systems. This is one reason why policy makers never seem to take account fully of the people affected by their decisions.

1.4.2 The design of procedures

The increased importance of standardised informational support for both machines and operators has led to the concept of procedures as a separate design issue within a system (Fig. 1.30). Much of this information can be incorporated in computer programs but there is also a need for extensive printed paper for the use of the operator. This takes three main forms: checklists, routines and knowledge-texts.

The terminology in this field is not standardised. Software might be restricted, as in this book, to computer programs but it is sometimes used as the generic term to include all sources of information. Procedures is sometimes used for what are here called routines and sometimes to indicate all the operator's information support except software. The situation is further confused when some but not all the operator information support is itself computer-based. Sometimes the term firm-ware is used. However whatever the terminology used there is a requirement for design effort.

The quality of procedures would be much improved if designers followed some simple guide-lines (Table 1.16). Many documents are written on the implicit assumption that the reader is much like the writer in terms of expertise

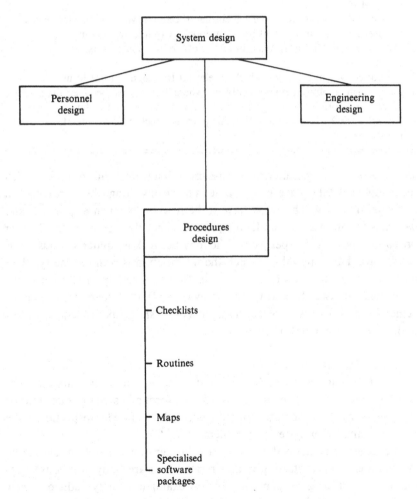

Fig. 1.30. Procedures as an integral part of system design.

Table 1.16. *Guidelines for procedures design*

---

1. Consider procedures design as an integral part of the total system-design problem. Procedures are the main communication channel between the designer and the user.
2. Allocate the total communication between the vehicles shown in Fig. 1.30.
3. Design the Task Analysis programme on the basis that Task Descriptions are the source of procedures as well as other ergonomic issues such as interface consoles and training.
4. Consider the relevant characteristics of the average user: what does he already know, what does he need to know, in what forms does he need particular knowledge?
5. Consider the conditions under which the procedures will be consulted, e.g. will the user be in a hurry, might he be in poor environmental surroundings?
6. Do not assume that a user is a junior or otherwise inferior version of a designer.
7. Do not convey information which is relevant to design but not to use.
8. Distinguish carefully between problems where the user can be given the solution and those where he can be given information to enable him to find a solution.
9. Always evaluate a procedure. For this purpose check with a population of users not designers.

---

and style of thinking. Similarly it is assumed that the conditions under which the reading will take place are the same as those of writing which are usually a clean well-lit office. They may have to be read in the open air, in rain and darkness or within a plant under oily, cramped, poorly lit conditions. The user probably has limited expertise and he may be working under various stress conditions. The material on which the information is printed, the typeface used, the sequence, the structure and the format generally should reflect the conditions of use, (Easterby and Zwaga, 1984). All these things can be achieved if it is acknowledged that all procedures should be validated by users under the normal conditions of use.

Checklists

Checklists are used in the pre-start mode, for routine maintenance and for fault-finding. They normally take the form of a series of questions or statements which the operator uses to guide and structure his inspection of the hardware and other system components.

The sequence is dictated by the optimal order in which actions should be taken, for example in starting up an aircraft. There are many situations where the order is of no great consequence, for example a safety audit of a new machine, and in this latter case some logical structure is needed. As mentioned above, the logic of the design may not be the optimal basis if the way the operator thinks and acts is different.

Baker (1984) suggests that four kinds of shortcoming emerge when checklists are validated in the real situation. The operator may deviate from the listed procedure because it may require excessive moving about or because he is interrupted by the requirements of other tasks. Systematic use of a checklist often reveals faults in work design such as inadequate access, visibility and labelling. The checklist itself may be inconsistent, incomplete, imprecise or ambiguous. Finally the checklist may have reprographic limitations such as inadequate vertical or horizontal structure, poor typefaces and insufficient linking of requirements, descriptions, remarks and tick-off points.

The International Ergonomics Association developed a general ergonomics checklist which is reproduced in Edholm (1967). There is a deceptive simplicity about such lists which requires extensive effort to ensure a comprehensive but coherent content. The context is, of course, the context of ergonomics as conceived by the designers of the list.

Routines

A routine is the most common form of instructional material. The reader is required to follow a series of steps which might, for example, introduce a change in the performance of a complex system. Normally routines are single chains of instructions although it is possible to have some conditional branching.

Each step should be simple and complete in itself – preferably with some indication that successful completion has been achieved, for example the appearance or the change of colour of a signal light, or the noise of a motor starting or a change of pressure which indicates that there has been a change in the flow of some material. As mentioned earlier a routine can often be regarded as a written task description.

By definition and design intention routines are inflexible. The user is intended to behave exactly according to their instruction. No great skill or intellectual effort is required, which is one way of saying that the human operator is being under-used, but the purpose of a routine is usually to avoid common human error such as omitting a step or reversing steps. In general the value of formal routines is precisely that the operator, left to himself, will not normally function in such a systematic sequential manner.

Knowledge texts

Knowledge is contained in documents which may vary from single sheet presentations to large manuals. As instructional material it is indirect in that the reader is not necessarily told what to do, as in a routine. Rather he is informed about the situation and the purpose of informing him is to provide a knowledge base from which he can work out his own actions. Nevertheless, the relevant action remains important and the knowledge provided should be carefully and stringently selected. It is too easy to follow the academic tradition and provide knowledge for its own sake. The 'need to know' criterion is crucial because unless it is applied, the operator can be overburdened with unnecessary material. Correspondingly the material should be structured in terms of how it is most likely to be used. In this context the operator requires a guide for action and not a scientific text-book. It is invariably better to provide material diagrammatically, systematically or at least in well-structured short paragraphs rather than in flowing prose.

Consider for example how readily information about the relative position of streets is available from a map of a town centre rather than a verbal description of all the streets. Such a map will enable the reader to work out for himself how to get from one location to another within the town. Note the enormous flexibility compared with a routine which would tell him only how to get from one particular point to another. A second important difference is that if he misses his place in a routine he will be totally lost, whereas if he happens to go in the wrong direction while using a map he is still able to make whatever correction is necessary. However the map does require more intellectual effort than does the routine not only in making decisions about how to proceed but also in filtering out the required information from the massive irrelevance (for a particular task) which is equally available. Thus, one would expect the use of the maps to be slower than the use of routines with the human performance being more versatile but less predictable.

With two-dimensional representations such as maps it remains important to avoid too much homogeneity and provide substructure in the form of main roads and key buildings or other features such as rivers. See, for example, Fig. 5.3

Manuals which may contain maps, schematic diagrams and other materials warrant separate consideration.

1.4.3 The design of manuals

A manual is usually in the form of a book or booklet which is sent with the hardware from the maker to the customer. It is part of the communication package from the designer to the user. Thus it is a particular form of job aid which provides the operator with information on a system and its performance.

The standard of manual design has traditionally been very low for several

Table 1.17. *The contents of a manual*

	Inclusions
1. Orientation	Required inputs
	Expected outputs
	Schematic diagrams
2. Setting-up	Procedural list
	Checks of successful completion
	of particular stages
3. Operation	Standard functions
	Ways to switch functions
4. Maintenance	Faults: Reasons: Remedies
5. Parts List	Drawings with) Names
	) Numbers
	) Notes
6. Glossary	All specialist terminology
7. Index	

reasons. For this purpose, the designer is too familiar with the product and he rarely takes the trouble to find out what the user really needs to know. Often the manual has to be provided hurriedly at the end of a project when the budget is running out, and it is regarded as a tiresome chore still required after the essential design work has been completed. The problem is particularly acute for computers. Manuals for cars, machine tools and so on are poor but at least it is possible to observe the mechanisms and their functions. Most computer operators do not know or wish to know about the mechanisms, and in any case these are not accessible to vision and manipulation. The computer operator is entirely dependent on the manual, at least in the early stages of gaining familiarity with the system and its functions. He is usually very badly served although the principles of manual design are well known.

For most systems the manual is best divided into parts as indicated in Table 1.17. The first part should be a general introduction which orientates the readers towards the system, its purpose, its functional structure and mode of operation and its performance limits. This should be followed by a separate section on how to set the system up in the first place and how to check that it is working properly. If it is fairly small it may be necessary to describe how to unpack it, fix it into position, connect it to power supplies and start it up. If it is large, the emphasis will be on the start up procedure. The section describing the operation of the system should cover not only how the system operates but also how the user can operate it. Extensive use of line drawings, schematic diagrams, algorithmic lists is desirable, and where prose is used this also should be structured into short sentences with meaningful separation into paragraphs.

The maintenance section should indicate what, if anything, the operator is expected to do and the symptoms which indicate that more specialist maintenance skills are required. Tables subdivided into Faults/Reasons/Remedies can be extremely helpful. Parts lists including description reference numbers and sometimes drawings are necessary if the user is expected to deal with his own replacements. A standard fault is to assume that the reader is familiar with the jargon which the designer habitually uses. A glossary of terms and acronyms used can be very helpful not only to the reader but also to the writer who is forced to consider carefully how he is using various technical terms. Finally, all manuals should end with an index which supplements the table of contents at the beginning.

References

Annett, J., Duncan, K.D., Stammers, R.B. and Gray, M.J. (1971). Task Analysis. Department of Employment Training Information Paper No. 6. London: H.M.S.O.

Baker, E. (1984). Applications of instruction design principles to nuclear power plant operating procedures manuals. In Easterby, R. and Zwaga, H. (eds.). *Information Design*. Chichester: Wiley.

Battersby, A. (1970). *Network Analysis*. London: Macmillan.

Bytheway, C.W. (1977). FAST diagram for creative functional analysis. *Value Engineering*. **6**. 10.

Chapanis, A. (1959). *Research Techniques in Human Engineering*. Baltimore: Johns Hopkins Press.

Crawley, R. and Spurgeon, P. (1979). Computer assistance and the air traffic controller's job satisfaction. In Sell, R.G. and Shipley, P. (eds.). *Satisfaction in Work Design*. London: Taylor & Francis.

Davis, L.E. and Cherns, A.B. (eds.). (1975). *The Quality of Working Life*. New York: Free Press.

Davis, L.E. and Taylor, J.C. (1972). *Design of Jobs*. Harmondsworth: Penguin.

Duncan, K.D. (1975). An analytical technique for industrial training. In Singleton, W.T. and Spurgeon, P. (eds.). *Measurement of Human Resources*. London: Taylor & Francis.

Easterby, R.S. and Zwaga, H. (1984). *Information Design*. Chichester: Wiley.

Edholm, O.G. (1967). *The Biology of Work*. London: Weidenfeld & Nicolson.

Edwards, E. and Lees, F.P. (eds.). 1974. *The Human Operator in Process Control*. London: Taylor & Francis.

Emery, F.E. and Trist, E.L. (1960). Socio-technical systems. In Churchman, C.W. and Verhulst, M. (eds.). *Management Science, Models and Techniques*. London: Pergamon.

Fitts, P.M. (1951). Engineering psychology and equipment design. In Stevens, S.S. (ed.). *Handbook of Experimental Psychology*. New York: Wiley.

Giles, W.J. and Robinson, P.F. (1972). *Human Asset Accounting*. London: Institute of Personnel Management.

Hick, W.E. and Bates, J.A.V. (1950). *The Human Operator in Control Systems*. London: H.M.S.O.

I.L.O. (1979). *Introduction to Work Study*. Geneva: International Labour Office.

I.P.M. (1972). *Company Practices in Man-power Planning*. London: Institute of Personnel Management.

Jordan, N. (1963). Allocation of functions between man and machine in automated systems. *Journal of Applied Psychology*. **47**. 161–5.

Klein, L. (1979). Some problems of theory and method. In Sell, R.G. and Shipley, P. (eds.). *Satisfaction in Work Design*. London: Taylor & Francis.

Lupton, T. and Tanner, I. (1980). Work design in Europe. In Duncan, K.D., Gruneberg, M.M. and Wallis, D. (eds.). *Changes in Working Life*. Chichester: Wiley.

Maynard, H.B., Stegmerton, G.J. and Schwab, J.L. (1956). Methods–time measurement. In Maynard, H.B. (ed.). *Industrial Engineering Handbook*. New York: McGraw-Hill.

Patten, T.H.Jr. (1971). *Manpower Planning and the Development of Human Resources*. New York: Wiley Interscience.

Shaw, A.G. (1952). *The Purpose and Practice of Motion Study*. London: Harlequin Press.

Shepherd, A. and Duncan, K.D. (1980). Analysing a complex planning task. In Duncan, K.D., Gruneberg, M.M. and Wallis, D. (eds.). *Changes in Working Life*. Chichester: Wiley.

Sheridan, T.B. and Johannsen, G. (eds.) (1976). *Monitoring Behaviour and Supervisory Control*. New York: Plenum.

Singleton, W.T. (1964). A preliminary study of a capstan lathe. *International Journal of Production Research*. **3**. 213–25.

Singleton, W.T. (1967a). The systems prototype and his design problems. In Singleton, W.T., Easterby, R.S. and Whitfield, D. (eds.). *The Human Operator in Complex Systems*. London: Taylor & Francis.

Singleton, W.T. (1967b). Ergonomics in System Design. *Ergonomics*. **10**. 541–48.

Singleton, W.T. (1974). *Man–Machine Systems*. Harmondsworth: Penguin.

Singleton, W.T. (1987). The design of design teams in high-technology industries. *Applied Ergonomics*. **18.2**, 111–14.

Singleton, W.T. and Crawley, R.C. (1980). Changing jobs and job demands in Europe. In Duncan, K.D., Gruneberg, M.M. and Wallis, D. (eds.). *Changes in Working Life*. Chichester: Wiley.

Swain, A.D. and Wohl, T.G. (1961). Factors affecting the degree of automation in test and check-out equipment. Dunlap & Associates. TR60–36F.

Tainsh, M. (1985). Job process charts and man-computer interaction within Naval Command systems. *Ergonomics*. **28.3**. 555–65.

Trist, E.L. and Murray, H. (1948). Work Organisation at the coal face: a comparative study of mining systems. *Tavistock Institute of Human Relations*. Document 506.

Wulfeck, J.W. and Zeitlin, L.R. (1962). Human capabilities and limitations. In Gagne, R.M. (ed.). *Psychological Principles in System Development*. New York: Holt, Rinehart and Winston.

2 Skill and training

2.1 Concepts

2.1.1 Developmental aspects

Most laboratory and field studies of human behaviour involve taking a situational snap-shot at a given time in a given place. It is easy to overlook the continuously changing nature both of people and of work situations.

When the skilled manager encounters what, on the face of it, is an intolerable set of work practices, attitudes and performance he does not necessarily take drastic action, he identifies the natural processes of change and accelerates them. In a remarkably short time changes in procedures, products and workload, promotions, resignations, retirements and so on can transform any situation.

The changes within an individual are even more inexorably continuous. Again it is easy to develop the illusion that a worker is a constant factor in a changing situation particularly for a person in the middle period of working life. This was encouraged by the traditional view of a skilled man as one who learned his trade by the age of 21 and thereafter practised it for more than forty years until he retired at 65. This was never the case and in the current working world it is even less so because of developing technology which has its impact on almost all jobs and also on the social context of work. For example, because of employment levels there is currently an emphasis on earlier retirement from and later entry into the working world. These trends are particularly marked in manufacturing industry where the work force is falling and the capital investment per worker is rising rapidly. For these reasons industry is moving towards a concept of the ideal worker as a physically fit adaptable young person. The labour force is becoming more like the military with the use of a limited age range and the screening out of anyone with any kind of disability who might not be able to work at a pace and with the flexibility and precision which will maintain the return on the very large capital investment.

Even so, it remains true that the performance of the individual is a function of the way he developed skills in his earlier more formative years and the way in which his capacities and skills are still changing in the work environment. Human development can be described in terms of three attributes: capacities, skills and aspirations (Singleton, 1981). The healthy, well-adapted individual keeps them in balance in a dynamic equilibrium. His natural endowment consists of a particular range of capacities: physical strength, mobility, vision, hearing, intellect and so forth. These form the basis for the development of a repertoire of skills dictated partly by capacities and partly by environmental circumstances such as the particular family, community and region he is born into and the available facilities for play, education and training. The balance and integration of capacities and skills is achieved by the third attribute of aspirations. These are partly determined by and partly determine the other attributes. The individual is in difficulties if his aspirations do not match his capacities and skills but most people are sufficiently realistic and have sufficient self-knowledge to keep these attributes in line. The most flexible attribute is the skills, these can be developed or changed in line with capacities and aspirations. A well-ordered civilisation demands standard basic skills of a physical kind: mobility and manipulation, and also of a mental kind: reading, writing and arithmetic. On the basis of these standard skills there is enormous flexibility for the individual to develop his own identity and to express it through his specialised skills.

As the individual gets older, he continues to acquire new skills for two reasons. Firstly, the passage of time provides more and more experience and this is inevitably reflected in the skill repertoire. Secondly, the ageing individual suffers a steady diminution of capacities, for example the decrease in adaptability to lower lighting levels and the decrease in physical stamina. Skills develop and change to compensate partially for the changing capacities. It follows, of course, that decreasing capacities as such are not direct predictors of decreasing performance. This is true not only for ageing but also for the onset of disabilities (see Chapter 7).

2.1.2 *Human skill*

Skills are the residues of learning. To describe behaviour as skilled is to say no more than that it has been influenced by training and experience. There is often an implication that skilled means highly skilled although this connotation confuses the concept of existence and level. Unskilled is also used to imply a low level of skill rather than its absence. Level of skill is usually assessed in terms of extent of formal training although this is only one of the relevant factors: others include length of experience and degree of integration.

Foundation skills are acquired in the first five years of life. These include not only perceptual-motor skills but also the basic language and social skills. Thereafter the educational system supplements the interaction with family and friends in providing facilities and exemplars for further symbolic and social

Table 2.1. *Examples of basic skills*

Perceptual-Motor	Perceptual	Symbolic	Social
Head Control	Vision	Colours	Parental interaction
Eye Control	Vision ⎱	Letters	Family/Friends interaction
	Hearing ⎬ co-ordination	Words	
Hand and Grasp Control	Tactile ⎰		
	Distance assessment	Reading	Organisational interaction
Crawl	Topological models	Writing	Rules and Procedures
Walk with aid	Switch between	Arithmetic	
Stand	inside/out		
Walk alone	and outside/in		

skill development. More details of all these skills are contained in Table 2.1. The specific skills which a person acquires whilst earning a living are combinations and developments of the standard skills of the normal healthy adult. This is not to denigrate the uniqueness and quality of working skills. They are often underrated because the universal characteristic of high skill is that, to an observer, the performance does not appear to be very difficult. This is because the skilled individual is normally working well within his capacities, he does not have to search desperately for information because he knows exactly what to look for, his movements are not hurried because they are integrated into smooth chains and he does not react suddenly because he anticipates what is going to happen. In general, he works on the principle of minimal effort to achieve the required objectives in terms of both speed and quality.

The importance of skill theory is that it relates human performance to systems concepts and to individual differences. The performer is pursuing an objective and the great variety of his activity has meaning in relation to his objective. Skill is a functional concept aimed at the understanding of how it is done without recourse to the detail of underlying physiological mechanisms. Individual differences are obviously a consequence of the particular past experience of each person who has thereby acquired a unique set of skills based on a natural endowment which was also unique. Skill theory also emphasises the closely integrated nature of behaviour in real situations, it is not readily susceptible to analysis into discrete components.

The internal representation of a skill is called a schema. A schema is an internal model which can be used to relate external events to a current purpose (Head 1920). It is modified continuously as external data is received and transformed into information. Schemata may be person centred or situation centred. For a more extensive discussion of schemata, how they differ and how they function, see Singleton (1981).

2.1.3 *Acquisition of skills*

Skills are acquired by a process of trial and error but the trials are not entirely random as is assumed in classical trial and error learning (Thorndike, 1911). However, the more primitive the skill the more there must be an element of chance. For example, one of the skills developed in the first few years of life involves the integration of data arriving through the different sensory channels. The fact that a visually observed impact between two bodies in the physical world is normally associated with a particular sound has to be learned. Hence the importance of play in hitting, say, tins with spoons – the visual, auditory and tactile impressions are being integrated. Similarly the kinaesthetic sensation of a limb moving has to be associated with the visual sensation obtained by observing the limb – hence the countless hours which babies spend just watching their own limbs move. This is how manipulative skills begin, but it will be noted that even these are not purely 'motor', they are mainly 'perceptual'. Greater precision is achieved by more definitive selection and guidance. Unskilled activity is to do everything rather than to do nothing.

The concept of motor skill is associated with the development of longer and more complex patterns of activity which can be reeled off following a single trigger and which are monitored on the basis that only feedback which indicates errors needs attention. Industrial training for manual operations is designed to encourage this kind of development (Seymour, 1966).

Perceptual skills by contrast are developments to do with the greater selectivity of information needed to monitor situations and guide actions. These begin from an appreciation of the complementary nature of data arriving through the different sensory channels and expand by the acquisition of concepts such as the continuity of the physical world, e.g. a person who walks behind a screen has not vanished, it is accepted that he is still there even though temporarily there is no sense data to confirm it, but a hypothesis will be generated which supposes that, if he walked behind a screen at a constant speed, he ought to reappear at a given time at the other side of the screen. Similarly it is soon accepted that the 'ostrich' theory of closing one's eyes and assuming that thereby either oneself or things in the environment will actually disappear is not tenable. In this phase babies and young children enjoy 'peep' type games.

There is an important stage at which the person-centred world is superseded or rather supplemented by the world of which the person is one part. Incidentally this is analogous to the distinction between displays which are 'inside looking out' and those which are 'outside looking in' (p. 251). The perceptual system can function either way which is, of course, why each of the two types of display has its utility. This development is one utilising pictorial skills as distinct from enactive skills. The latter are based on the body, its extensions and images, the former are based on internal 'pictures' of the world which are one kind of schema or mental model (see next section). Social skills are in principle more complex than perceptual-motor skills because the latter assume (correctly) a passive world which will react neutrally, according to the laws of physics. In spite of occasional feelings to the contrary, usually described as good or bad luck, the physical world is neither for nor against the actions of the individual (except in the robotic sense of Le Chatilier's principle which states that whenever a constraint is placed on a system in equilibrium, the equilibrium is altered in such a way as to annul the efforts of the constraint). In social situations it has to be recognised that there is at least one other sentient being present who has his own objectives which might accord with or oppose those of the first person. Thus, social skills involve assessing the skills of the other person, a process known as mutual construing. The evidence about the constructs of another person is indirect and may have been deliberately obscured or falsified.

Nevertheless, it is true for all skills that a person developing skills is indulging in a process of constructing models of what is happening externally. These models develop continuously while attempting to modify the external situation (physical or social). What seems to happen is that an individual, given his arrival in a situation, reviews it in the context of his own objectives and decides that if he takes certain actions, the situation will change in the direction of his objectives. He then takes the action, observes the changes and compares them with his stored version of those expected. If they correspond, then all is well, his concept of the situation is confirmed and he can progress to the next step in the context of his objectives. If, however, the observed changes are not what was predicted, then he has made an error but he has also learned because he must now modify his view of the situation accordingly. For example, I might decide the angle of light on my desk is not as I require it on the basis of assessing the illumination and the lamp which is the source of it. I hypothesise that if I move and turn the lamp in a particular way I will get the result I want. So I reach out, move and turn the lamp and check the result. If the result is as intended there has been no learning but equally none was needed because I understood the situation, I achieved my objective and I can move on to other problems. In a more complex case I might sit in on a discussion within a committee but begin to consider that it is not moving in a direction that suits me. I therefore form a hypothesis about an appropriate contribution based on the proposition being considered, the associated facts and logic, the personalities of my fellow committee members and my own standing within the committee. I then state my proposition and observe its effects. If I get the result I wanted there is consolidation rather than extension of my committee skills, but if I do not get the result I wanted then I have learned something and I form a new hypothesis about my next interjection strengthened by this new learning.

It will be noted that errors are the basis of further skill acquisition. Facilitating the acquisition of skill is a matter of providing situations where the skill can be practised with adequate, sometimes enhanced, feedback so that there can be learning from mistakes. The necessary conditions for learning are feedback and motivation, the result of actions must matter to the individual. All this is quite generally true, it applies equally to motor skills, perceptual skills and social skills.

2.1.4   *Mental models*

The principles of perception indicate that the human operator does not react unambiguously to stimuli which arrive via the sensory mechanisms (p. 196). To assume that he responds directly to data from the real world is to oversimplify the relationship between his inputs and outputs. The skill model described above implies that, except in highly restricted artificial situations, his information processing must be described in terms of patterns of stimuli related to patterns of responses. It is also true that responses are a function of enormous differences between and within individuals. To encompass all these parameters, it is currently fashionable to describe the person as responding in terms of his mental model of the situation rather than to the situation itself. The idea is that any person in any situation builds an internal model of the situation which is being reported to him, as it were, by sensory data. He uses each perceptual datum to update his model of the situation. The model is his picture of what is going on outside him and it is essentially an hypothesis based on the available evidence. This theory explains nicely why he sometimes does not react in tune with his own interests, that is, he gets it wrong. In these circumstances he is considered to have developed a model which does not bridge the gap between reality and his aspirations.

These models are most easy to visualise in pictorial terms – the human operator has his internal picture which topographically matches the real world. Models can, however, be simpler than these and can take the form of rules or they can be more complex in that symbolism can be used. Thus a model can be entirely abstract using symbols which have no pictorial quality as in the use of language and mathematics. Even when a picture is used, it is not complete, it takes the form of an icon which contains what the perceiver considers matters at the time.

For example, a person working in a room with or without other people can easily develop the misconception that he has a complete picture in his mind of the physical environment. In fact the picture is complete only in the sense that it contains the details which are relevant to his activity in that room, it certainly does not contain all the detail which is available to the senses. This is readily demonstrated by asking him to close his eyes and answer questions such as 'is there a picture on the wall on the left?' or 'what colour are the eyes of the person you are talking to?' This is the kind of data which is not relevant to his objectives and thus it is not recorded in his model. On the other hand he will be able to answer questions such as 'is the door behind you to the left or to the right?' because he has used that door and needs to use it again. He knows where it is even though he cannot currently see it.

Thus the visually-based mental picture is invariably an icon in the literal sense of a 'symbolic representation' rather than a complete reproduction. At a more abstract level the mathematician or scientist will perform manipulations within a set of symbols which follow certain rules but neither the symbols nor the rules need have direct representation in reality. Indeed any attempt to relate them prematurely to reality may restrict the development of the model. However, at some stage he will return to reality and say, for example, 'what this means in practice or in terms of my next experiment . . .' The skilled thinker has an extraordinary facility not only to develop varieties of abstract models but also to switch rapidly between them and between them and reality. The switching takes place up and down a hierarchy of abstraction and generality.

Consider for example the maintenance engineer operating as a diagnostician. He will look at a piece of equipment to try to detect signs which indicate what is wrong. Is there a gap or a hole which indicates a leak? Is there a part which is too hot? Most of this information comes not so much from what is happening but from what is not happening. Basically the thing is not working as it should, the outputs are not as they should be so he will probably begin by checking that the inputs are present, that is the electric power or fuel or other materials are available. He will then envisage the designed chain of events between input and output and look for the hiatus, he may do this by rules, by a pictorial model or by a model involving some symbolism such as expected voltage levels. He will shift very rapidly between different representations of the equipment; the thing itself, his maintenance instructions, the manual, the drawings of the system, verbal discussion with a colleague, his recollection of what has happened to it in the past and so on. He may think in terms of bits of equipment, flows of material, flows of energy or flows of information. He will shift through levels of generality and levels of abstraction until he has formulated an hypothesis which takes the form of 'if I do this – that should happen'. He will then perform an action and check its results. There are many interesting facets of this complex diagnostic process and three are worthy of re-emphasis: firstly most of his information comes not from positive signals, stimuli or cues but from their absence, secondly he is relying on a hybrid model – a mixture of rules, mental pictures and symbolism, thirdly it all happens without very much conscious guidance – one mental or physical event leads to another and each event in the chain plays its part before handing over to the next one. There is some analogy with a control system used in early naval warfare. There was not one ship permanently in command, the particular ship in most direct contact with the enemy was in command until the leading position was taken over by another ship which then assumed command as well as action.

The working situation is different from the training school and even more from the educational system. However it does seem that mental models can be developed in the abstract without the need to resort to action, in other words it is possible to learn while sitting passively in a class-room. Education or abstract learning does seem to take the form mainly of symbolic modelling and the relating of these models to reality awaits later practical experience. The great asset of symbolic modelling is just this, learning does not have to depend entirely on practice and it is possible for collective knowledge to accumulate. This knowledge is communicated between people by the use of shared models. Conversely, abstract communication cannot take place without the development of appropriate models.

For example, the technical teacher is trying to convey various models to his pupils , some of the models will be physically based as in describing particular machines or systems and some will be functionally based as when he talks about thermodynamics or communication. What the teacher is trying to do is to guide each pupil into developing a set of mental models which have been found by experience or experiment to be useful in understanding technical processes. Having developed these models the pupil is in a position to communicate much more readily with other technical people who can manipulate similar models. Conversely, this communication between specialists will be incomprehensible to those who do not have the expertise which resides in this particular set of models. Even between technical peers as in a design team there can be difficulties in communication because the models which individuals are using are not identical. Debate, demonstration and other communications take place until a common modelling is accepted. When there is disagreement, there is much to be said for retreating specifically to consider the model rather than the problem. Correspondingly, when there is a complex situation to discuss there can be considerable dividends in attempting to get an agreed model 'on the table' before considering specific issues. This is what briefing sessions are intended to accomplish.

This approach also explains why engineers and ergonomists sometimes have difficulties in reaching agreement. The former is likely to be using mechanism-based models with people as ancillaries while the ergonomist will be using models of people with mechanisms as ancillaries. For good cooperation it is essential that the engineer has some grasp of ergonomics and that the ergonomist understands at least in general terms the technical situation in the particular industry. There can of course still be disagreements even when there is clear mutual understanding because underlying values result in the assessment of very different priorities.

In summary, communication, whether between a person and the physical world or between people, involves each person in developing and manipulating a mental model by interacting with the situation. Modelling the physical world and modelling other people's models share the same developmental procedures. Understanding what a person is doing requires an appreciation of the kind and content of the models that that person holds.

2.2   Knowledge
2.2.1   *Individual differences*
Capacities, abilities and aptitudes
It is useful to discriminate between a *capacity* which is a natural endowment and an *ability* which is a competence to act. A capacity relates to an ability through an intervening phase of education, training and experience. Thus an ability represents what a person can do now, whereas a capacity is essentially a potential. An *aptitude* is demonstrated by success in learning which results in the acquisition of an ability. An aptitude is therefore a capacity plus an inclination or interest.

Ability and skill are often used interchangeably although ability is the wider term. An ability is made up of a repertoire of skills and is thus a higher level skill. Ability and capacity are often confused for several reasons. Human resources might be expressed in terms of either since capacities can be transformed into abilities by training. Strictly we can only measure abilities but much psychometric testing aims to infer capacities from the measured abilities, e.g. intelligence tests.

All three terms are attributes of individuals intended to describe their distinction from other individuals. All are used loosely because there are no taxonomies which are either comprehensive or rigorous. That is, it would be unduly ambitious to claim to be able to describe a complete range of human abilities and the descriptors used for particular abilities are not always separable. The same is true for capacities and aptitudes. The best known attempt to provide a comprehensive structure of human abilities is that due to Guilford (1967). His model contains about 120 different abilities, it is not currently very popular with psychometricians.

The only unambiguous categorisations of people are by physical size, age and sex. None of these is uniquely related to abilities but nevertheless age and sex are useful parameters. Age in particular at least correlates with some of the parameters which affect choice of work and performance at work.

Intelligence and personality

There is no agreed definition of intelligence although a century of experience has accumulated in attempts to measure it (Friedman *et al.*, 1981). Intelligence defined as that which is measured by intelligence tests is obviously circular and also variable as the fashions in intelligence testing change. For example, the attempt in the past thirty years to incorporate more divergent factors changes the emphasis towards inductive and creative abilities. This supplements the consideration of deductive and logical abilities measured by the traditional convergent questions for which there are unique correct answers.

In spite of the absence of a sound theory, the concept is operationally useful. Intelligence is a descriptor of the quality of mental functioning, the ceiling of intellectual manipulation to which the individual can rise. High achievers in technically demanding fields are always intelligent although the converse is not true. That is, there are many intelligent individuals who are not high achievers. It follows that a particular score from an intelligence appraisal can be a useful cut-off point in that those who do not attain the cut-off should not be expected to cope with the demands of the particular task. However, a high score does not necessarily predict success in a high level job. The intelligence test can be a useful source of evidence about individuals who are considered for lower level jobs. For more senior jobs individuals will have already demonstrated an appropriate level of intelligence by their educational standards and successful work experience. In line with the principles of defining the relevant abilities in terms of reliable test measures, intelligence can be divided into verbal ability, arithmetical ability, reasoning ability and spatial ability. For more extensive discussion see Eysenck (1979).

There is a long established distinction in psychology between cognitive and conative aspects of behaviour. Cognition is to do with the rational domain:

logic, reasoning and problem solving uncomplicated by irrational behaviour. Conation is to do with the emotional domain: feeling, caring and striving. Intelligence is connected with cognition but personality incorporates conation. Thus Freudian theory is regarded as a personality theory. Clearly if we wish to describe the whole person conative aspects must be included. Unfortunately personality testing is much less well developed than intelligence testing. The best known personality tests are the Minnesota Multiphase Personality Inventory (M.M.P.I.), Catell's test (16 P.F.), and the Eysenck Personality Inventory (E.P.I.). For details see Kline (1976). These are self-report inventories where the testee has the possibility of cheating in that he can respond with an answer which he considers will give him a good score rather than providing a completely truthful one. Such manipulation of answers is less feasible with *projective* tests where the testee is asked to respond to a highly ambiguous situation and his response is presumed to reflect his personality as well as the situation. The presentation might be a picture (thematic apperception test), an ink-blot (Rorschach test) or prose (sentence completion test). The difficulty about using these tests is how to score the responses with any reasonable hope of reliability let alone validity.

There are other tests which relate indirectly to personality, namely interest tests. Here the testee is presented with a set of questions or checklists which steer him into trying to think carefully about his own interests. The best known ones are the Kuder Preference test and the Strong–Campbell interest inventory. They are particularly useful in occupational guidance (Nelson-Jones 1982).

Age differences

The extremes of the age range, children and old people, are outside the scope of this book. The working age range is 15 to 65 years. This is not to suggest that those outside this range never work, but rather that in advanced countries gainful employment is considered to be mainly the responsibility of those in this particular age band of 50 years. This band is currently contracting even further in European societies. Because of the rise in unemployment it is now becoming standard that almost all those in the 15–18 age range are in education or training schemes and retirement is increasingly common from 55 years upwards, particularly from manufacturing industry.

Nevertheless, from both physiological and psychological viewpoints, ageing is regarded as a continuous process so that considerable changes can be expected between 18 and 55 years. Using the information processing model of receptor, central and effector processes (Welford, 1958; Birren and Schaie, 1977), changes occur in all these processes. The receptors diminish in efficiency: there are consistent changes in visual acuity and changes in sensitivity to light, the threshold of hearing increases particularly for higher frequencies. The effector processes become slower and less powerful but these effects are not so marked or so consistent. The main change in central processes seems to be decreased short-term memory which results in performance which is less rapid and more deliberate; measured intelligence falls slightly but not very much within the working age range. This may seem to be a gloomy picture but it must be noted that, in relation to work, age is not a large aspect of individual differences compared with natural endowment, and that increases in ability can more than compensate for small decreases in capacity. Welford (1979) suggests that work on the shop-floor is likely to peak in the thirties – those in their twenties lack experience and social skills, those in their forties are beginning to notice the effect of sensory changes and are less tolerant of fast or very heavy physical work. On the other hand, from the forties onwards there is likely to be greater stability in the sense that individuals are more settled in their jobs and ambitions and are supported by less rapidly changing domestic and leisure situations.

The effectiveness of training can be maintained if the training scheme incorporates features such as smaller learning steps and 'discovery learning' where the trainee proceeds at his own pace using his own strategies (Belbin 1965).

For more senior positions there are more subtle attributes such as self-knowledge and the ability to see 'the big picture' which increase with age, these are the reasons why most institutions and societies rely on older leaders (Singleton, 1983b).

Sex differences

There is surprisingly little research on the differences in work performance which are traceable to sex differences, and the situation is complicated in many countries by the inclusion of sex as one of the variables where discrimination is legally inadmissible. Incidentally, in this book 'man', 'he' and 'him' are used as generic terms covering both sexes.

There can be no argument that, on average, women are physically smaller than men, and there are other features such as the greater proportion of fatty tissue which give men the advantage in relation to tolerance of heat stress and physical effort involving fast or heavy work or awkward posture. On the other hand in Russia, for example, where so many males were lost in two world wars women do do much heavier work than is traditional in Western countries. Similarly there seem to be many cultures in tropical countries where the women get on with the necessary work while the men sit around discussing matters.

There appear to be no important differences in performance on intelligence tests in the working age range and as the influence of physical effort in work becomes less important so it is more feasible that jobs can be performed equally well by either sex. The overall situation was reviewed by Hoiberg (1982). Equal opportunity legislation exists in most advanced countries but this is not yet reflected in equal pay rates. The average wage of women workers is two-thirds that of men. Part-time work seems to be a prerogative of women presumably as a consequence of their central role in the home. Educational opportunity varies, depending mainly on family attitudes. In some cultures sons are given priority, others give daughters priority, following the McIver principle 'when you educate a man you educate an individual: when you educate a woman you educate a whole family'.

Ethnic, cultural, climatic and economic differences

This is a sensitive topic on which to conduct research or establish principles with the consequence that, in spite of the extensive effort (Triandis *et al.*, 1980) there is not a great deal of knowledge established beyond argument.

Climate and economics need to be included because these factors may well determine features which at first sight might be attributed to ethnic or cultural factors. Clearly the work that people do is determined by the level of technology which is related to overall wealth. Ways of working and locations of work are also affected by climate. For example, in a tropical country shoes may still be made in the open air by a craftsman who uses his feet as well as his hands to hold and manipulate materials. In a temperate country shoes are made in a factory by workers who are process controllers rather than craftsmen, and they touch the materials only when loading or unloading machines. For these and many other reasons the practice of ergonomics in developing countries is different from that in advanced countries (p. 155).

The acquisition of skills is governed by the current needs of particular societies and by the adaptation of individuals within the societies in which they happen to find themselves. Research on the influence of cultural factors on intelligence testing and test results have been conducted on a wide scale and the results are endlessly discussed because of the inextricable mixture of technical and value judgments. As Crombach puts it in the foreword to Irvine and Berry (1981) 'the progress is as much in the psychology of the investigators as in the investigations being reported'. As in other fields of behavioural study there are three phases. In the first phase techniques and theories are developed in the West. In the second phase Western practitioners try out their ideas in other cultures and many new insights emerge by comparisons and contrasts, in particular it becomes clear that some of the principles thought to be valid for 'man' turn out to be valid only for man in Western cultures. In the third phase scientists from other cultures acquire these concepts, develop them further in their indigenous environment and provide penetrating comments on Western ideas and their application from an external viewpoint (Crombach and Drenth, 1972).

The dominant influence of culture on the direction of human development implies that descriptions of human abilities cannot be context free. Specific cultures are themselves dynamic, in particular they change under the influence of technology. Ergonomics cannot be simply the adaptation of technology to suit invariant properties of 'man', people change with technology.

2.2.2 *Learning*

Learning has been a major topic within academic psychology for the past century or so. The nineteenth century work of Pavlov on the conditioned reflex generated vain hopes that psychology, and in particular learning, might be studied by a rigorous methodology closely allied to physiology. It was assumed that all learning could be reduced to a series of conditioned reflexes. There was extensive research in this behaviourist tradition (Hilgard and Marquis, 1940) mostly on the laboratory rat. So called verbal learning in man was studied by a similar process of scoring repetitive performance. Reliance on such data produced the systematic behaviour theories of Thorndike, Hull and Skinner. There was a parallel although less popular theoretical development based on Gestalt psychology which resulted in the field theories of Lewin, Wheeler and Tolman (Hilgard, 1948). There were many attempts to devise taxonomies of learning which used particular theories as descriptive of different kinds of learning (Melton, 1964). At this stage there seemed to be little connection between the vast experience of learning in practice within educational and training systems and learning as conceived by psychologists on the basis of laboratory experiments. The psychologists attempted to polarise various issues such as massed versus spaced learning, whole versus part learning and transfer of training which had some face validity in appearing to identify general principles, but in practice it always seemed that the generalities vanished into the enormous variety of specific issues. The answer always differed with the particular situation. Gagne (1970) attempted to produce a theory which was germane to educational problems by switching the emphasis from categories to conditions of learning. The deliberate attempt to link learning to the design of instruction provided the necessary discipline to treat learning as a practical as well as a theoretical issue. The eight types of learning which Gagne distinguishes are shown in Table 2.2. Gagne also separated four

Table 2.2. *Gagne types of learning*

Signal learning	An automatic but diffuse usually emotional response to a familiar signal
Stimulus–Response	A specific adaptive reaction to a stimulus which is understood
Chaining	Connecting together a series of Stimulus–Response units
Verbal association	Connecting together words which have related meaning
Discrimination learning	Identification by patterns of subtle distinctions
Concept learning	The abstraction of generalisations by common features applicable to a variety of situations
Rule learning	Connecting together two or more concepts
Problem solving	Creating a higher order rule by connecting established rules

phases of a learning sequence; apprehension, acquisition, storage and re-trieval. The apprehension phase includes attending and perceiving, that is accepting new information. Acquisition is not easy to separate from either apprehension on one side or storage on the other, but it implies that learning has taken place in that something new can now be done if appropriate. The distinction from apprehension is necessary to incorporate the phenomenon that it is possible to understand a situation in one sense without knowing what to do about it. Correspondingly acquisition is different from storage in that the latter implies a formal recording possibly in short-term or possibly in long-term memory. Finally retrieval is a separate process because of another familiar phenomenon that it is possible to know something, that is it must be in storage, but not actually succeed in retrieving it at a particular time. These phases and the difficulties of separating them reflect the fact that mental processes are not subject to clearly defined distinctions and boundaries. In common with all educational psychologists Gagne is also restricted by reliance on evidence which comes mostly from laboratory experiments, usually on lower animals, with all the limitations and artefacts which this implies. More subtly he is also restricted by attempting to set the knowledge in another artificial situation, the educational process of sitting in classrooms learning by rote leavened by some understanding and being examined and tested in standardised situations.

Thomas and Harri-Augstein (1985) attempt a more autonomous approach to learning in two senses. That is, learning need not be restricted to the orthodox educational system and also that learning, as a process, is essentially self-centred, and self-organised. This approach follows the tradition of Rogers (1951) who developed client-centred therapy and Kelly (1955) who developed personal construct theory. The emphasis is on the individual who inevitably has a unique view of the world which he continuously modifies in the light of experience. Each view of the world can be described using personal constructs which can be elicited by the use of a Repertory Grid. The individual reflects on his own experience and is thus continuously involved in both internal and external conversations. Learning takes place as a result of these conversations. Traditional distinctions between teaching, training and therapy disappear, so also does the conceptual distinction between cognition and conation. One attractive aspect of this theory is that it highlights the way in which formal instruction can inhibit learning by not allowing sufficient scope for self-expression and self-development – alienation following submission to being taught rather than learning how to learn. The emphasis on self does not limit the application to individual activity, shared meaning can be negotiated and developed within groups, this is group learning. Correspondingly the teacher is not redundant, a competent teacher is a learning manager and so also is every parent, manager or counsellor, their task is to provide the conditions and facilitate the process of self-development.

If learning is defined as the improvement of specific performance following experience of that performance then organisations as well as individuals can be said to learn. Paradoxically much of the more abstract work on the mathematical theory of learning curves has its application at least in principle in the requirements of accountants and production engineers. The process of making anything from a switch to a civil airliner is subject to improvements in speed, quality and cost reduction which follow the characteristic learning curve. It is obviously important to the managers of such organisations to be able to predict by how much the process will improve after particular lengths of time and numbers of products made.

Conversely, because of the universal very steep learning curves with early experience, any novel enterprise is bound to have extensive teething troubles, which should be allowed for in general even though they are not predictable in particular. Experiments, trials, prototypes and the running in parallel of old and new systems are all valuable, almost essential procedures – when something radical is being attempted on any scale from a new car suspension to a new educational system. Technology and society generally is continuously in trouble because this elementary principle is forgotten or ignored by enthusiastic innovators.

2.2.3 *Memory and thinking*

Thinking is essentially an internal activity although of course it is stimulated and aided by interaction with the external world including other people. Since it takes place 'inside' it must be related to memory. This is one of several complications of the simplistic view that memory is just a store. Another is that a store is useless without means of access and egress. In other words there must be processes of recording and retrieval and the underlying mechanisms must be closely integrated with the mechanism of the store. The store or stores are almost certainly active rather than passive records of events and knowledge so that these also are best considered as processes.

Early studies of memory by psychologists concentrated on apparatus such as the memory drum which was used to measure the ability to associate verbal items. In the pursuit of generality these items were often nonsense syllables. This is another example of the way in which the attempt to standardise human performance can negate the purpose of study. There is a built-in assumption that memory is about association and a removal of any possibility of demonstrating that memory might be dependent on meaning.

Other early studies of memory attempted to measure capacity by data such as the length of a number series which could be accurately reproduced after one presentation. The answer turns out to be about seven (Woodworth, 1938). These studies of immediate memory span are of more than historical interest because the fact that there is such a severe limit is important in the design of information presentations of technical data – a standard ergonomics problem.

Other significant phenomena which have emerged from such studies are that simple reversals of the numbers are a common form of error, accurate reproduction is facilitated by deliberate grouping in twos or threes and the ends of a span seem to be less prone to error than the middle. With the advent of information theory (Attneave, 1959; Edwards, 1964) other interesting issues arose such as whether the performance of the store could better be measured in terms of bits of information or chunks of material (the bits-versus-chunks controversy (Miller, 1956)) and the possibility that memory processes might distinguish between content and order. The simple memory span measure confounds these variables.

Clearly there is more to memory than the reproduction of numbers or lists and another distinction which has arisen is between episodic and semantic memory. The former is concerned with specific events and the latter is relatively context free (Baddeley, 1976). A parallel but not identical distinction is between short-term and long-term memory. Short-term memory has capacity limits and is readily purged, it probably keeps a record of the current situation, whereas the long-term memory is the repository of principles and strategies. Both these distinctions imply that registration in storage continues long past the time of reception of information. Whether or not this implies shifting to different stores is not known. In functional terms there do seem to be storage facilities relatively near the entry channels through the senses, those for the visual and auditory systems are called respectively the iconic store and the echoic store (Wickens, 1984). These stores have available a literal record of the stimulus so that the observer can, as it were, internally inspect them but such impressions decay very rapidly, typically in less than ten seconds.

In an elegant series of experiments Conrad (1964) demonstrated that in transposing visually presented data the errors are more likely to be in numbers or letters of similar sound rather than those which are of similar appearance. This suggests that this short-term store is auditorally rather than visually based even when the task is visual-motor. The effect diminishes if there is irrelevant articulatory activity at the time, this raises the possibility that there may be pre-output stores as well as post-input stores, almost literally memory in the fingers. If an experienced operator of a complex console of switches is asked where a particular switch is he will often touch it and check what he has touched, the action precedes the recall and recall precedes recognition.

The distinction between recall and recognition is clearly an important one, in that the human memory is so much superior in the latter function. We may be totally unable to recall an event or a fact but recognise it and all its context immediately if it is presented. Again there seems to be a distinction between what and when. Any busy person will recall that he has a particular engagement but will have only a sparse internal record of when this commitment will arise, hence the importance of a diary. If asked to recall a date such a person will proceed by inference rather than by a direct introspective search, e.g. 'it cannot be next week but it must be within the next month' or 'this kind of event is always on a Tuesday' and so on.

This is one illustration of the process which Bartlett (1932) called 'turning round on one's own schemata' – 'I am in this state therefore this must be so' rather than the direct retrieval from a store. In Bartlett's view long-term memory involves the reconstruction of events, such remembering is subject to bias and distortion not only from idiosyncracy but also from the context and even the culture. It is in this sense that memory is a consequence of the continuously modified record of experience (p. 100) rather than a separate function.

The analogy of the ego or self, the internal little man consulting personal records is attractive but misleading. One dubious consequence is that the short-term memory, of limited capacity compared with the virtually infinite capacity of long-term memory, is conceived as the internal stage on which exhibits from the store are manipulated. This is one view of thinking but again it is thinking restricted by the limitations of the laboratory situation where the problem must be easily assimilated and the proposed solution is readily measurable.

Psychological research on thinking has been the province of the field theorists, in particular the gestalt psychologists (Humphrey, 1951). There was considerable debate within this school about the overlapping concepts of motive, determining tendency and set. Some such concept is required to explain why different individuals reach different solutions in diagnosing and providing remedies for particular situations. These ideas have recently been revived by the concept of 'mind-set' to describe why errors are made in coping with complex system failures. Craik (1943) considered that thinking paralleled reality in that within the mind there must be a model of reality which can be manipulated independently of the outside world. The advantages of such a mechanism are clear, it is possible to manipulate the model and thus understand the outside world in the sense of predicting what will happen without the potential costs of attempting to manipulate the real world and allowing things to happen, some of which might be considered to be unfortunate. Using technology, this process can now be partially externalised in that, for example, a simulation of a situation can be run in parallel with a real situation and can be manipulated independently of what happens in real time. Bartlett (1958) regarded thinking as a form of skill in that it has the characteristics of organising information. A situation can be structured and comprehended so as to indicate a direction for proceeding. In technological situations there is often also a timing characteristic, evidence is developing and at some point in the future, which itself has to be determined, something will have to be done. One attribute of thinking as opposed to perception is that the evidence is relatively less complete, gaps have to be filled either within or beyond the available data. This is achieved on the basis of past experience and interests. Inevitably the product of thinking is a function of the thinker as well as of the situation. Past experience is brought to bear on a new situation by a categorisation, a process regarded as central to thinking by Bruner and his colleagues (1956). Classification must be a function not only of the situation but also of the existing internalised classes and their relative accessibility. Bruner (1957) discusses the classical problem of determining tendency as 'perceptual readiness' and notes also the problem that the first classification can mask a more appropriate classification. This relates to a currently important limitation in fault diagnosis for technological systems where a first hypothesis about the cause of the problem can inhibit flexibility in considering other possible causes.

The above ideas were generated mainly on the basis of experiments and it is not surprising that many of the key characteristics of thinking in real situations were not given sufficient weight. These include the use of evidence arising from the absence of events rather than their presence, the cost-effectiveness criterion in pursuing evidence and reasoning processes based on extensive experience rather than intellectual analysis. More recent work on observation of, rather than experiment with thinking (Johnson-Laird and Wason, 1977) goes some way to restoring the balance in appraising all the relevant parameters in a real situation where thinking is taking place.

There is also a dearth of evidence about thinking by groups. This is surprising in view of the time which people spend in committees, task forces and the like. There is experimental work on issues such as kinds of group organisation, e.g. autocratic versus democratic versus laissez-faire (Sherif, 1948) and on the group dynamics of people interactions (Lewin, 1935) but little work on the process of problem solving by groups. The collective mind in action is clearly an important topic but it seems to be a challenge which psychologists have not yet taken up. It is important in education as well as in gainful employment (Singleton, 1983a).

2.2.4 Language

There has been extensive work on the psychology of language (Campbell and Smith, 1976; Gerver and Sinaiko, 1978), but with a greater emphasis on language as an interpersonal communication vehicle rather than language as a supporter of thinking. The work of Piaget (1950) and Chomsky (1957) is essentially about thinking and language or psycholinguistics, but these authors did not concern themselves with the level of problem which arises when, for example, a physiologist and a psychologist attempt to exchange mutually supportive ideas. Herriot (1970, 1974), however, makes some interesting suggestions about the relationship between language, schema, strategies and deep structure. As he sees it, deep structure is represented in schemata which relate non-linguistic and linguistic thinking. Language and indeed behaviour generally is necessarily ordered and is represented internally as strategies, schemata are not inherently sequential and thinking can thus be concerned with context before the constraint of achieving is introduced in order to generate an output.

Thinking regarded as internal manipulation of events and ideas does not necessarily depend on language, but if it is not entirely ego orientated, that is not concentrated on the relationship of the person to the scheme of things, then it usually invokes iconic representation. Designers of computer based support for thinking beyond the level of merely providing additional information will hopefully begin to simultaneously use and develop these ideas. Effective computer support must be matched to human thinking so that communication is readily established and yet different in providing functions which supplement human thinking (p. 233).

2.2.5 Learning and memory

The learner must have the drive to learn and he must also have knowledge of the results of his activities.

1. Behaviour at a higher skilled level is characterised by selectivity in choice of inputs and outputs and by increasing influence of the past and the future rather than the immediate situation.

2. Learning is an activity of an individual, no one else can do it for him. Educators and trainers can do no more than provide the conditions, the content and the materials.

3. Social skills and communication generally depend on the detection and definition of mutually agreed internal models of reality.

4. The human memory, in common with every other store, has to be positively consulted before it will function. This is not a limitation, it is essential for coherent behaviour, there would be chaos if material emerged without prompting. The trigger is usually some external stimulus, not necessarily an obvious one. It might be a particular smell, a particular melody or a brief glimpse of a person resembling one of the actors in an event which is then recalled. This facility for associations which are neither obvious nor apparently logical is extremely valuable in creative thinking and problem solving. The converse of positively trying to recall some fact such as the name of a person is subject to curious blockages which are not understood.

5. Given the alternative of storage internally in the mind or externally in a file (paper-based or computer-based) external records are much superior for literal reproductions at least in western societies (there is anecdotal evidence concerning illiterate traders in other cultures who seem to have remarkable memories for detailed facts and numbers connected with their personal business). The capacity and flexibility of desk-top computers is now such that the optimal sharing of processing, storage and presentation of material between computer and operator may well be quite different from the traditional combination of human memory and material on paper. This topic is too recent for there to be many guidelines available but for a particular topic the designer can assume that he need not be inhibited in allowing his imagination to run to many kinds of novel solutions.

6. There is a considerable art in developing the most effective combination of external and internal stores and reminders which every highly skilled person

deliberately cultivates. For example, there is no need to write in a diary 'check in-tray and consult secretary', these actions take place as routine following arrrival at the office. On the other hand a diary entry such as 'ring X' is effective and if the entry is some way in the future it may be necessary to amplify with a trigger of the form 'ring X re Y' and to have easily accessible some factual data such as the X telephone number and some data re Y. In a different context a car driver will develop a strategy to ensure that he does not run out of petrol, he may rely on a light which appears when the tank is nearly empty or he may calculate from his expected travelling that he need not concern himself about the issue until at least the next weekend, or he may programme himself to react to the fact that he is approaching a particular garage.

This self-programming goes on continuously with an implicit acknowledgment of the need for triggers and the relative advantages of various kinds of stores and stored materials.

7. This self-organised work design has its parallel in designing tasks for others. In studying an elaborate sequence of events within a task the designer will systematically consider the need for appropriate triggers for the memory at specific points in the task. In particular he will never rely on the operator spontaneously remembering to do something which has no natural place in the developing task (p. 56).

8. There are at least three and probably many more levels of storage. The sensory stores decay very rapidly, items are lost in less than ten seconds. The short-term store has a limit of about twenty seconds unless there is opportunity for rehearsal, e.g. this is the maximum time available between looking up a telephone number and then dialling it unless the operator repeats it to himself. Some kinds of long-term memory seem to endure indefinitely even though they have apparently been lost for a long time, e.g. an older person may find it easy to recall childhood events with great clarity even though there has been no use of the material for fifty or sixty years.

9. There seems to be a memory for elaborate patterns and sequences which takes a long time to develop. For example a chemist will learn about compounds by laboriously memorising as a student the properties of each one separately but eventually sets of compounds are perceived as a pattern and thereafter all the relevant material is readily available because it fits together neatly.

The corollary for the trainer is to look for patterns which exist in complex material and introduce the trainee to the patterns as well as to the separate facts. Similarly an information presentation will be more readily comprehended if there is a detectable structure such as the 'christmas tree' method of working through a checklist.

10. Errors in recall can be similar for different individuals. For example the propensity for simple reversals within a number sequence. It follows that attempting to reduce error rates by one person checking another's performance or automatically comparing the output of the individuals simultaneously performing the same task is not as effective as it would be if errors in the sources were independent (Chapanis *et al.*, 1949).

2.3 Principles, methods and procedures
2.3.1 *Interviewing*

An interview is a formal conversation in which there is a non-reciprocal relationship between the parties. It is formal in that there are purposes which define the reasons why the transaction is taking place. There is conversation which is usually face to face but may sometimes involve telecommunication. It is non-reciprocal in that the two parties are never equivalent; one is the interviewer who has the initiative, the other is the interviewee. The interviewing party may be a group facing one interviewee, e.g. a selection board. The interviewed party may be a group facing one interviewer, e.g. a group of witnesses facing a reporter. Any transaction involving two groups or two equivalent individuals is regarded as a negotiation rather than an interview. The interview can be initiated by either side, e.g. by the interviewer when a more senior person calls a subordinate or by the interviewee when a patient calls a doctor. The information transmission will inevitably be two-way but the main purpose may be transmission from interviewer to interviewee as in an appraisal interview, from interviewee to interviewer as in an opinion survey, or it may change direction during the course of the interview as in a patient–doctor interview. In this last case the interviewee begins by providing information which facilitates a diagnosis and the interviewer thereafter provides information about possible causes and remedies.

In view of the universality and range of the interview situation it is not surprising that there has been extensive research, but for the same reasons the research is of little operational consequence. Checks of interview effectiveness by, for example, having the same list of candidates ranked independently by two selection boards invariably indicates rather poor consistency. On the other hand no manager willingly accepts a new member of staff without the use of a selection interview, no doctor will express a confident diagnosis without an interview with the patient, and no counsellor could function without meeting his clients face to face. The key to the issue is that interviews except in the simplest case of surveys, to be discussed later, are not about acquiring factual evidence. This is best obtained by asking interviewees to complete standard forms or to take tests before or between interviews. Information obtained during an interview is about assessable but unquantifiable attributes such as attitudes, motivation, reliability, integrity, social ease and so on.

In skill terminology the interviewer uses the interview to create a model in his mind which he can use to predict the behaviour of the individual interviewee in a work situation, a stress situation, an illness or whatever an interview is about. Obviously he can create a better model if he knows what the interviewee looks like, how he dresses, talks and responds non-verbally. Equally the interviewee forms a model of the interviewer(s) and this can be a considerable aid to his decision-making about whether he can respect, trust, work with or tolerate guidance from the interviewer. This interaction may or may not achieve a successful conclusion for both sides depending on their level of skill. Attempting to do research on the interview *per se* is doomed to failure because the skills of the actors will dominate the success or otherwise of the proceedings. It should be remembered also that the interview is only one incident within a series of communication functions which aim towards one objective. For example, a work placement involves trawling for candidates, testing and form-filling and preliminary sifts before the interview followed by induction and training after the interview. Those responsible are interested in an effective total process not just an effective interview and all the stages in the process interact.

For these reasons it is difficult to generate principles of interviewing, there are always alternative viewpoints and exceptions. For example:

1.	Always try to put the interviewees at ease. For senior posts it can be instructive to do the opposite to see how far the candidate can cope with the stress.

2.	Always ask open-ended questions. If the interviewee is very nervous it can help to ask some questions which can readily be answered with a yes or no, this provides the opportunity to adjust the tension.

3.	Do not make jokes. Sometimes the interviewee exhibits too much respect creating a communication barrier, a demonstration that the interviewer is only human by a weak joke can remove this barrier.

4.	Always structure the interview to ensure that all essential points are covered. On the contrary a free-wheeling interview with direction changes as key points emerge can yield unexpected but valuable evidence.

5.	Assess the interviewee under various headings to obtain a comparable profile score. Part of the skill of the interviewer is in extracting different salient points from individuals and appropriately weighting totally disparate facets.

On the other hand it must be acknowledged that there are many bad interviews and, as always, improvement is possible by design, consideration of procedures and training.

The design of the situation and the process should adhere to standard practices which have been found to be helpful by experience and commonsense.

1. Obtain all the relevant factual data (biography and testscores) before the final interview.
2. Provide a waiting room which has accessible toilet facilities including mirrors.
3. The interviewer should collect the interviewee, not have him sent for from the waiting room.
4. Provide the interviewee with a written job aid which indicates the name and function of the interviewer(s).
5. The relative positioning of the two main interactors and the direction of lighting are significant. The obvious 'third-degree' lighting should be avoided but not being able to see the inverviewee clearly is equally deleterious. Face to face is the most formal, side by side the least formal, seating at right angles is often a suitable compromise.
6. Provide the interviewee with opportunities to make points which have not been covered in questions and to ask other questions on matters important to him. This is not mere courtesy, what the interviewee regards as important can be very revealing.
7. Provide clear if indirect indications that the interview is ending.
8. Tell the interviewee what the next stage in the process will be and when.
9. Escort the interviewee at least to the door, again the behaviour at the parting point can be significant.

In view of the above discussion training of interviewers and interviewees must necessarily be based on principles of training (p. 121) rather than principles of interviewing.

Role playing and case studies are often used and they can be effective in reducing self-unease (self-awareness and self-analysis are necessary attributes of the good interviewer in action) and highlighting idiosyncratic features such as mannerisms and biases. The most powerful tool of the interview trainer is the closed circuit television system. So powerful that it needs to be used circumspectly to avoid reducing self-confidence. Normally the trainer will go through a reproduced interview and discuss the good and bad points which are usually clearly evident. This provides salutary knowledge of results of the interview itself if not of its degree of success in terms of a real objective. Randell (1978) suggests that an interviewing at work course can reasonably take two days covering 'unfreezing', conceptual analysis, technique development and practice with feedback. Rutter (1979) devised an interview training programme for medical students involving a history taking scheme and two videotaped 15 minute diagnostic sessions one week apart, with discussion feedback based on a nine-point method of scoring information elicited. These scores were also used to validate the training by comparing experimental and control groups.

2.3.2 *Psychological testing*

The design and development of tests is a well established formal procedure involving checking for internal consistency and absence of ambiguity, efficiency of administration and marking procedures and the production of norms for definitive populations. There is a comprehensive list and description of available tests in the '*Mental Measurement Yearbook*' which is updated at intervals of a few years.

The *reliability* of a test is measured by correlation between the test scores, obtained at two different times, between different forms of the same test or between samples of questions in different parts of the same test. The interpretation of this measure of consistency is not as straightforward as it seems at first sight. For example, it has been pointed out that one person cannot be asked the same question twice, the second time he is not the same person because he has already been asked the question once.

The *validity* of a test is an even more complex concept. It refers in general to the confidence the tester can attach to decisions based on the test scores. There are at least three kinds of validity: construct validity which refers to the degree to which the test seems to be based on psychological theory, content validity which describes how well the test measures what it is intended to measure and criterion validity which indicates its value as a predictor using as criteria other measures of relevant performance.

The problems of criterion validity nicely illustrate the difficulty of finding any solid foundation on which to construct a psychometric measure. Suppose that the purpose of a particular test is to predict success in a particular job. Even with hindsight this is not easy to determine. The measure of success in a training course depends on the validity of the training course itself, supervisors' opinions based on experience of job performance are subject to distortion by various biases and measured performance such as productivity is subject to many vicissitudes independent of the ability of the producer.

Faced with all these uncertainties the strategies adopted in the U.S.A. and Europe are in general different but usefully complementary. The American approach is to be as formal and rigorous as possible with insistence on systematic sampling, correlating and so on. The European approach is less tidy and more humanistic with continuous questioning of philosophies and methodologies. A good example of the latter is Heim (1970) in which intelligence and personality testing is discussed in the context of the meaning of intelligence, creativity, personality, test taking as a skill and the different but inseparable limitations of speed and accuracy based measures. For further discussion of these elusive topics see Super and Bohn (1971), Drenth (1978) and Jessup and Jessup (1975).

The aim of psychological measurement is optimal discrimination between individuals, for this purpose the difficulty of the test should match the range of abilities of the testees. For example an intelligence test may be too easy so that all testees have almost perfect scores, or too difficult in that all testees have very low scores, in both cases discrimination will be poor. One answer to this problem is *tailored testing* in which questions are computer-based and the test is adaptive in focussing the range of presented questions at about the level of success/failure which is appropriate for each testee. In this way discrimination is much improved without excessively lengthening the test time (Killcross and Cassie, 1975).

The value and extent of the use of tests is subject to other changes in the history of the particular community. Obviously testing can be extensively utilised in war-time when many people are changing jobs both in military and civilian life. In peace-time the selection ratio, the ratio of applicants to available jobs is a key feature, there tends to be more testing in times of economic depression when jobs are scarce and also in post-war periods when there is extensive experience of using tests.

The use of tests is not, of course, confined to selection procedures. Indeed there is currently much greater utilisation in guidance and therapy.

2.3.3 *Surveys*

In common with tests, surveys are required to be as reliable and valid as is feasible in the circumstances. Surveys are however different from tests in their objective: a test is usually carried out to find out about an individual, a survey is carried out to find out about an issue which is across people.

The issue itself must be specified as precisely as possible usually in terms of both what we want to know and why we want to know. 'Why' will clarify 'what' and will also contribute to the practical question of how much to spend on finding out.

For reasons of economy the population of individuals approached is usually a small sample of the total relevant population. The size of the sample is less important than its structure. The first rule of sampling is that each member of the relevant population must have some chance of being included. If the probability of being included is equal for each member of the relevant population then the sample is said to be a random one. Often the relevant population is stratified to ensure that the sample will be more representative in certain respects. For example a survey of hospital staff would not usually be carried out by selecting names at random from the total staff list, it might concentrate on doctors, nurses or cleaners only, or might sample medical, paramedical, administrative and support staff in proportions of their total numbers depending on the purpose of the survey.

Sampling might also be carried out progressively involving different stages. For example a survey concerned with the whole National Health Service staff might begin by separating the hospital and the general practice services, then sample key regions of the country, separate urban, suburban and rural services and then select within organisations as mentioned above. Sampling might also involve time phasing as in attempting to detect opinion trends leading up to a general election. It is possible to estimate sample sizes required if the tolerable error is known and vice versa (Yates 1960).

Data may be obtained purely by observation but usually involve asking questions. The design of questionnaires is itself an art with certain ground rules. Clearly the questions must be such that the relevant population can be expected to understand them and to make informed responses. The questions must avoid ambiguities which is not as easy as it might seem, it is desirable to obtain several opinions about the interpretation of each question from the same kind of people as those who will be in the survey. The sequence of questions may bias the answers e.g. a likely alternation of Yes/No answers is more 'natural' than a uniform series of Yes or No answers. The style of the question can also be unintentionally 'loaded' towards a particular response. There is a temptation to put in questions which will check against each other but this can irritate the responder who will easily detect redundancy. There is also the temptation to make the questionnaire too long in the hope of getting just that little bit more information, this can more than defeat its object by reducing the response rate. A new questionnaire should always be piloted, that is tried out on a small sample, before it is finalised.

The main factor influencing response rate is whether the survey is postal or personal. The response rate to a verbal questionnaire can easily be 90% or more but a mailed questionnaire can have a response rate as low as 30% even with follow-up reminders. A low response rate is serious particularly if there is reason to suspect that persons likely to give particular kinds of answers might be less or more likely to respond than others. Telephone based surveys are currently popular as a reasonable compromise, this increases the speed of data collection rather than the insight which is revealed by personal interviews.

Table 2.3. *The survey method*

1. Define what is required
2. Consider why it is required
3. Determine sampling techniques
4. Determine sample sizes
5. Determine any stages and phases
6. Consider administration (personal, postal, telephone)
7. Design questionnaire
8. Pilot questionnaire
9. Administer questionnaire
10. Determine response rate and assess consequences
11. Code and structure data
12. Consider data handling
13. Prepare report
14. Present to users

Large scale impersonal surveys can be supplemented by more personally based interviews either with individuals or groups.

The inference from samples may be deductive or inductive. Deductions can be made by statistical comparisons of samples to determine whether they are from different populations. Inferences from samples to populations can be made within quantitative confidence limits.

Much of the labour which used to be involved in manipulating and presenting data can now be delegated to specialised computer software but the basic issues of coding and structuring data still depend on the skills of the analyst.

The survey is the most extensively used method of obtaining generalisations about people. It can vary in precision from quantitative anthropometric surveys to attempts to describe the attributes of products which particular users prefer. The systematic survey is the antidote to excessive reliance on personal experience which is usually biased by exposure to idiosyncratic samples and by selective perception. The required systematic process is summarised in Table 2.3.

2.3.4 Task training

The distinction between task training and skill training is one of degree rather than kind. In task training the objective is to guide the trainee into following rules and essentially to make the performance more automatic. In skill training the opposite can apply, the trainee is persuaded to be flexible

Table 2.4. *Task training and skill training*

Task Training	Skill Training
System oriented	Person oriented
Procedures based	Purpose based
Measured by sequential performance	Controlled by conditions/guidelines
Based on task analysis	Based on skills analysis

and to orient himself towards the end rather than the means. The difference between the two kinds of training is not as great as would appear at first sight because it turns out that task training has in common with skill training an emphasis on the perceptual side of human functioning. Even in what appear to be straightforward motor skills the changes in learning are associated with greater selectivity and more economical use of the evidence needed to guide performance. These distinctions are summarised in Table 2.4. Task training is often called operator training or industrial training.

The essential principles are:

1.   The trainee must wish to learn, nothing can be achieved unless the trainee is adequately motivated.

2.   The learning must be steered by adequate knowledge of performance.

The behavioural characteristic which facilitates both of these requirements is knowledge of results. This is the most potent and consistent performance shaping factor ever uncovered by psychologists. It simultaneously promotes motivation and performance. Knowledge of how well one is doing will not provide the basic motivation in that the performer must care about his performance but if this is established, knowledge of performance is a most vigorous factor in developing and maintaining the will to perform. Carmichael and Dearborn (1950) demonstrated that continuous reading was likely to result in increased failure of concentration within an hour, but if the performance of the reader was checked and confirmed by asking questions at half-hour intervals then performance could continue for six to eight hours without signs of fatigue. Mackworth (1950), within his classical studies of vigilance, showed that without knowledge of results the proportion of detected signals decreased in succeeding half-hours compared with the first half-hour, but for subjects given knowledge of results there was no deterioration compared with the first half-hour through the full two hours of the study.

Correspondingly the effectiveness of performance will improve with knowledge of performance. This is as much a logical as a psychological principle. Clearly if a person has no knowledge of the success of performance the performance cannot improve because there can be no guidelines to steer the improvement. There have been many experiments demonstrating the validity of this principle and exploring detailed variables such as the timing and quality of feedback. For details see Welford (1968), Bilodeau (1969), Annett (1969). Miller *et al.* (1960) formalise it into what they call the TOTE principle (Test – Operate – Test – Exit). The first test is a review of the situation, operate is the action which follows, the second test is a check as to whether or not the desired result has been achieved and this is followed either by another operation or by an exit if the desired result has been achieved. The TOTE is regarded as a fundamental unit of behaviour.

Broadly speaking the more immediate the feedback the more effective it is except that there comes a point at which, to use Miller's (1953) distinction, learning feedback becomes action feedback, the latter improves the current response whereas the former improves succeeding responses. There is a risk that what is intended to be an aid only during training can become an undesirable crutch in that performance comes to depend on it but this is rare and can be avoided by using a suitable time delay, thus ensuring that it is really learning and not action feedback. The accuracy of the feedback need not be greater than the discrimination ability of the trainee but equally its value will diminish if it is too approximate. Feedback of the discrepancy between desirable and achieved performance is superior to feedback of absolute performance. Holding (1965) distinguished between successive sub-classifications of feedback into intrinsic/artificial, concurrent/terminal, immediate/delayed, non-verbal/verbal, separate/accumulated.

The superior value of direct, rapid, unambiguous feedback dominates the choice of length and content of learning periods. There was an extended controversy between supporters of part and whole learning (Blum and Naylor 1968). The advantage of whole learning is that the connections between the parts are also learned simultaneously. However the advantage of part learning is that the feedback can be of much higher quality. An excellent compromise is the progressive-part method (Seymour, 1966) in which parts are learned separately but combined in groups within a tree-like structure which converges on the total task. See, for example, Singleton (1959), King (1964).

The identification of the sub-tasks which are appropriate for intensive training with feedback is achieved by task analysis. Unfortunately there is confusion in the literature and the required procedures may be referred to as either skills analysis or task analysis (Seymour 1968, Singer and Ramsden 1969, Miller 1962). In the terminology used in this book task analysis is the correct description of this activity.

It will be evident from the dates of most of these references that this kind of training and the supporting research flourished in the 1960s. The need for it has reduced but has not vanished over the past twenty years. Technology has shifted the general allocation of function slightly both in industry and in defence. Many processes have changed so that there is less direct human involvement in the production cycle, e.g. metal working, highly repetitive cycles can be conducted by robots and similar devices, e.g. in car assemblies, and the human operator gets better support even when still involved directly, e.g. the word processor as a substitute for the typewriter. Nevertheless within most jobs there are at least some tasks which are amenable to this kind of training and the benefits are considerable. If task training is neglected the larger job may be interfered with, e.g. the manager attempting to use a personal computer with inadequate key-board and data search performance.

Key-board manipulation is a skill relevant to many tasks and is typical of psycho-motor skills in that the perceptual elements of identify and select dominate the motor element of actual key pressing. As mentioned earlier improvements in speed and accuracy result from changes in the control of performance.

2.3.5   Skill training

The simplest criterion for the distinction between a skill and a task is that a skill description is susceptible to individual differences but a task description is not. Skill implies idiosyncratic performance and as such can transfer between many tasks whereas a task meets a particular requirement within a system activity.

Thus it follows that skill training is more generalised and generalisable and is better fitted to the overall role of human operators. Education is the ultimate form of skill training where no attempt is made to specify the particular purposes for which the skills might be utilised. This limits the potential rigour of design because the anchor of skill training is the specification of the objectives. Incidentally this accounts for the interminable debate about education, since objectives are not specifiable the content can only emerge as a consensus within the current *zeitgeist*.

Skill descriptions are generalisable in that human operators have characteristic abilities and limitations and therefore have tendencies to perform in the same way. Differences in level of skill are partly but not wholly attributable to different locations on a learning curve which has some uniformity for that particular skill.

Skills cannot be transferred directly from a trainer to a trainee, the function of the trainer is to provide conditions and guidelines which will facilitate learning. To do this the trainer must have a coherent model of the form of the

Table 2.5. *Task analysis and skills analysis*

Task analysis	Skills analysis
Derived from system	Derived from person
Assumes standardised performance	Assumes idiosyncratic performance
Assumes monitoring by organisation	Assumes self-monitoring
Assumes basic skills only	May depend on specific education, training, experience
Assumes guidance is available in unusual circumstances	Assumes that exponent can cope with obstacles and changes of direction

skill, this is attained by skills analysis. Inevitably skills analysis is more general and less definitive than task analysis although many of the same procedures for extracting evidence might be used. Skills analysis may also involve experiments to study more closely how the required objective is achieved (Drury and Fox, 1975, Singleton, 1978). It requires a broader approach than task analysis in that it often involves tracing the acquisition of the skill starting from the kind of persons who undertake training (the selection criteria) through the training procedures to the end product (the training success criteria). Such training often has an emphasis on features such as style and quality rather than mere speed of activity. This can extend beyond skill training to attitude training (see below). These differences are summarised in Table 2.5.

There is emphasis on the end purpose or objective with relatively less attention to the means, partly so as to allow for individual differences and partly because the evidence accumulating in particular cases may change the direction of progress. For this reason skill training is sometimes called strategic training. Such activities are found in the broad range of tasks concerned with diagnosis. These can vary from dealing with faults in equipment (Tilley, 1967) to dealing with patients in a surgery or clinic (Rutter, 1979). In all cases although the reason for the activity is clear cut the means of achieving the desired end vary widely in terms of the path taken and the time required. The medical interview has much in common with counselling (Joanning *et al.*, 1979) and occupational guidance (Davis and Shackleton, 1975).

Medical diagnosis involves social skills (Melhuish, 1979) but as discussed earlier the basis and development of these skills is not dissimilar from other cognitive skills and correspondingly the training can follow the same principles (Singleton *et al.*, 1980; Argyle, 1981).

2.3.6 *Attitude training*

Attitudes are much more difficult to change than are skills and there can be ambiguity about what constitutes an improvement. Attitudes involve values which vary between individuals, societies and cultures. For example 'brain washing' is a form of attitude training which attempts to change the beliefs and values acquired within a particular culture (Biderman, 1967). The extreme techniques of isolation, starvation and other forms of stress induction give some indication of the pressures required to positively change attitudes. Generation of standard useful attitudes has always been one of the main purposes of military training. The objective is to cultivate the willingness to accept or ignore personal risk (Page, 1987).

In the civilian context the purposes of attitude training are to do with care about quality and safety. Apprenticeship training is essentially about ensuring standards of workmanship and characteristically it appears at first sight to take an unconscionably long time. A common fallacy is the attempt to assess apprenticeship schemes in terms of task and skill training. Safety training is also about attitudes and such schemes rarely have the hoped for success because the difficulty and time required are invariably underestimated. This is also the reason why road accidents are so difficult to approach by training, safety on the road is much more to do with attitudes than with driving skill (Parry, 1968).

In summary, we have no useful theory about the design of attitude training and success in practice is based on indirect traditional procedures.

2.3.7 *Skills analysis*

It will be appreciated from the earlier sections of this chapter that skills analysis is not reducible to simple procedures or recipes. In principle it is impossible because skills are by their nature totally integrated and interactive so that they cannot meaningfully be separated into independent parts. Nevertheless, as in many other situations the analyst, himself a skilled performer, has some success in practice.

A skill description relates to how a task is performed and what is achieved rather than what actions are taken. The reference is to the end and the means is described in person terms rather than task terms. This is because the end is more consistent than the means. Although there may be considerable idiosyncracy in the actions the situation is not anarchical. The human operator has characteristic ways of doing things and detection of these is one aspect of the skill of the skills analyst.

There are differences in skills analysis procedure depending on the kind of skill. For the skills of interacting with the physical world the procedure summarised in Table 2.6 is appropriate. This involves observation of the skill in practice and during training and discussion with practitioners and trainers. There are useful ways of focusing such observation by contrasting good/poor performers and experienced/inexperienced performers. Discussion with practitioners can be focused by asking them to talk while performing and by jointly discussing performances observed on film or tape.

For management skills there is greater emphasis on the objectives and how they are arrived at. Objectives in an organisational context are subject to many constraints. Some such as financial resources are easily specifiable, others such as not contravening the mores of the organisation are more elusive but a key aspect of these skills is sensitivity to limitations and obstacles as well as positive assets (Singleton, 1981). The variety of management tasks is often so great as to warrant a task analysis with separate skills analyses of particular tasks or groups of tasks. At this level the practitioner is often the conscious monitor of the practice and facility in self-monitoring is a useful indicator of skill.

Social skills can involve not only self-monitoring but also monitoring of what another person is thinking as well as doing. For example, analysing a transaction between two skilled negotiators requires the study of the overt interaction and the identification of what each one is thinking about what he himself is doing and what his opponent is probably thinking about in the context of what he is saying (Singleton, 1983a).

There are no standard formats for skill descriptions but usually they can be separated into two parts: the performance and the antecedents to the performance. That is respectively the key aspects of behaviour which contribute to success and the kind of education, training and experience normally required. At high levels of idiosyncratic skill (flair see p. 245) analysis is particularly difficult because the practitioner may have little conscious awareness of how or why he achieves unusual success. In fact it almost seems to be a condition of such performance that the exponent must not proceed logically but must temporarily inhibit his conscious critical faculties and accept control by intuition. This has been graphically described as 'switching on the autopilot' (Drasdo, 1979). The commonsense view that to proceed with care is to proceed slowly can also be reversed in high level skills, there are instances where speed seems to be an essential accompaniment of delicate discrimination (Lacy, 1978). Thus, the observer cannot simplify his task by asking the practitioner to go more slowly nor can he rely on the introspection of the skilled performer.

Skill is demonstrated by persistent and efficient pursuit of an objective and

Table 2.6. *Skills analysis procedure* (from Singleton 1979)

1. Observation of the skilled activity in the normal context on a sufficiently long-term basis to detect any changes in rhythm, possibly over days or even weeks, to note individual differences and the consequences of fatigue and learning
2. Clarification and unification of hypotheses developed during observation using prococol methods, good/poor contrast, critical incident techniques and so on
3. Study of the development of the skill during the training phase with examination of the reasons for particular training practices and assessment procedures
4. Analysis of the structure of the skill: the dimensions of perceptual activity, decision making and action strategies
5. Checking of hypotheses by specific experiments or field performance measurement
6. Validation of the success of any innovations in system design, training or work design introduced as a result of the appraisal.

the skill can usually be understood although not necessarily written down with any great precision in terms of a goal and the path towards that goal. The path is generated by navigating through a conceptual map containing landmarks and decision points (key features of the skill) and by the avoidance of obstacles and misleading features which have been sensitively detected.

2.4 Applications
2.4.1 Selection and guidance
These processes are variations on the general theme of matching a worker to an appropriate job. In the case of selection the given point is the job and the population is searched to find the most appropriate worker, in the case of guidance one worker is the starting point and the range of jobs is searched to identify the best one. The two complementary processes are shown in Fig. 2.1. They can usefully be considered together because they are similar and interactive. Thus, in the selection situation the process involves not only analysing and describing the job but also considering the availability of potentially appropriate workers. In the guidance situation the process involves analysing and describing the worker and consideration of the availability of suitable jobs.

At the point of a successful match the worker is described in terms of the kinds of job he could do and the job is described in terms of the kind of worker needed to do it, Table 2.7. For most people and jobs the whole process takes place within a localised community. For the highest level jobs a whole country or even an international community might be considered, but in European countries most workers attempt to find jobs which do not require either moving house or excessive travelling, and such proximity has corresponding advantages for the potential employers. Thus, the selection process involves

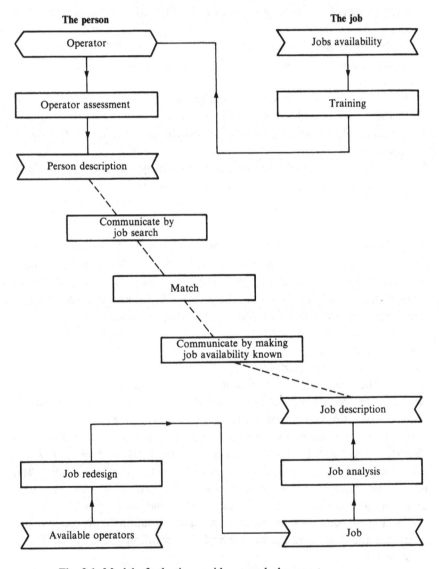

Fig. 2.1. Model of selection, guidance and placement.

Table 2.7. *Matching job and operator descriptions*

e.g. Secretary/Typist

Person oriented description	Personable, tactful, literate, conscientious, probably female, interested in office work
Work oriented person description	Trained in shorthand and audio-typing, word-processing, filing and office routines. Demonstrates facility in social skills
	Match
Worker oriented job description	Skilled in shorthand and audio-typing, word-processing, filing and office routines. Good appearance and ability to communicate
Task oriented job description	To deal with correspondence including producing letters and reports. Making appointments and coping with inquiries and visitors

describing the job first by analysis (task and skills analysis) and then the translation of these data into worker relevant terminology. Consideration of the potential worker availability may lead to a redesign of the job either by the use of a different task combination or by introducing different technology. It is then necessary to communicate with the market by publicising the available job usually by advertising. This is itself an important stage in the process because a well prepared advertisement will enable the recipients to engage in self selection which does not, at this stage, involve further selector resources. To this end it is useful to have a multi-stage process as shown in Fig. 2.2. Having developed some interest on the basis of a necessarily brief advertisement a potential candidate can apply for further written details which should contain a comprehensive description of the job, the task and skill content, the responsibilities, the salary and the details of the organisation including its history and anticipated future, and an application form. A name with job title and telephone number should be included so that informal interaction and discussion of details of particular interest to the candidate can take place before the commitment to transmission of the application form. All this can be done at minimal cost. If the job description has been properly constructed there should not be an excessive number of applicants so that the next stage of a paper sift is also economical.

There then follow the more expensive stages of final selection which may involve testing and interviewing as described earlier. The choice of the interviewers and the interview process depends on the particular job. At one extreme it may be one company representative, at the other extreme there may be a series of interview boards. The interview board can have covert purposes where the senior person who is the chairman of the board will use the opportunity to orientate the precise expectations from the post to be filled including settling differences of opinion between his subordinates who are also members of the board. Ideally this should be done before candidates are interviewed but it can happen that differences in preferences for candidates reveal different opinions between board members which the chairman can detect and deal with.

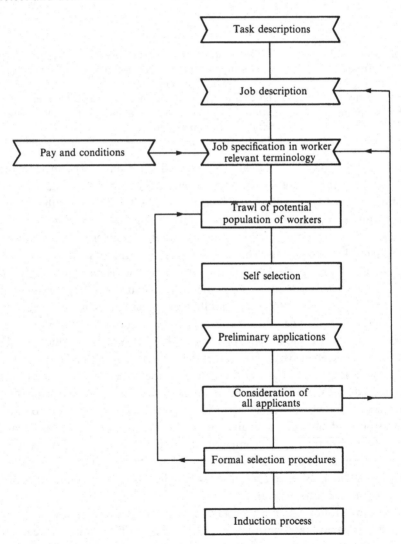

Fig. 2.2. Relating jobs and people.

Guidance also involves testing and interviewing but this is invariably a two person situation of a counsellor and client. The problem is that most clients have only the vaguest, undefined ideas about the most suitable choice and direction of career. The counsellor can help by identifying the client's job-relevant characteristics and by contributing his knowledge about occupations (Fig. 2.3.). The former may be supported by testing although test results are essentially evidence to enable the individual to clarify his own self concept. The latter may start from national classifications of occupations such as the

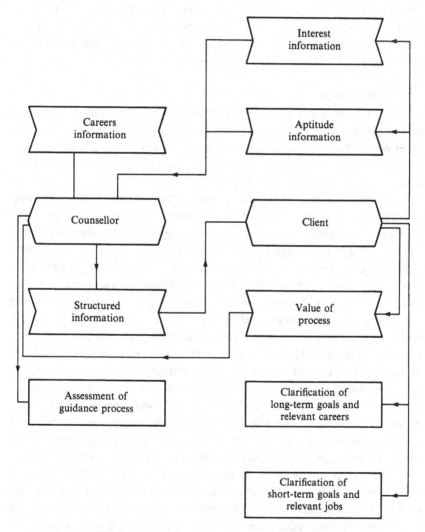

Fig. 2.3. The Guidance process.

American Dictionary of Occupational Titles (DOT) and the British Classification of Occupations and Dictionary of Occupational Titles (CODOT), but the counsellor's suggestions are likely to converge very rapidly into a more comprehensible repertoire of possibilities using evidence about the particular client (Singleton, 1975).

This process can be supported by a computer with which the client may interact alone or it may be used by the counsellor as a database and prompter.

A guidance episode necessarily takes place at one point in time within the developing skills and experience of the client. To emphasise the continuous nature of career development and the changing aspirations of people at different ages Super has proposed a division into five stages: Growth (0–14 years); Exploration (15–24 years); Establishment (25–44); Maintenance (45–64 years); and Decline (65 onwards) (Super and Bohn, 1971).

2.4.2 Placement

Placement is a mixture of selection and guidance, a process of mutual matching takes place within a known range of persons and jobs. The problem arises when a batch of recruits enter military service or when a large company takes on a new set of graduates. It is one application of psychometrics to manpower planning (see previous chapter).

It becomes of particular significance within the currently fashionable company policy of separating core and peripheral employees. Given the vagaries of the market and rapid changes in processes and products stimulated by changing technology the strategy has evolved of taking on many employees for a short term only. These may be production workers but they may also be senior people; managers hired for a fixed term and technologists and others used as consultants. The placement task is to describe the requirements and the appropriate sources of individuals with the relevant skills (Fig. 2.1). For the core workers who are permanent staff again there may well be a mixture of people at all levels and here there is more emphasis on career progression and job satisfaction. Core employees are given written annual assessments which can be discussed with the immediate senior who is probably the writer of the assessment. For this purpose he is provided with a well-structured form by the personnel department who will also advise on the timely use of in-house or external courses to extend the range of skills of a particular employee. By contrast the peripheral employee is judged entirely on his past record or that of the consultant company which employs him on a semi-permanent basis. He is hired to undertake a specific task without reference to longer term features such as job satisfaction or career development. The peripheral employee will be compensated for his disadvantages by a much greater pay rate per hour and the company gains by reduced overheads and greater work-force flexibility.

The whole strategy works very well for younger workers with well documented training and experience. This reinforces the view, developed in the previous chapter, that manufacturing industry in particular is following the Armed Forces in relying more and more on fit, skilled, mobile workers.

Psychometrically the problem is to develop appropriate descriptive taxonomies so that a person's actual or potential contribution to an organisation is succinctly expressible. These remain primitive in that, on the whole, non-technical English is used with all the possibilities of ambiguity and communication at cross purposes which this implies. The accountants are ahead of the psychologists in developing ideas such as profit centres applicable to small groups or even to individuals.

The increased awareness of the importance of the individual worker to profit and success generally, particularly at higher levels in the organisation, has stimulated the growth of a specialist placement profession colloquially known as the head hunters. These are companies which specialise in assisting a client in clarifying what kind of person they need and how to locate him within the potentially suitable worker population. They may also start with an individual and search for a location. This also is done mainly by interview although some use is made of psychometric tests, profiles and rating scales.

2.4.3 The design of training schemes

Designing and conducting training schemes is expensive and is not undertaken without good reasons. Among possible reasons are:

1. An inadequate reservoir of competent workers for particular tasks
2. A workforce sufficient in numbers or supply but not in skill level as evidenced usually by quality of work and less frequently by failures to meet production targets, danger to people and damage to equipment
3. Changes in technology which result in changes in required skills
4. An organisational commitment to continuous improvement of the skills of members
5. To meet statutory requirements in certain dangerous industries and services
6. As a service to customers buying equipment
7. As a service to the community paid for by public funds

The remit of the training scheme and those responsible for it may end at the transition point to operational activity or may continue in those periods of work regarded as a continuation of training and supervised as such. In either case there needs to be close liaison between those responsible for training and those responsible for operations.

On the other hand training is always vulnerable because the benefits are long-term and it often needs protection from the demands of management and operations where there are other priorities. The simplest protective barrier is a geographical one, namely to conduct the training away from other centres of activity within the organisation. Sometimes a separate room is sufficient, in other situations a different part of the country may be chosen to provide adequate isolation.

The essential vulnerability reinforces the requirement that the starting point of design should be a clarification of objectives followed by a consideration of the criteria of assessment that the objectives have been achieved. None of this need be numerical, sometimes numbers are used to provide a pseudo precision which can be counterproductive because the validity of the numbers can so easily be questioned. Precise verbal statements and descriptions avoid this pitfall.

The sensitivity of training regimes to external pressures is demonstrated by the erratic interest and activity in this area observable at the national level. Inevitably there was a burst of activity during and immediately after World War II as shown for example by military research and development (Wolfle, 1951) and by the 'Training within Industry' (TWI) movement (War Manpower Commission, 1945). Although research continued the next burst of application in the U.K. took place following the Industrial Training Act of 1964 (Robinson and Barnes, 1968, Barber 1968). The Act concentrated on training oriented by industry, the other possibilities considered were occupations and geographical regions. It resulted in the creation of a Central Training Council and a comprehensive range of Industrial Training Boards. Each Board was financed by a levy on the relevant industry. Not surprisingly this created a demand for experienced trainer manpower which could not be met, there was some disillusion and retrenchment in the 1970s. In the 1980s there has been another resurgence of activity following the realisation that the country is simultaneously suffering from a high rate of unemployment and a shortage of workers with specific skills. Extensive government resources are channelled by the Department of Employment through the Training Commission into the Youth Training Schemes, job training, skill training and so on.

The objectives and criteria of success of any training scheme are best described in system terms. The next step is to translate these into a person oriented description of what the successful scheme graduate will have acquired. This is more than skills because the total expertise will include also rules, knowledge and contextual information. This last will vary from some acquaintance with the parent company to the basic technology behind the tasks. Together these make up the content or syllabus of the course.

Decisions are then needed on how to train, which will include whether or which parts should be on-line or off-line, whether the operator is required to

Table 2.8. *Training scheme design procedure*

Inputs	Function	Outputs
Task Descriptions	Define objectives	Criteria of success
Skill descriptions	Consider content	Syllabus
Role descriptions	mix of	
Company culture	−roles	
	−skills	
	−knowledge	
Experience of operational activity	Consider mix of programmed- and concept-type required functions	Curriculum
Precedents from similar training	Consider mix of on-line/off-line training	
Available technological resources	Consider use of training aids	
Task/Skill descriptions of instructor	Define Instructor requirements	Instructor selection criteria

function in a mainly programmed (i.e. rule-following) mode and how far he may need to function in a conceptual (i.e. actions based on understanding) mode.

Consideration will be given to the use of training aids such as technical notes, schematic diagrams, video tapes, closed circuit television and simulators. The most important training aids are the instructors, the selection and training of these is a vital secondary scheme supporting the primary scheme.

These many facets of training scheme design are shown in Table 2.8.

2.4.4   Programmed instruction

The origins of this movement are in the teaching machines first developed systematically about 1960. These consisted of film strips with associated projection devices and control panels which enabled the student to examine a particular screen presentation and respond by moving to another frame. The succeeding frame might take up another topic or might contain answers and comments on questions posed on the previous one. There was some scope for interaction in that the series of presentations was determined by the student's choice of responses. If the student demonstrated by his choices that he did not fully understand a particular point then the programme could send him round an additional explanatory loop. This was called a branching programme as distinct from a linear programme which contained no loops.

It will be appreciated that this technique of automated teaching seemed to have enormous potential. Classroom teaching is inherently skilled man-power intensive. There are obvious benefits in allowing each student to go at his own pace. It is not surprising that teaching machines had considerable appeal to the military and to large scale industry. Some years of intensive research and development resulted in a more realistic view (Glaser, 1965; Wallis *et al.*, 1966, Kay *et al.*, 1968). It became clear that the quality of the programme was the key to degree of success. The machine itself and its style of operation was incidental, in fact it was possible to achieve the same procedure if not quite the same discipline on the student by using programmed books with directional references to other pages at the end of each page. If a well-structured book is the answer then we have gone full-circle and back to the benefits of a systematic text-book.

In research terms the study of programmed instruction was instrumental in encouraging a more systems view of the teaching/training process with associated trends towards greater consideration of objectives, task analysis, cost/benefits and so on. Correspondingly from a practical training viewpoint there developed a more systematic approach to taxonomies of training and of instructional methods together with their inter-relationships. Tables 2.9 and 2.10 are examples from an overview of military training.

Regarded in systems terms, programmed instruction cannot be an isolated continuously developing activity because it depends on the skills of the programme writer and these skills can only be developed on the basis of experience in the classroom. On the other hand teaching machines are one way of utilising the skilled teacher on a larger scale than his personal activity in the classroom.

There is a different form of automatic teaching device called a pacing machine which can facilitate the development of motor skills. It consists of a machine which emits bleeps at timed intervals. The intervals are predetermined by the elements of a motor task or more simply by the target cycle time of a task. The trainee performs his task and tries to keep in phase with the bleeps which are intended to pace his performance. The required rate of work can be increased by shortening the time intervals.

The second main phase of programmed instruction became feasible with the development of low cost computing. Computer aided instruction (C.A.I.) strictly should cover other techniques such as simulation and computer based procedures but it is usually intended to mean a situation where a student sits in

Table 2.9. *A taxonomy of instructional methods*

(adapted from Wallis *et al.*, 1966)

Self instructional student centred methods	Programmed instruction Private study 'On-the-job' learning Role playing, group dynamics
Instructor centred methods	Expedition training Classroom teaching Supervised practical/laboratory work Formal instruction in occupational setting Illustrated presentation Guidance training
Equipment centred methods	Procedural trainers Simulation using real equipment Simulation generated synthetically

Table 2.10. *A taxonomy of training areas*

(adapted from Wallis *et al.*, 1966)

Descriptor	Examples
Physical fitness	In normal and extreme climates
Procedural and routine skills	Drills, assembly operations, clerical routines
Perceptual skills	Monitoring and recognition tasks
Control skills	Crafts, operations, data transposing
Acquisition of information	Assimilating theory and background knowledge
Intellectual skills	Diagnosis, navigation
Character building	Self-reliance, initiative
Managerial skills	Leadership, decision-making, committee activity
Identification with group	Positive attitudes towards organisation
System activities	Working teams

front of a screen on which the presented formats relate to his developing cognitive activity as expressed by his manipulations of the associated keyboard. Even with this restricted interface there is enormous flexibility and the training tasks can vary from reading and simple arithmetic to diagnosing faults in the complex plant used in process industries.

The use of computer aided instruction in primary schools has created a new generation of what have been called 'television children'. They regard the screen/keyboard interface as no more unnatural than a book is to earlier generations. This has far reaching consequences at the cultural level not only for learning but also for the design of jobs and even for leisure pursuits which increasingly depend on the same kind of interface.

Many of the earlier forms of computer aided instructions used a central computer facility and a set of work-stations where a whole class of trainees could function simultaneously. The development of micro-computers resulted in the use of more isolated dedicated systems for just one trainee. In either case it is feasible to collect data about a trainee's performance and modify the presented information accordingly. It is also possible to collect learning data and feed it to an instructor either on-line or off-line. The widespread use of computer based learning and testing situations has stimulated the development of 'student modelling'. All the data about one student is collected into one bank which changes dynamically with his learning achievements (and failures). In this way a student model containing a profile of attainment together with a history of progress to date can be made available to the trainer and to the trainee. However, communication links between the trainee and the trainer via a computer are not a substitute for the two-way conversation and observation which normally takes place in a class-room. Computer programmes are notoriously literal in their requirement for and response to operator responses. Trainee–computer communication failures for very simple reasons can lead to a complete hiatus unless they are detected and restored by an experienced trainer who can explain to the trainee why the system is failing to respond adequately.

The third phase of programmed instruction called Tutorial Expert Systems (TES) involves artificial intelligence (see p. 234). To a trainee at the interface this may not seem very different from a teaching machine or computer aided instruction but the logic or architecture of the driving system is different so that even more flexibility is available. Instead of responding directly by logical rules and paths which have been envisaged and stored by the programmer an expert system training programme contains a knowledge base and an inference engine which can consult the knowledge base and respond more adaptively to the idiosyncratic needs of the trainee. It can also explain why it is proposing a certain strategy and why the detected strategy of the trainee is appropriate or not, and, if not, why not. From the user's point of view these systems are usually menu driven, that is the operator can select his path of consultation by choices within ranges of possible choices which are presented to him. Technically the task of the programme designer is made easier by the use of training skills and declarative programming languages. A training shell is a generalised tutorial system which can operate with a variety of knowledge bases. A declarative programming language is one which can accept statements of relationships or rules for relationships contrasting with more traditional languages which encompass only step by step logic.

It will be appreciated that this rapidly developing field of expertise contains extensive new jargon. At this stage the jargon is an obstacle in that anyone wishing to find out about the field has first to interpret the jargon. This is doubly difficult in that there is much overlap in terminology and concepts and specialists are not consistent with each other in the use of these new terms. No doubt the field will eventually clarify and mature and the terminology will be designed with precision so that meaningful concepts, tools and methods are unambiguously clarified and distinguished but this has not yet happened.

From a behavioural standpoint the issues are the same as in any other field where technology is simultaneously providing many new facilities for supporting and measuring human performance.

1. Technology provides trainer aids not trainer substitutes. Thus computer assisted instruction (CAI) is more aptly descriptive than computer based training (CBT).

2. Technology enforces rigorous thinking to the point of revealing embarrassing gaps in learning, teaching and training theory. On the other hand technology also opens up new possibilities for monitoring and measurement which should support the development of better basic theory.

3. It is essential to develop the basic taxonomies behind the learning situation. For example any diagnostic task can be aided by a taxonomy of symptoms and a taxonomy of causes together with connections between them.

4. The need for interdisciplinary approaches is reinforced but the abiding difficulties of interdisciplinary communications remain at every level from different values and concepts to different terminologies. Communication between information technologists and behavioural specialists is a continuous struggle which can eventually be rewarding.

5. The design of the man–machine interface (MMI) or the human–computer interface (HCI) or more simply human interfaces (HI) remains one of the most difficult design problems but a crucial one in that poorly designed interfaces will wreck the performance of any system.

6. Evaluation is an essential procedure within the implementation of any new system. For training systems this can be very expensive because of the requirements to monitor the learning process and compare procedures which are anyway never completely comparable. Apparently extraneous variables such as trainee motivation and trainer expertise continue to dominate other factors such as differences in technology and differences in learning tasks.

7.   Pedagogically the need to be much clearer about what is being taught and why is a mixed blessing. The formal discipline can sometimes tidy up muddled thinking but at other times it can interfere with the creatively developing interaction between trainer and trainee.

In general, programmed instruction is most useful for tasks which can be comprehensively specified. This implies tasks based on rules for example arithmetic, or on logic, for example fault finding.

2.4.5 *The use of simulators*

When serious consequences can follow from human errors, e.g. in flying an aircraft, or when on-line operation is too expensive to be trusted to the hands of trainees, e.g. in process control, there is obviously a case for providing training devices which simulate the performance of on-line systems. In this way risks and costs are reduced, the performance of trainees is more easily measured and the presented situation is precisely controlled by the trainers. It is feasible to provide adequate exposure to events which in practice might be rare but very serious. High fidelity simulation is an interesting challenge to technological design. Simulators can provide demonstrations which always impress visitors.

With all these advantages it is not surprising that a great deal of effort and resources go into the provision of simulators for high technology industry. Paradoxically the more advanced the technology the easier it is to provide good simulation. For example, a process control plant which consists of dials, charts and visual display units responding to activation of switches is much easier to simulate than, say, an opponent in a game of tennis.

The perfect simulation which has been suggested but not yet implemented in process control, power generation and air traffic control would be to have two identical control rooms and two crews coming on duty. One crew would control a real system and the other would think they were so doing but would in fact be in a control room driven by software. This seems to be the only way of avoiding the main snag of simulation, namely that the trainee is aware that his performance is not important in that reality out there is not changing as a consequence of his actions. However, he will always know that his performance on a simulator is being assessed and, except for the business of risks, he may well take more care than he would in a real plant. In many if not most industries where simulators are used the benefits to training are not confined to dynamic system control and fault diagnosis. The control function is exercised by a team and the efficient interaction between the team members is also subject to improvement with practice (see p. 95).

Transfer of training from a simulator to a real situation is never complete and does not necessarily increase with degree of fidelity. Simple simulations can be as effective for training purposes as more elaborate ones and can certainly be more cost effective. Degree of transfer is not easy to measure and needs to be carefully defined. For example, in training manually guided missile operators the degree of transfer is appropriately measured by 'first shot' success whereas in training and retraining flight deck crew the long term contribution to safety is the appropriate measure. Gagne (1962) provides an excellent review of earlier work in this field. More recent experience is reviewed in Stammers (1983). For details of experimental studies using large scale defence simulations see Parsons (1972). Moraal and Kraiss (1981) contains chapters dealing with simulations of a ship entering harbour, car driving, tank driving, the flight deck and air traffic control. MSC (1986) reviews the current use of simulators in twenty U.K. industries.

As a research tool the simulator provides a happy medium between the precision of laboratory studies and the realism of field studies. It is not widely used for research outside the military because of the cost of high fidelity simulator time. A complex dedicated simulator can cost several million pounds and it needs its own crew of skilled operators. On the other hand standard micro-computers have considerable potentiality for quite elaborate simulation and effective simulation training on procedures may only require simple static mock-ups.

Simulator development has been driven by technology rather than by the behavioural sciences with the standard result that there is a high reliance on face validity with relatively little resource devoted to systematic evaluation. Key features such as the timing and extent of simulator usage are based on experience in particular industries rather than on more formal evidence. The ergonomics approach to their use is shown in Fig. 2.4 but it must be admitted that this is as yet rarely followed in practice.

Simulation should be regarded as one tool within the repertoire of the training specialist. There are other uses of simulators. They can be used for assessment independently of training. Data collected during simulator trials is a useful source of risk and reliability data. In the nuclear power plant design they are also used as the final stage of pre-construction design evaluation (Williams and Story, 1987). They can also be used as a resource for checking operating instructions and for conducting detailed task analyses. For these purposes the simulator must be available before the main control room is constructed. The full range of potential simulator usage is summarised in Table 2.11.

Table 2.11. *Uses of simulators*

1. Training in dynamic plant control
2. Training in diagnostic skills
3. Team training
4. As a dynamic mock-up for design evaluation
5. As a test-bed for the checking of operating instructions
6. As an environment in which task analyses can be conducted, e.g. on diagnostic strategies
7. As a source of data on human errors relevant to risk and reliability assessment
8. As a vehicle for the testing/assessment of operators

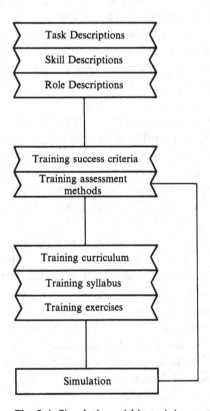

Fig. 2.4. Simulation within training methodology.

References

Argyle, M. (ed.) (1981). *Social Skills and Work*. London: Methuen.

Annett, J. (1969). *Feedback and Human Behaviour*. Harmondsworth: Penguin.

Attneave, F. (1959). *Application of Information Theory to Psychology*. New York: Holt.

Baddeley, A.D. (1976). *The Psychology of Memory*. New York: Harper and Row.

Barber, J.W. (ed.) (1968). *Industrial Training Handbook*. London: Iliffe.

Bartlett, F.C. (1932). *Remembering*. Cambridge University Press.

Bartlett, F.C. (1958). *Thinking*. London: George Allen and Unwin.

Belbin, E.M. (1965). *Training methods for older workers*. Paris: O.E.C.D.

Biderman, A.D. (1967). Life and death in extreme captivity situations. In Appley, M.H. and Trumbull, R. (eds.). *Psychological Stress*. New York: Appleton Century Crofts.

Bilodeau, E.A. (ed.) (1969). *Principles of Skill Acquisition*. New York: Academic Press.

Birren, J.E. and Schaie, K.W. (1977) (eds.). *Handbook of the Psychology of Ageing*. New York: van Nostrand Reinhold.

Blum, M.L. and Naylor, J.C. (1968). *Industrial Psychology*, New York: Harper and Row.

Bruner, J.S. (1957). On Perceptual Readiness. *Psychological Review*. **64**, 123–52.

Bruner, J.S., Goodnow, J.J. and Austin, G.A. (1956). *A Study of Thinking*. New York: Wiley.

Campbell, R.N. and Smith, P.J. (1976). *Recent Advances in the Psychology of Language*. New York: Plenum.

Carmichael, L. and Dearborn, W.F. (1950). *Reading and Visual Fatigue*. New York: Houghton Mifflin.

Chapanis, A., Garner, W.R. and Morgan, C.T. (1949). *Applied Experimental Psychology*. New York: Wiley.

Chomsky, N. (1957). *Syntactic Structures*. The Hague: Manton.

Conrad, R. (1964). Acoustic comparisons in immediate memory. *British Journal of Psychology*. **55**, 75–84.

Craik, K.J.W. (1943). *The Nature of Explanation*. Cambridge University Press.

Crombach, L.S. and Drenth, P.J.D. (eds.) (1972). *Mental Tests and Cultural Adaptation*. The Hague: Manton.

Davis, D.R. and Shackleton, V.J. (1975). *Psychology and Work*. London: Methuen.

Drasdo, M. (1979). The Rock Climber. In Singleton, W.T. (ed.) *Compliance and Excellence*. Lancaster: M.T. Press.

Drenth, P.J.D. (1978). Principles of Selection. In Warr, P.B. (ed.) *Psychology at Work*. Harmondsworth: Penguin.

Drury, C.G. and Fox, J.G. (1975). *Human Reliability in Quality Control*. London: Taylor and Francis.

Edwards, E. (1964). *Information Transmission*. London: Chapman and Hall.

Eysenck, H.J. (1979). *The Nature and Measurement of Intelligence*. London: Springer.

Friedman, M.P., Das, J.P. and O'Connor, N. (eds.) (1981). *Intelligence and Learning*. New York: Plenum.

Gagne, R.M. (1962). Simulators. In Glaser, R. (ed.) *Training, Research and Education*. New York: Wiley.

Gagne, R.M. (1970). *The Conditions of Learning*. New York: Holt, Rinehart and Winston.

Gerver, D. and Sinaiko, H.W. (eds.) (1978). *Language Interpretation and Communication*. New York: Plenum.

Glaser, R. (ed.) (1965). *Training, Research and Education*. New York: Wiley.

Guilford, J.P. (1967). *The Nature of Human Intelligence*. New York: McGraw-Hill.

Head, H. (1920). *Studies in Neurology*. Oxford University Press.

Heim, A. (1970). *Intelligence and Personality*. Harmondsworth: Penguin.

Herriot, P. (1970). *An Introduction to the Psychology of Language*. London: Methuen.

Herriot, P. (1974). *Attributes of Memory*. London: Methuen.

Hilgard, E.R. (1948). *Theories of Learning*. New York: Appleton Century Crofts.

Hilgard, E.R. and Marquis, D.G. (1940). *Conditioning and Learning*. New York: Appleton-Century.

Hoiberg, A. (ed.) (1982). *Women and the World of Work*. New York: Plenum.

Holding, D.H. (1965). *Principles of Training*. London: Pergamon.

Humphrey, G. (1951). *Thinking*. London: Methuen.

Irvine, S.H. and Berry, J.W. (eds.) (1981). *Human Assessment and Cultural Factors*. New York: Plenum.

Jessup, G. and Jessup, H. (1975). *Selection and Assessment at Work*. London: Methuen.

Joanning, H., Brock, G.W., Avery, A.W. and Coufal, J.D. (1979). The educational approach to social skills training in marriage and family intervention. In Singleton, W.T., Spurgeon, P. and Stammers, R.B. (eds.) *The Analysis of Social Skill*. London: Plenum.

Johnson-Laird, P.N. and Wason, P.C. (eds.) (1977). *Thinking*. Cambridge University Press.

Kay, H., Dodd, B. and Sime, M. (1968). *Teaching Machines and Programmed Instruction*. Harmondsworth: Penguin.

Kelly, G.A. (1955). *The Psychology of Personal Constructs*. New York: Norton.

Killcross, M.C. and Cassie, A. (1975). The potential use of tailored testing for allocation to army employments. In Singleton, W.T. and Spurgeon, P. (eds.). *Measurement of Human Resources*. London: Taylor & Francis.

King, D. (1964). *Training within the Organisation*. London: Tavistock.

Kline, P. (1976). *Personality: Measurement and Theory*. London: Hutchinson.

Lacy, B.A. (1978). The Tea Blender. In Singleton, W.T. (ed.). *The Analysis of Practical Skills*. Lancaster: M.T. Press.

Lewin, K. (1935). *A Dynamic Theory of Personality*. New York: McGraw Hill.

M.S.C. (1986). *Simulation in Training*. Sheffield: Manpower Services Commission.

Mackworth, N.H. (1950). *Researches on the Measurement of Human Performance*. London: H.M.S.O.

Melhuish, E.C. (1979). An approach to teaching doctors social skills. In Singleton, W.T., Spurgeon, P. and Stammers, R.B. (eds.). *The Analysis of Social Skill*. London: Plenum.

Melton, A.W. (ed.) (1964). *Categories of Human Learning*. New York: Academic Press.

Miller, G.A. (1956). The magical number seven, plus or minus two: some limits on our capacity for processing information. *Psychology Review*. **63**, 81–97.

Miller, G.A., Galanter, E. and Pribram, K.H. (1960). *Plans and the Structure of Behaviour*. New York: Holt.

Miller, R.B. (1953). *Handbook on Training and Training Equipment Design*. U.S. Air Force. *quoted in* Holding, D.H. (1965).

Miller, R.B. (1962). Task description and analysis. In Gagne, R.M. (ed.). *Psychological Principles in System Development*. New York: Holt, Rinehart and Winston.

Moraal, J. and Kraiss, K-F (eds.). (1981). *Manned Systems Design*. New York: Plenum.

Nelson-Jones, R. (1982). *The Theory and Practice of Occupational Counselling*. London: Holt, Rinehart and Winston.

Page, M. (1987). Risk in Defence. In Singleton, W.T. and Hovden, J. (eds.). *Risk and Decisions*. Chichester: Wiley.

Parry, M.H. (1968). *Agression on the Road*. London: Tavistock.

Parsons, H.M. (ed.). (1972). *Man–machine System Experiments*. Baltimore: Johns Hopkins Press.

Piaget, J. (1950). *The Psychology of Intelligence*. London: Routledge and Kegan Paul.

Randell, G.A. (1978). Interviewing at work. In Warr, P.B. (ed.). *Psychology at Work*. Harmondsworth: Penguin.

Robinson, J. and Barnes, N. (1968). (eds.). *New Media and Methods in Industrial Training*. London: B.B.C.

Rogers, C.R. (1951). *Client-centred Therapy*. Boston: Houghton Mifflin.

Rutter, D.R. (1979). A programme of interview training for medical students. In Singleton, W.T., Spurgeon P. and Stammers, R.B. (eds.). *The Analysis of Social Skill*. London: Plenum.

Seymour, W.D. (1966). *Industrial Skills*. London: Pitman.

Seymour, W.D. (1968). *Skills Analysis Training*. London: Pitman.

Sherif, M. (1948). *An Outline of Social Psychology*. New York: Harper.

Singer, E.J. and Ramsden, J. (1969). *The Practical Approach to Skills Analysis*. London: McGraw-Hill.

Singleton, W.T. (1959). The training of shoe machinists. *Ergonomics*. **2.2**, 148–52.

Singleton, W.T. (1975). The role of the computer in vocational guidance. In Singleton, W.T. and Spurgeon, P. (eds.). *Measurement of Human Resources*. London: Taylor & Francis.

Singleton, W.T. (ed.) (1978). *The Study of Real Skills. Vol. 1: The Analysis of Practical Skills*. Lancaster: M.T. Press.

Singleton, W.T. (ed.) (1979). *The Study of Real Skills. Vol. 2: Compliance and Excellence*. Lancaster: M.T.P. Press.

Singleton, W.T. (ed.) (1981). *The Study of Real Skills. Vol. 3: Management Skills*. Lancaster: M.T.P. Press.

Singleton, W.T. (ed.) (1983a). *The Study of Real Skills. Vol. 4: Social Skills*. Lancaster: M.T.P. Press.

Singleton, W.T. (1983b). Age, Skill and Management. *International Journal of Aging and Human Development*. **17.1**. 15–23

Singleton, W.T. (1983c). The university teacher. In Singleton, W.T. (ed.). *The Study of Real Skills. Vol. 4: Social Skills*. Lancaster: M.T.P. Press.

Singleton, W.T., Spurgeon, P. and Stammers, R.B. (eds.) (1980). *The Analysis of Social Skill*. New York: Plenum.

Stammers, R.B. (1983). Simulation in training. In Kvalseth, T.O. (ed.). *Ergonomics of Work Station Design*. London: Butterworth.

Super, D.E. and Bohn, M.J. (1971). *Occupational Psychology*. London: Tavistock.

Thomas, L.T. and Harri-Augstein, E.G. (1985). *Self-organised Learning*. London: Routledge and Kegan Paul.

Thorndike, E.L. (1911). *Animal Intelligence*. New York: Macmillan.

Tilley, K.W. (1967). Fault diagnosis training for maintenance personnel. In Singleton, W.T., Easterby, R.S. and Whitfield, D. (eds.). *The Human Operator in Complex Systems*. London: Taylor & Francis.

Triandis, H.C., Lambert, W.W., Berry, J.W., Lonner, W.J., Heron, A., Brislin, R. and Draguns, J. (eds.). (1980). *Handbook of Cross-cultural Psychology*. Boston: Allyn & Bacon.

Wallis, D., Duncan, K.D. and Knight, M.A.G. (1966). *Programmed Instruction in the British Armed Forces*. London: H.M.S.O.

War Manpower Commission. (1945). *Training Within Industry Report. 1940–1945*. Washington: War Manpower Commission.

Welford, A.T. (1958). *Ageing and Human Skill*. Oxford University Press.

Welford, A.T. (1968). *Fundamentals of Skill*. London: Methuen.

Welford, A.T. (1979). Skill in aging. In Singleton, W.T. (ed.). *The Study of Real Skills. Vol. 2: Compliance and Excellence*. Lancaster: M.T. Press.

Wickens, C.D. (1984). *Engineering Psychology and Human Performance*. Columbus: Merrill.

Williams, J.C. and Story, D.T. (1987). Ergonomics and Control Room Design. *Nuclear Energy*. **26.4**. 225–31.

Wolfle, D. (1951). Training. In Stevens, S.S (ed.). *Handbook of Experimental Psychology*. New York: Wiley.

Woodworth, R.S. (1938). *Experimental Psychology*. New York: Holt.

Yates, F. (1960). *Sampling Methods for Censuses and Surveys*. London: Charles Griffin.

3 Needs and organisations

3.1 Concepts

3.1.1 *Social factors*

Activity involving others

It is rare for a human being to do anything in isolation for very long. It is possible to think of examples such as the tractor driver who may be alone for a working day, and there are unusual tasks such as single-handed yachting where the person may be alone for several weeks. Nevertheless, the obvious rarity of these illustrations emphasises the point that people at work are usually interacting with other people.

This may involve the interdependence of tasks, in which case there is a team or crew involved or it may be that people happen to be working in the same location and the interaction is social rather than operational. Many, perhaps most, tasks are of an intermediate kind where there is some common purpose linking the tasks, but nevertheless individuals are working more or less independently and their interaction is mainly social. They may chat at intervals, they share rest periods and meals and they may travel to and from work together. This is the common situation in industry and commerce. The social interaction is very highly prized, it is often mentioned as the main reason for enjoying going to work. A different kind of interaction occurs when one person is providing a service for a second person, for example the shop assistant or the dentist. There is yet another kind of interaction where one person seeks the cooperation of a second person, for example the salesman or the market researcher. None of these necessarily involves the complication of different status. When one person is in some way guiding or instructing another, then we have a different interaction currently difficult to discuss in Western societies because of taboos based on some underlying beliefs in democracy and equality. A century ago this was much discussed in an uninhibited way as the master–servant relationship. Even the concept of leadership has been clouded by these social norms for the past twenty years or so, although it is now becoming more fashionable again. An efficient, complex natural system such as the human body is inherently hierarchical, and this must be true also for the man-made systems we call organisations. To maintain order and direction there must be dominance and precedence or to use other terms authority and responsibility.

Conceptual approaches

The study of people in organisations can be considered starting either from the people or from the organisation. People approaches can begin with individual attributes of behaviour such as attitudes and motivation or with the phenomena of people interaction in groups. Organisational approaches begin with the properties of organisations – centralisation, flatness, integration and so on, or with a systems approach to task allocation, communication and decision-making. Intermediate approaches include the study of social skills and leadership.

In trying to classify the complex of relevant theories there is much to be said for taking a systems approach. An organisation is created to achieve an objective, this objective in turn is related to some real or imagined human needs and purposes. The purpose or objective is achieved by converting a range of inputs into a range of outputs as shown in Fig. 3.1. If this enterprise is to be reasonably effective there must be a control system. The resources of the system are space, energy, materials and people. The origin of the control and operating systems is influenced by all the behavioural theories listed above, although it must not be forgotten that people are only one of the resources and

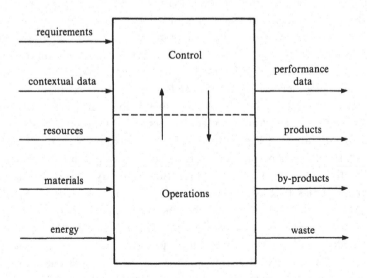

Fig. 3.1. Objectives described as inputs and outputs.

organisational design must depend also on the others, in particular technology. Hence the concept of the socio-technical system (p. 32).

However, organisation theories naturally concentrate on the people aspects. For both the organisation itself and the people within it the basis must be human needs and the closely related human aspirations.

3.1.2 *Human aspirations*

The importance of context

It is a natural consequence of human physiology that energy is generated continuously within each person by metabolic processes which cannot be switched off except by starvation, disease or death. Within the healthy individual this energy is channelled into a variety of activities which are associated with particular purposes. The purposes emerge from the context of the community of which the individual is a member.

What an individual wishes to achieve is modulated by his natural endowment of capacities and his skills acquired throughout his life, but probably most of all by his social relationships – his membership of a family, his friends, acquaintances and colleagues, and his membership of other groups to do with either his work or with his leisure activities. This is not a situation where it is possible to identify unidirectional cause–effect relationships. Rather it is a continuously developing interactive phenomenon.

What an individual aspires to, and what satisfies him when that achievement is realised, is limited by what is normally possible at a given time within the community of which he is a member. For example, the tremendous rise in prosperity which has taken place in West European countries over the past forty years has resulted in a corresponding change in the standard of living which the ordinary person regards as satisfactory, but no more than adequate. The normal human adaptive processes ensure that any improvement rapidly becomes an essential component of a reasonable life-style. If needs are restricted to necessities then there are relatively few defined by the requirements for survival but aspirations and satisfaction match current living standards.

It is, of course, much easier to allow these things to rise than it is to reverse the process unless the reversal takes place for the whole community. For example, in wartime it is not difficult for people to adjust to severe rationing of all commodities providing that the system is seen to apply to everyone and the reason for it is agreed. It is much more difficult to adjust to restrictions made necessary by unemployment when others remain in jobs with the associated higher standard of living, and few people are prepared to accept that any reduction in quality of life is caused by any faults in themselves. It is much easier to blame the system, the politicians, the management or the trade unions.

In this, as in many other fields of behaviour, people seem to behave as comparative devices. Standards which are normal in that community are acceptable to the individual. Thus the study of these behavioural factors is almost entirely context dependent, and the transfer of theories or principles to other communities, countries or ways of life should only be attempted with extreme caution. What follows has been explored and delineated mainly in Northern European/North American communities and may not be valid in other parts of the world.

Terminology

Traditionally, two main features of behaviour have been distinguished as cognitive aspects and conative aspects respectively.

Cognition is the process of knowing, of comprehending the external world by perceiving, remembering, imagining and reasoning. It is assumed to be essentially rational and similar for different individuals so that agreement about any situation ought to be possible. As discussed in Chapter 2, the picture of the external world built up by an individual is called a *cognitive map*. Another currently fashionable topic is *cognitive ergonomics* which is to do with mental activity as distinct from bodily activity, the study of which is also part of ergonomics. It is analogous to the distinction between this book and the earlier one entitled *The Body at Work*.

Conation, by contrast, covers the volitional and emotional processes. It means literally 'striving', and thus covers issues to do with purposes, goals and objectives. Paradoxically it is more to do with the inner world and yet arises in situations involving people interaction. Concepts and theories are immature enough in cognition (see Chapter 5), but they are even more confused in conation. Many terms are used but they are never precisely defined and consequently there is extensive overlap and ambiguity. For example, it is not easy to distinguish between motives and drives. *Motives* govern orientation and arousal. A *drive* is a motive force or source of energy, an innate drive is also called an *instinct* and is assumed to have a direct physiological basis. Instinct is also used in relation to the form of congenital behaviour as well as its origin. For terminology within conation there is confusion between the origin and impulse, the direction and the end-point. Typically, *need* refers to a felt necessity to act and a particular terminal effect, e.g. hunger and food. Formally instincts, motives, needs and drives are not distinguishable except that motives, needs and drives can be mixed, inherited and acquired, whereas instincts can only be inherited.

Attitude and *set* both refer to a disposition to expect a particular kind of stimulus or generate a particular kind of response, but attitudes are rather more permanent than sets. However, attitudes are not unchangeable, it is feasible to consider attitude training which is sometimes not respectable as in 'brainwashing' but can be respectable in relation for example to safety (p. 287). The term 'mind-set' is currently popular as an explanation for failure to switch hypotheses adaptively in diagnosis and problem-solving, but it is a label rather than an explanation. There would appear to be redundancy in that there can hardly be a set which is not to do with the mind, but perhaps the purpose is to distinguish this phenomenon from an orientation reflex which is a postural attribution associated with stress (p. 163). A *belief* is a cognitively accepted attitude, an *opinion* is a stated belief.

A *culture* is characterised by a group who share common attitudes, knowledge, institutions and organisations. The *status* of an individual denotes his position within a culture and his relationship with respect to other individuals in the same culture.

The fact that the terminology is vague and diffuse, and the interactions and manifestations are obscure, is not a sufficient reason for ignoring the phenomena. The effects are extremely potent and in practice can dominate the surface phenomena of cognitive behaviour to which the greater part of this book is addressed. The main obstacle to study is *rationalisation*, the use of cognitive facilities such as reason and verbal communication to justify decisions and actions which are based on more fundamental human characteristics and interactions. The decision or belief was arrived at, its pseudo-logical explanation is secondary and comes later. Fortunately this is not so valid for man–machine communication, it applies to interpersonal activities and most clearly to those where the individual is personally involved. It is possible to be reasonably logical about other people's problems, but intervention needs to be cautious because that is not the way they will see it.

This position would not have been accepted by nineteenth century theologians and educational theorists, e.g. Newman (1873). Their support for education was based on the belief that it would free mankind from the muddle of tradition and superstition, the universities in particular were seen as monuments to rational man. The case has not yet been proved, it can be argued alternatively that intelligence and education merely provide improved facilities for even more elaborate rationalisation. Either way it is possible to pursue understanding of human interactions provided that they are those of people other than oneself.

3.2 Knowledge
3.2.1 Small groups

Small groups consist of more than two people and less than thirty or so. The key characteristic is not the number but the principle that each member retains his personal identity and is recognised as an individual by other members of the group. A pair (often called a dyad) is not a group in this sense because the possibilities of multiple, graded interactions are too restricted. A group may be defined either by its purpose or by its boundary, these are described respectively as formal groups and informal groups. All groups develop the equivalent of 'territory' which is regarded as private to members of the group and within which non-group members who enter uninvited are regarded as trespassers. The territory may be geographical (a home which is the family group territory), or functional (the activities of a particular working-party or committee), or discipline based (a company medical group which will resent suggestions on one of their topics from anyone not medically qualified). This automatic rejection of ideas from outside the group is known in industry as the 'not invented here' reaction (see also page 311).

Groups also develop norms which reinforce their cohesiveness and identity (Sherif, 1948). These cover such diverse features as clothes and other aspects of appearance, attitudes and beliefs, modes of interaction and methods of working (Argyle, 1972). Deviation from these norms is regarded as extremely serious and deviants may be punished by expulsion from the group, again either physically or functionally, e.g. by refusing to consider their point of view. This is one reason why groups are not highly innovative, creativity is a function of the individual uninhibited by group norms. Within the group, conflicts of opinion are mediated by relative status, either formal or informal, and by other norms of interaction which help to maintain stability. In these ways also the position of an individual as a group member is defined. This is his role. A role is a position within a particular group and there can be role conflict if there are incompatible expectations from an individual who is a member of several groups. Individuals are usually members of about five main groups: work, professional, leisure, domestic and so on. There can, of course, be groups within groups.

One of the earliest classification of groups was the distinction between the autocratic, the democratic and the *laissez-faire* (Lewin *et al.*, 1939). These terms are descriptive of temporary styles of activity rather than permanent characteristics of groups. A competent leader or chairman can change the style to suit a particular topic or objective.

The T-group (training group) method is intended to increase awareness of group behaviour by encouraging sensitivity to others and their attempts at communication. There is extensive discussion of the way the structure of a synthetic group evolves encouraged by the trainer. Usually the synthetic group meets regularly during the training period, and indulges in what might be called group introspection.

There have been many studies of communication within groups sometimes

as observed, as deliberately manipulated (by setting up communication channels in line, in circles, or like the spokes of a wheel or whatever), and as
examined by discussion with participants of relationships between group
members (sometimes called sociometry). Selections from the extensive literature are contained in Smith (1970) and Furnham and Argyle (1981).

The study of small groups is frustrating in that although the effects are real
enough any rules and principles which can be generated are always notable by
exceptions which are often complete reversals. For example, the opinions of a
non-group member may be welcomed if the outsider is sufficiently remote (the
'prophet from a distant country' effect), an obviously deviant member can
sometimes be tolerated and accepted as an eccentric (a kind of mascot), small
groups can be creative – usually when there is a gifted autocratic leader (e.g. a
research group), the opinion of a recognised junior member may be suddenly
accepted ('we must give the boys a chance sometimes'), and a T-group
graduate may find his performance ruined rather than enhanced by his
increased sensitivity because he pays too much attention to why something is
said as distinct from what is said. Attempts to deliberately manipulate a group
(e.g. by putting a controversial item late on an agenda in the hope that
everyone will be too fatigued to discuss it, or by a too obvious attempt to push
something through using a sub-group deliberately scattered through the
assembly) can backfire if the main group detects what is happening.

3.2.2 *Large groups*

The size distinction from small groups is incidental, the key difference
is that in a large group the individual loses his identity and with it his moral
restraints. This is why they are known as mobs (Le Bon, 1895) and herds
(Trotter, 1916). Their most notorious manifestations are in street violence,
lynchings, damage to property and attacks on the established authorities such
as the police and the army. Their behaviour can be oddly coherent without
necessarily being directed by an obvious leader, in this sense they behave like
flocks of birds with each member being influenced by others in proportion to
their distance from him. Nevertheless they can react strongly to leadership, a
demagogue is a leader who can appeal skilfully to the prejudices of a large
group. All groups change their objectives and orientation in time, sometimes
with alarming speed, the study of such changes and their origin is called group
dynamics. This covers large and small groups.

Le Bon hypothesized that, within a mob, an individual regresses to more
primitive behaviour where the emotions dominate the intellect. Trotter also
would support the view that individuals in large groups behave in a much less
rational fashion in that objectives and even opinions are formulated by the

group, and the intellect is used to justify a belief already accepted. This is what he called rationalisation. It follows that such beliefs are not susceptible to rational argument. He stresses the evolutionary advantages of gregariousness not only in providing for the basic needs of self-preservation, nutrition and sex, but also in the immortality which the group can achieve which is patently not possible for the individual. From this point of view the group is superior to the individual in the same way that multicellular organisms are superior to single-celled organisms. The group, like the multi-celled organism, will only function effectively with very close and efficient intercommunication. To achieve this state the individual must subordinate himself to group objectives and the interactions within the group are qualitatively different from those with others outside the group. This intercommunication is not heavily loaded with new ideas, its purpose is rather to strengthen bonds within the group.

The large group is thus a paradoxical combination of more primitive human attributes together with potentiality of robustness and achievement which is far beyond that of the individual. All leaders of large groups, such as generals and managing directors, pay a great deal of attention to morale and morale is essentially the willingness of the individual to pursue collective objectives if necessary at cost to himself. In short, subordination to the group. It is not accidental that insubordination is a serious crime in all military groups.

Experience of membership of a large group in action is highly exhilarating even when there is considerable personal danger. Military organisations are based on this human facility to subordinate individual needs and drives to those of the group. Hence the importance which armies attach to highly cohesive group membership in terms of standard clothing, modes of interaction and methods of working, including highly formalised status within the organisation. Industrial organisations are more diffuse and often incorporate the split loyalty of membership of the company and membership of a trade union. Behaviour in management/trade union conflict seems inexplicable to those outside both groups. There can also be role conflict between work and the family and the balance of these loyalties changes with the culture (that is, the norms of the very large group).

The fundamental human conflict is partly role conflict and partly the conflict between the needs of the individual and the needs of the various groups of which he is a member. This is not just an issue for the group member, from another point of view it poses an even more difficult set of problems for anyone with responsibility for leading a group.

3.2.3 Leadership

The standard approach to this topic is to identify what kind of leaders emerge and are successful in what circumstances. For example, Bartlett (1927) identifies three types of leader: the institutional, the dominant and the persuasive. The authority of the institutional leader depends on his status, he is essentially conservative and is a symbol of the social sentiments of the group, he emphasises rank and is strong on the 'social distance' which must be maintained between him and his followers. The dominant type is assertive, good at rapid decision-making and at taking action. Such leaders are most effective when there is strong competition between groups. The persuasive leader is the most civilised in his belief in taking thought and practising democracy – he 'expresses the group rather than impresses it'. This last is the least obvious manifestation of MacCurdy's (1943) dictum that leadership and privilege are inseparable.

More recently there have been many inductive and experimental approaches to leadership (Brown, 1965, Blum and Naylor, 1968). They have in common an emphasis on the multifactorial nature of leadership, and an attempt to provide a structure in terms of the main variables. For example, in the former category McGregor (1960) separates leaders who emphasise the goals of the organisation (Theory X) from those who emphasise the goals of the individuals (Theory Y). In the more experimental category Fiedler's (1967) contingency model distinguishes two dimensions: styles – task oriented or relationship oriented, and degree of control over the group and the situation – high, medium or low. Task orientation is associated with high or low control, a relationship orientation with moderate control. Fiedler *et al.* (1975) also suggest that historically neither experience nor training seems to have increased leadership performance. This would be highly unusual if it were so; it would indicate that leadership is innate or that it is only a minor variable in group activity, or that to be effective training must be matched closely to the required style and the situation. Fiedler supports this last view, he also considers the impact of the leader in achieving his goals outside the group. This point obviously gets neglected if the emphasis is on study of the activity within the group, yet it is clearly an important part of his role to represent the group within the larger group (Singleton, 1981).

3.2.4   Organisation theory

Theories of organisations inevitably parallel changing industry and culture in Western societies. The earliest theories were essentially economic with an emphasis on allocation of work, chains of authority and financial incentives. In the 1930s the Human Relations approach began to develop triggered by the work of Mayo (1933), and in particular the seminal Hawthorne experiments in the Western Electric Company from 1927 to 1939 (Blum and Naylor, 1968). These started with an experiment in which lighting levels were manipulated, and went on through extensive interviewing to try to identify all the variables affecting production with an emphasis on social and behavioural factors. This movement redeveloped after World War II and was supplemented then by the systems approach with its emphasis on communication and modelling (Johnson *et al.*, 1973). A useful comparison and contrast of these three approaches is contained in O'Shaughnessy, (1966).

More recently, with the extensive development of management courses, a more empirical approach has been adopted with an emphasis on how to manage and how to reorganise a company (Drucker, 1977; Child, 1977). There are some variations between kinds of industry and the rise of the international organisations has created new problems, but it is surprising how much consistency can be detected in the useful principles and practice. The staff of any company or any industry naturally regard their problems as unique and uniquely difficult, but management and organisation consultants who move across many industries are more impressed by the sameness of the problems and solutions. This is no doubt because, in a particular economy and culture, the people are similar in attitudes and aspirations, the technology is always changing rapidly and the organisation environment, mainly set by the government, the financial institutions and the markets, is also the same. In detail it is possible to detect differences in centralisation of authority, configuration, e.g. length of management chain, standardisation and formalisation of procedures and degree of role specialisation, and to relate these to system environment variables such as origin, history, kind of ownership, size, products and technology (Payne and Pugh, 1980). However the dramatic changes in manufacturing industry over the past decade seem to have overlaid these more subtle effects with the dominating influences of technology and market forces. The traditional small scale industries still survive (see applications below) and there are many new ones. In all of them the dominant behavioural problems are the interactions between small numbers of people in the management group. Even in larger scale industries, where the technological communications revolution has radically altered appearances in terms of computers and other office machines, the source of the effectiveness of the organisation is still in the relationship within a group of key people.

3.2.5   *Motivation theory*

The concept of motive is necessary to explain why individuals react differently to what is ostensibly the same stimulus or causal situation, and why they voluntarily place themselves in very different situations. Motives are related to incentives which are external directors of choice and activity, and to internal needs which are assumed to underly motives. The study of motivation is more than usually difficult because, although an attribute of the individual, it is determined not just by himself and his needs, but also by his membership of various groups. There are many attempts to apply theories of motivation to the working situation (see, for example, Warr, 1976; Duncan *et al.*, 1980), but there seem to be only two theories which have emerged in the post-war period which are relevant to organisational problem solving and which make sense when explained to people who work in industry. These are due respectively to Maslow and Herzberg.

Maslow (1943) suggested that needs can be arranged in a hierarchy of five sets: physiological (e.g. nutrition), safety, love, esteem and self-actualisation (self-fulfilment). The essential point about the order of this series is that there is prepotency. The needs at the lower levels have priority, the higher levels are unimportant if the lower levels are not met, and when the lower levels are met the higher levels become important. Thus there is no point in considering self-actualisation for a worker who is starving, but for a worker who is adequately fed, housed and domestically supported esteem and self-actualisation become critical.

Herzberg *et al.* (1959) separated factors which relate to job satisfaction into two categories: *hygiene* factors which include pay and environmental conditions, and *motivators* which include achievement, recognition and responsibility. The innovative proposition is that hygiene factors are essentially negative, and only motivators are positive. Absence of appropriate hygiene factors will lead to dissatisfaction, but they never become satisfiers, satisfaction can only be generated by motivators. The positive/negative aspects are not to be taken too arithmetically, the two sets are not opposites, they are entirely different.

Taken together these ideas form a useful background to the strategy of a consultant concerned with management and productivity from a behavioural viewpoint. There is a considerable contrast between the issues which arise in developing and developed countries. In terms of the behavioural norms of large groups countries can be very different in attitudes to authority, acceptable differentials, standards of education for particular jobs, work-space designs and so on, e.g. in tropical countries many tasks involve female hard manual labour, on the other hand many secretaries are male university graduates. The key problems in developing countries are at the lower end of the Maslow needs hierarchy, effort at work is a function of nutrition, fatigue due to inadequate domestic and travel facilities, chronic diseases and so on. In developed countries the need for motivators is paramount. What might be called the E.A.R. theory of motivation applies. The organisational design problem can be summarised in the requirement to ensure that effort, achievement and rewards are closely and manifestly related.

3.3 Principles, methods and procedures

3.3.1 Group decision making (committees)

The above discussion provides some explanation of why this universal practice in current communities has been the subject of so little productive research. Committees are sub-groups within large groups, they may behave like large groups or like small groups. At one extreme they can assemble the intelligence of their members, at the other extreme they can be entirely irrational at least from the point of view of an outsider. Usually they occupy some intermediate position depending on the separate skills of the members including their social skills in collective communication. More particularly their effectiveness depends on the skills of the chairman. His problem is that he must function with a combination of conative and cognitive sensitivity. He will not be effective unless he can sense the emotional problems of the group, but equally he will not retain their respect unless he can understand and collate their intellectual debate. His authority is based partly on his status within the organisation, and partly on his perceived personal competence. He must acknowledge the relative status of members of the committee, which again is partly organisation-based and partly expertise-based. A normal committee meeting usually has agenda items which require different treatments and a good chairman will behave accordingly: for some items he will merely disseminate information and observe the reaction, for others he has already decided how the committee ought to respond and he will steer it accordingly, for yet others he is genuinely interested in the democratic reaction to the choice. Unless there is spare time (which ought to be unusual), he will not normally allow a committee to search for alternatives, these should be enumerated either by himself or a resident expert, and the committee's task is to weight them. Committees are useless unless they have access to resources – there is no point in making decisions without the facilities to implement them. The implementation may be long-term, and the minutes of a committee should record decisions with reasons as well as any immediate actions, this avoids the need to reconsider matters already dealt with.

The procedure for arriving at a decision varies from democratic to autocratic. The democratic process of one man – one vote is useful in correcting bias due to an excessively vocal minority, and voting systems based on the degree of interest of representatives (as measured for instance by share-holding) have the advantage of equity. On the other hand they can be used by a weak chairman to reduce personal responsibility. An autocratic system where a competent chairman closes an item by delivering his decision in the context of discussion has much to commend it. The worst systems are those found in bureaucracies where membership of committees is the main source of power, committee activity becomes an end in itself and issues are shunted up and down committee hierarchies by groups seeking to avoid or to cancel decisions unacceptable to themselves. These are found in large organisations where cost-effective criteria are remote and responsibilities are diffuse, e.g. civil services, local governments, universities and the military in peace-time (Singleton, 1981). The remedy is to locate responsibilities definitively with individuals and to apply cost-benefit criteria to administration including committees.

3.3.2 *Role analysis*

This is related to task analysis but the emphasis is on the relationships within a group or team. The group may collectively perform a unitary task (e.g. a crew flying an aeroplane) or they may have many tasks within a diverse responsibility (e.g. controlling a factory). It is important because it is clear from experience that errors often arise at the interfaces between people, and lack of role clarity can be a source of personal dissatisfaction. Role analysis and consequent role definitions can make the difference between an effective team and a team which is inefficient and a source of hazards.

Role analysis can also contribute to the clarification of staffing issues. How many men are needed in a team has a simple answer but is none the less a very difficult question. It is not easily approached by measurement of work-loads, but it can be approached indirectly by examining the responsibilities of individuals and their relationships with each other.

An interconnected tree of management titles is one simple form of role analysis with the vertical dimension indicating relative status. The titles are not highly informative and such a chart needs to be supplemented by statements of responsibilities – to whom and for what.

As with task descriptions, there is no universal way of producing or presenting role descriptions. By definition they cover more than one person, and there are often overlapping responsibilities, responsibilities are conditional on particular situations and relative status/authority may be variable. For example, in conducting a role analysis for a process control team the relationships and roles differ in the quiescent phase, the starting up/shutting down phase, the normal operations phase and the emergency phase. A role analysis of a busy man and his secretary could show that he will dictate letters to her for typing and she will provide him with cups of tea and coffee at appropriate times or even act as a private bar waitress when he has visitors. On the other hand she will allocate his time both to appointments and to tasks which she detects are getting neglected. She controls his diary and monitors what he does much more closely than he monitors what she does.

Roles may be defined by designers within technological systems but they evolve within management systems and change with the skills and experience of team members. There can be no objection to this providing that those affected are clear about what is happening. In senior management it is not unusual to deliberately appoint a successor who has different capacities, skills and aspirations from those of the incumbent. In this way it is hoped that some matters which may have been neglected for one period of office will be taken up again during the next period, there may be some productive changes of direction and the roles of his subordinates will change in support of his aptitudes. Correspondingly a senior manager may deliberately change his roles as one or more of the people for whom he is responsible change.

Detecting such processes and presenting them on paper is a useful discipline. A role description usually takes the form of either Venn diagrams which nicely indicate overlapping roles, or path/node diagrams with individuals at the nodes supported by descriptions not only of the responsibilities and tasks at the node, but, at least equally importantly, what the paths are designed to indicate.

Role reversal can be used to clarify the relationship between two people, each attempts to imagine himself in the role of the other and to examine the attitudes and beliefs which naturally emerge from this position. *Role playing* applies to a group where each member is asked to behave as though he did occupy an extreme role not normally familiar to him. This may sound rather juvenile at first sight but it can be extremely effective in providing insight into human attitudes and relationships. It can be used to explore multi-disciplinary situations and is popular also in group therapy.

3.3.3 Job analysis

This is more widely used and understood than is role analysis because it is the standard personnel psychology procedure (e.g. Anastasi, 1964). It is a method of providing evidence which can be used to generate selection and training criteria to provide promotion and job enlargement/enrichment indications, and as part of the documentation concerned with negotiating rates of pay (Fig. 3.2).

Jobs exist. Workers apply for them, spend their time within them and get paid for doing so. In principle they are designed by managers, but there are strong elements of custom and practice, they evolve over time as organisational requirements change and individual worker expertise develops.

A job analyst has plenty of source material from earlier documents, observation of and discussion with workers, consultation with supervisors and with technical experts. His first problem is that there are bound to be inconsistencies between his data sources, and his own experiences and judgments are needed to reach a valid consensus. His second problem is that he is engaged in a political act, the results of his deliberations matter to quite a large range of people – the workers themselves, the management and various specialists. Job descriptions are a recorded version of part of a complex communication process which

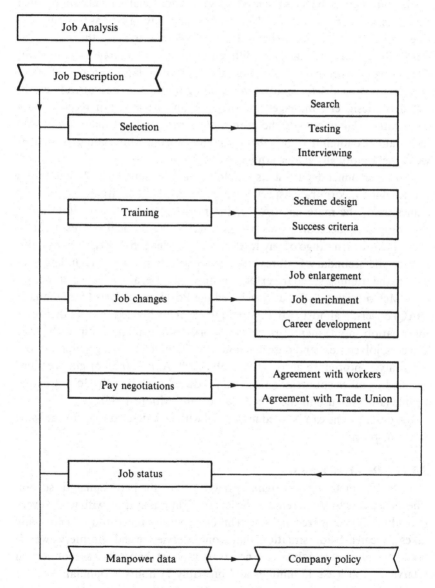

Fig. 3.2. The uses of job analysis.

someone has deemed necessary. The first requirement of the analyst is that he must be clear about what he is trying to do, for whom, why, in what context, with what objectives and with what resources and limitations. The context may have political, legal and social connotations in addition to the informational aspects. For example, a senior person may decide that job analysis shall be carried out because he feels the need for some additional evidence for his own superiors, his peers or others with whom he is negotiating such as trade unions. The workers whose tasks are being analysed will want to know the reasons for this activity, and may react very differently depending on how they interpret why the work is being done. The analysis may be mandatory because of safety regulations. Socially the analyst is intruding into a situation already established by designers, managers or workers, and he may not receive ready cooperation. He is outside the groups concerned and not many people are secure and broadminded enough to welcome someone who is going to put their work metaphorically under a microscope.

Many personnel departments develop their own standard job description forms which incorporate aspects such as the working environment, the machines used, the materials treated, the range of tasks, the relationship to preceding and succeeding jobs within a series, the particular stressors, any critical features, a range of pay rates and so on. The job description may also include the secondary features such as the selection criteria including education, the training standard externally and in-house, and avenues of promotion. McCormick (1979) has developed the Position Analysis Questionnaire (PAQ) covering almost two hundred job elements divided into six divisions: information input, mental processes, work output, relationship with other workers, job context and miscellaneous. It is intended to be a general purpose job analysis procedure although it is obviously American in origin. Versions adapted to other countries have been produced including the Job Structure Profile (JSP) for use in the U.K. (Patrick and Moore 1985).

Job descriptions can be used in parallel with task descriptions for the same range of purposes.

3.3.4 Depth interviews

This method was originally developed by the psychoanalytic school. The objective is to try to remove the layers of rationalisation with which every individual is encumbered and reveal his basic beliefs and attitudes. It normally takes place in a dyadic situation, that is one interviewee and one interviewer. It takes much longer to achieve the necessary rapport than is the case for normal interviews – at least 45 minutes and probably $1\frac{1}{2}$ hours is optimal.

Skilled depth interviewers are rare. A sympathetic approach, complete integrity and the ability to submerge one's own personality are required. The interviewer gently steers the interviewee to talk at length about his opinions or his problems, and responds only to indicate understanding. It should not be used lightly, it can be dangerous in revealing vulnerabilities unanticipated by both parties.

It can be used by a senior person such as the company medical officer or personnel officer to support his management colleagues who are often people who believe, probably mistakenly, that they must always maintain an impersonal front in relation to their peers and their subordinates. It is used also in market research in an attempt to reveal basic customer preferences and images of products. A good example of its use to trace the impact of automation on an industry is provided by Chadwick-Jones (1969).

3.4   Applications
3.4.1   *Batch production*
The glamorous large-scale manufacturing industries such as electrical assembly, car assembly and chemical processing, are dependent on parts which are produced in much smaller companies where things are usually made in batches. In the clothing industry wearing apparel, shoes, gloves, accoutrements and so on are also made by the same kind of production organisation. Many of the newer small companies providing specialist services such as printing work on the same principles. Such a company may have a staff of anything from 20 to 400. Up to this size it is possible for one person at the top to have fairly complete control, although there will be two or three levels of management below him. Beyond this size we get into quite different management structures, with promotion ladders, career planning, specialist personnel, training and accounts functions and so on. The small companies have to rely on external specialists and other consultants because they cannot have the complete range of required expertise in-house. A behavioural science consultant can make a valuable contribution.

The decision to call him in may have been triggered by a particular problem such as skill shortages, quality complaints, or inadequate performance in meeting delivery dates, but it is normally possible to widen the remit and persuade the customer that his company needs an overall appraisal.

The first step is to identify how and why the company survives. This usually turns out to be the management skills of a small group, plus the production skills of a loyal labour force. The key management skill can differ over a wide range even between companies making the same products in the same quality range. It may be purchasing, selling or leadership of the production team. All are important of course, and there will be competence in all these fields, but excellence perhaps in only one. It is appropriate to conduct a semi-formal skills analysis of each member of the management team, and a role analysis which indicates how they share and delegate responsibilities. It is not unusual to find that the role separation is far from optimal and is itself the source of disagreements and conflicts which occur regularly. Some tactful redefinition of roles can result in much smoother cooperation. Again this can differ quite widely. Typically there may be three levels: Director, often a member of the family which owns the company, Manager and Foreman. The Director may rarely go in to the production shops or, at the other extreme, he may be the *de-facto* foreman with the titled foreman acting as his assistant. He can have some intermediate role where, for example, he fixes piecework rates but leaves the production control to the foreman. The Manager will often look after all the personnel and general office functions including all the paperwork. The Foreman's basic task is control of production which is mathematically an impossible problem, but he does it by working to a set of rules he has formulated for himself, e.g. try to make sure that each operator has several hours of work waiting, always try to have several operator/machine systems which can perform any one task, encourage operator versatility. The amount of work in progress is a key optimising problem, too little and some work stations will have idle periods, too much and the average throughput time will be too high, plus the accentuation of the control problem of where everything is. A detailed job analysis with separation into tasks and rating of performance on each task is the basis for suggesting any changes. The Foreman is also a leader, and the group dynamics of the production shop incorporate rapid fluctuations from smooth homogeneous activity to phases of edgy temperamental collective alienation (Singleton, 1978).

There are often physical environmental issues of how to combine reasonable lighting and temperature with sufficient air circulation to maintain a fresh atmosphere and hopefully reduce the probability of cross-infection. In winter absenteeism mainly from colds, flu and the like can be 10–20%.

The layout of the plant also poses interesting problems (Singleton and Simister, 1957). The production flow and control issues have to be combined with consideration of motivation and group identities. The workers are often divisible into groups which have separate interests and topics of conversation, e.g. for female workers: the older family-grown-up group, the young marrieds with no children, and the youngest group between school and marriage. Some encouragement of sub-group identities can improve morale even though it can also produce minor 'them and us' symptoms. The youngest group in particular are often not properly identified and looked after. If they are withdrawn or rebellious it can be because no one is providing the appropriate combination of consideration, training, guidance and leadership.

There are also work-place design problems centring on lighting, posture and ease of manipulation. The feeders can be helped by real display design in storing and labelling materials which are thereby easily located.

3.4.2 Construction

Construction sites have three main problems: the weather, safety and control of highly heterogeneous operations. The weather, in Europe at least, is so unpredictable as to dominate the whole style of work with rapid adaptation and improvisation rather than the smooth conduct of a pre-planned operation. Snow and frost in winter and heavy rain in summer cause so much disruption it is surprising that more systematic protection is not provided, it is rather too easily accepted as inevitable, although there are trends now to improved sheltering and screening on a large scale. There are also clothing design issues which are too frequently left to the individual worker's discretion. Properly designed clothing from helmet to boots can be a considerable boon. Dry cold or heat are straightforward, but the typical European moderately cold, windy, intermittently damp weather is the most difficult to design clothing for. Provision of adequate personal storage, washing and hygiene facilities are also poor compared with those in, say, coal mines or process plant. The relative severity of these issues can be detected by site inspection, by any records of causes of delays, and by general human resource study including access and egress (e.g. transport facilities) as well as on-site operations.

Safety is always a problem because the basic process is the movement and manipulation of large quantities of heavy materials and operations at different heights. The work is energy intensive and dangerous for this reason alone (see Chapter 6). The industry is unusual in that safety precautions almost inevitably clash with immediate speed of operations (e.g. the need for elaborate scaffolding).

Motivation is not usually a problem because there is the intrinsic satisfaction of participating in causing things to happen on a large scale and in the visible results of effort. This can accentuate the safety problems because of priorities and degree of corner cutting tolerated by the management.

The site can easily degenerate in a muddle of equipment, stored materials and completed parts, and this adds greatly to the hazards. Good housekeeping is even more critical than in factories. There are more problems of pilfering and other consequences of dishonesty than is normal in a closed factory.

The leadership style is usually autocratic with the site manager as the key figure. He controls the distribution of the work force in relation to the required phasing of many tasks and constraints such as weather, machine availability and materials and components which do not arrive on time or do not match the requirements. There is always urgency because there is no return on the extensive investment until the work is completed and there may well be penalty clauses for lateness.

The scope for improvements is in the presentation of information to the site manager in relation to the vast range of situations about which he has to make decisions. There may be some scope for role analysis, not so much within the on-site organisation but in relationships to the parent company and the many site visitors: designers, sub-contractors, inspectors and so on.

3.4.3   *The management consultant*

There are of course many experts in management consultancy in specialist technology, accountancy etc., but the general purpose consultant will have to deal with many issues which are to do with the behavioural sciences. He is a job analyst writ large.

He will begin a new project by a tour of the premises and will often be able to arrive at a surprisingly accurate appraisal of the situation in a very short time. He may not know how he does it, but the cues he uses are the general state of the place in terms of cleanliness, the amount, condition and location of work in progress and stores, the number of people active, not active or unproductively active, e.g. walking about. Indications of overactivity are as ominous as those of underactivity, they suggest emergencies, lack of planning or perhaps merely a show to impress him and his escort. He will be very interested in the way people react to him, and, equally important, the way they react to each other. He will then ask for some documented data, its ease of retrieval and its relevance are as important as the data itself.

He will examine the ostensible case for calling him in, and try to look below the surface of this for reasons which have not been emphasised or even mentioned, but which may be critical to what he can do and how to do it. To this end a number of versions from individuals at different levels are useful, and useful also in his first analyses. These will be at two levels: the physical world in the sense of the resources, the inputs and outputs, and the behavioural world, a role analysis of how participants interact, some as individuals, some as groups. His preliminary report will be a compromise between the need to impress the customer that he has understood the situation sufficiently and the need to avoid generating alarm by revealing that he has understood it too well. This may sound rather devious but the experienced consultant is well aware of his impact as an outsider on an established group and, however serious their internal problems, they will close ranks against him if he seems immediately to be threatening the *status quo*. As in all skilled performance, when he does something is as critical as what is done. He will try to smooth the almost inevitable cycle of early suspicion followed by a swing to excessive expectations of what he can do, followed by a swing back again when there is some disillusion that neither he nor anyone else has a complete answer to a mixed individual/social/economic/technical problem.

People who regularly employ consultants are themselves not naive and they also may be aware of all these issues. It thus becomes a complex long-term negotiation where the consultant has a constructive role because of his specialist expertise including his experience of similar problems elsewhere. One of the key elements in his expertise is his ability to express clearly in a mixed verbal/diagrammatic fashion what is already known or at least suspected by some of the people he is dealing with. Depending on the particular case this can be any mix of the methods and procedures described in this book.

There is very little literature on this interesting and important topic, probably because those who have the experience are practitioners rather than academics. They have no incentive to make public what they know. One useful general survey is Kubr (1986).

3.4.4 Ergonomics in developing countries

The reasons for the importance of this subject are described in the companion volume *The Body at Work*. The more obvious benefits are to do with climate, energy expenditure, posture, and physical well-being generally, all topics in the earlier book. More recently reviews have been provided by Sen (1984) and Wisner (1985).

Within the scope of this book are matters such as how this subject might be developed, because communication between different countries with different cultures is required. There is extensive good-will in advanced countries, and it has been noted that aid in this expertise sense can be at least as beneficial as economic aid. There is, for example, a Centre of Ergonomics of Developing Countries at the University of Lulea in Sweden. From the scientific point of view there are benefits in the other direction in enlarging the view of the attributes of 'man' and correcting the tendency to view Western man as universal man.

On the other hand cross cultural communication is not easy. Rivers (1914) noted from his nineteenth century studies of communication of ideas in Polynesia that when a traveller moves to and fro between two islands he more readily takes ideas back from his host to his own country rather than giving ideas to his host, the principle applies generally to communication between groups and cultures. Even within a group the odds are weighted against action, as Cornford (1964) nicely put it in relation to academic discussions 'There is only one argument for doing something, the rest are arguments for doing nothing'. Within the arguments for doing nothing he includes the principle of the wedge (thin end of), the principle of the dangerous precedent, and the principle of unripe time.

It is a well-established consultancy adage that it is easier to improve already highly competent organisations than it is to do anything about the incompetent ones. This applies to developing countries where the range of organisational quality across companies is very large, from the extremely able to those where everything that could be wrong is wrong. What can be achieved by an outsider in a necessarily brief period is very limited, even when things happen whilst he is there they readily lapse to old ways after he departs. The blame lies partly with the consultants who do not always appreciate the gulf between their way of thinking and acting, and those of the indigenous managers and workers. This is to do with cultural norms and styles. One effective approach is to concentrate on staff training in principles and procedures, and hope that innovations in the operational systems will follow later as a consequence of this training (Singleton and Whitfield, 1968; Singleton, 1972). This is in line with the Rivers concept of transmission across group interfaces mentioned above. A valuable additional incentive is for the consultant to return after six months or a year to discuss progress.

The two United Nations Organisations with extensive experience of applications in the developing world are the International Labour Office and the World Health Organisation. They have interesting differences in programmes, partly of course because they have different overall remits.

Since 1976 the I.L.O. has been running the PIACT programme (International Programme for the Improvement of Working Conditions and Environment). The emphasis is on making work more human. There are five main spheres of activity: safety and health, hours of work, organisation and content of work, conditions of work including choice of technology, and the working and living environment. This last is a recognition of the importance of the necessary support for work from the domestic situation of housing, food, education, leisure etc. The 'Organisation and Content of Work' programme is a very ambitious one, including design of interesting jobs which provide self-expression, work satisfaction, promotion opportunities, worker participation and reduction of fatigue. It seems to be designed as a deliberate attempt to set very high targets in the hope that this will provide the incentive to at least make some progress in the desired direction.

A similar strategy lies behind the very different programme of the W.H.O. called H 2000 – 'Health for all by the year 2000'. This a broad programme which by its title is so ambitious it could be called romantic rather than logical. It was separated into more achievable objectives by a conference at Alma Ata in the USSR in 1978. The Alma Ata declaration includes safe water, adequate nutrition, basic sanitation, maternal and child care, and health education among the objectives. There is emphasis on working not only through governments but also through non-governmental organisations (NGOs) such as scientific institutes, charities and voluntary agencies. Again there is recognition that societal living conditions are a necessary basis for movement along the chain of quality of life from domestic conditions through work to standard of living.

References

Anastasi, A. (1964). *Fields of Applied Psychology*. New York: McGraw-Hill.

Argyle, M. (1972). *The Psychology of Interpersonal Behaviour*. Harmondsworth: Penguin.

Bartlett, F.C. (1927). *Psychology and the Soldier*. Cambridge University Press.

Blum, M.L. and Naylor, J.C. (1968). *Industrial Psychology*. New York: Harper.

Brown, R. (1965). *Social Psychology*. New York: Macmillan.

Chadwick-Jones, J. (1969). *Automation and Behaviour*. London: Wiley.

Child, J. (1977). *Organisation*. London: Harper & Row.

Cornford, F.M. (1964). *Microcosmographia Academica*. London: Bowes & Bowes.

Drucker, P. (1977). *People and Performance*. London: Heinemann.

Duncan, K.D., Gruneberg, M.M. and Wallis, D. (eds.). (1980). *Changes in Working Life*. Chichester: Wiley.

Fiedler, F.E. (1967). *A Theory of Leadership Effectiveness*. New York: McGraw-Hill.

Fiedler, F.E., Bons, P.M. and Hastings, L.L. (1975). New strategies for leadership utilisation. In Singleton, W.T. and Spurgeon, P. (eds.). *Measurement of Human Resources*. London: Taylor & Francis.

Furnham, A. and Argyle, M. (eds.). (1981). *The Psychology of Social Situations*. Oxford: Pergamon.

Herzberg, F.B., Mausner, M. and Snyderman, B.B. (1959). *The Motivation to Work*. New York: Wiley.

Johnson, R.A., Kast, F.E. and Rosenzweig, J.E. (1973). *The Theory and Management of Systems*. London: McGraw-Hill & Kogakusha.

Kubr, M. (ed.). (1986). *Management Consulting*. Geneva: I.L.O.

Le Bon, G. (1895). *The Crowd*. Reprinted 1960. New York: Viking.

Lewin, K., Lippit, R. and White, P.K. (1939). Patterns of aggressive behaviour in experimentally created social climates. *Journal of Social Psychology* 10, 271–99.

MacCurdy, J.T. (1943). *The Structure of Morale*. Cambridge University Press.

McCormick, E.J. (1979). *Job Analysis*. New York: Amacom.

McGregor, D. (1960). *The Human Side of Enterprise*. New York: McGraw-Hill.

Maslow, A.H. (1943). A theory of human motivation. *Psychological Review* 50, 370–95.

Mayo, E. (1933). *The Human Problems of an Industrial Civilization*. New York: Macmillan.

Newman, J.H. (1873). *Idea of University Defined*. Reprinted 1960. New York: Holt, Rinehart and Winston.

O'Shaughnessy, J. (1966). *Business Organisation*. London: George Allen & Unwin.

Patrick, J. and Moore, A.K. (1985). Development and reliability of a job analysis technique. *Journal of Occupational Psychology* **58**. 149–58.

Payne, R.L. and Pugh, D.S. (1980). Organisations as psychological environments. In Warr, P.B. (ed.). *Psychology at Work*. Harmondsworth: Penguin.

Rivers, W.H.R. (1914). *History of Melanesian Society*. Cambridge University Press.

Sen, R.N. (1984). Application of ergonomics to industrially developing countries. Ergonomics Society Lecture. *Ergonomics* **27**. **10**, 1021–31.

Sherif, M. (1948). *An Outline of Social Psychology*. New York: Harper.

Singleton, W.T. (1972). *Introduction to Ergonomics*. Geneva: World Health Organisation.

Singleton, W.T. (1978). The sewing machinist. In Singleton, W.T. (ed.). *The Analysis of Practical Skills*. Lancaster: M.T. Press.

Singleton, W.T. (ed.) (1981). *Management Skills*. Lancaster: M.T. Press.

Singleton, W.T. and Simister, R. (1957). The design and layout of machinery for industrial operatives. *Occupational Psychology* **31**, 26–34.

Singleton, W.T. and Whitfield, D. (1968). The organisation and conduct of a World Health Organisation. Inter-regional course on Ergonomics for Developing Countries. *Human Factors* **10.6**, 633–40.

Smith, P.S. (ed.) (1970). *Group Processes*. Harmondsworth: Penguin.

Trotter, W. (1916). *Instincts of the Herd in Peace and War*. London: Fisher-Unwin.

Warr, P.B. (ed.) (1976). *Personal Goals and Work Design*. Chichester: Wiley.

Wisner, A. (1985). Ergonomics in industrially developing countries. *Ergonomics* **28.8**, 1213–24.

4 Performance and job design

4.1 Concepts

One of the fundamental attributes of human behaviour is that it changes continuously along the time dimension. This fact is neglected by many experimental psychologists who are attempting to describe the behaviour of the human operator, the average man, the laboratory subject (actually labelled 'S' in some journals) or even the human organism (labelled 'O'). This is only defensible provided that it is recognised that whatever properties are adduced they relate to a static abstraction. The properties of this abstraction are described in Chapter 5 but as a preliminary to such studies the set of concepts which express what is known about dynamic behaviour are needed.

The constructive changes in time are generally put into the category of learning already described in Chapter 2. The analogous negative changes which occur in parallel are described as fatigue (in the short term) and ageing (in the long term). Ageing is also dealt with in Chapter 2.

There are several concepts which centre on the facility to change level of activity either voluntarily or involuntarily. This is described as arousal. Within arousal studies two sets of phenomena have been identified and investigated in great detail, particularly over the past forty years. These are stress and vigilance. Stress was adopted as a popular behavioural research topic because it seemed to have possibilities of easier measurement than fatigue which had its heyday from 1920 to 1950. Vigilance studies were stimulated by the practical need to understand behaviour in new tasks resulting from instrumentation technology – essentially the monitoring of displayed data.

The need to keep expensive equipment in continous operation has accentuated the requirement for working 'unsocial hours' which has renewed interest in the mental and bodily changes which occur over a twenty-four hour cycle – *circadian rhythms*.

All the phenomena in this chapter are characteristically humanistic, or at least organismic, in that there are no corresponding effects in the behaviour of hardware mechanisms.

4.1.1 *Fatigue*

Fatigue is broadly defined as a change within the organism resulting in changes in feeling and decrements in performance which are traceable to earlier performance. The essential measurable attributes are that performance worsens as a consequence of performance. This is accompanied in human behaviour by introspective changes usually regarded as undesirable, although in appropriate circumstances of achievement and the prospect of rest fatigue can be agreeable.

Fatigue is a broad descriptor covering a wide range from the reduced responsiveness of an isolated muscle preparation to feelings that some relaxation would be restorative after months of intellectual effort. As often happens with behavioural functions, the term is applied indiscriminately to measures of performance, performance criteria and the underlying presumed cause.

Many of the phenomena related to fatigue can be demonstrated by a simple ergograph in which the movements of a finger flexing against a weight are recorded (Muscio, 1920). The movements gradually decrease in amplitude, the decrement is more rapid for a higher load and is restored by rest. The greater the decrement the longer the required recovery time. The fatigue effect is not restricted to the finger in use but spreads to adjacent fingers. Recovery also takes place if the weight is reduced and if the weight stays the same but is apparently reduced. Thus, although there is an effect due to accumulation of the waste products of muscle activity in the intact human operator similar to that in a muscle preparation (where diminished reaction to an electrical stimulus can be restored by washing in a saline solution), there are complications not only in the spread of the effect but also in the direct influence of a belief (that the weight has been reduced) on a simple muscular action. Muscio eventually proposed that the term fatigue should, for scientific purposes, be abandoned. This in fact has happened. In neither of the two recent introductory textbooks of psychology in the U.K. (Taylor and Sluckin, 1982 and Lloyd and Mayes, 1984) is the term fatigue listed in the index. However, although psychologists can abandon a topic it does not vanish from everyday life, from manufacturing industry where 'fatigue allowances' are still much debated, nor from high technology tasks such as flight deck operations where considerations of potential fatigue dominate the determination of working hours.

The straightforward measures of performance decrement are a reduction in amplitude or rate of activity, responsiveness as measured by reaction time and accuracy (Singleton, 1953). These effects can indeed be measured in appropriate circumstances but there are many complications (Bartley and Chute, 1947; Floyd and Welford, 1953). In addition to performance decrement, performance disorganisation occurs. This is detectable in irregularities of order and timing; the right responses may be made but in the wrong sequence and responses may not be appropriately phased either in series or in response to external events. If this mistiming is sufficiently severe the performance may become more and more disorganised eventually leading to complete disruption. Corresponding changes occur on the input side, the perceptual field is subject to gradual disintegration so that events are treated in smaller units, and there is a tendency to concentrate on central aspects (physically or functionally or both) with a neglect of peripheral aspects, e.g. a fatigued pilot may continue to fly straight and level but doesn't notice a need to switch fuel tanks. Paradoxically, although the perceptual field narrows in the sense that there is increasing 'tunnel vision', there is also a greater awareness of task irrelevant stimuli, such as feelings of discomfort.

There may or may not be self-awareness of diminished effectiveness, but if there is the response can vary enormously. In studies of pilot fatigue (Davis, 1948; Bartlett 1943) it was noted that some subjects responded by withdrawal and inertia, others by aggression and irritability.

Most of these ideas were developed from military studies during World War II where the conditions were extreme. For example pilots were flying for up to 12 hours in cold, noisy, vibrating aircraft with a high probability of being shot down. Even so the effects were just an exaggerated version of those which can be noted either introspectively, by observation or by measurement on much less severe tasks.

4.1.2 Arousal

There is a spectrum of degree of arousal from coma and sleep to excitement and terror. Arousal is indicated externally by tenseness and alertness and there is some correspondence with internal states as detected by introspection and by physiological indicators. There is also some inconsistency in that a catatonic state of passivity may be due either to no internal activity or to such gross internal activity that there is no scope for accepting any more external stimulation, the coma to terror scale becomes circular. At a more normal level the human operator may fail to register a stimulus either because he is not sufficiently mentally active (drowsiness) or because he is overactive either in thinking about something else (anxiety) or in excessive and disorganised mental activity (terror).

From this context the concept has arisen that for a given task there is an optimum level of arousal. There is a so-called 'inverted U' relationship between efficiency and arousal, the apex of the inverted U indicating the optimum arousal level for that particular task. Performance falls off on each side of this optimum for reasons to do with inputs, processing and outputs. At the input level greater arousal seems to lead to greater selectivity so that attention narrows and cues may be missed for this reason, but they may also be missed because of reduced alertness. At the central level when arousal is too low there is not enough activity to cope with the information, whereas at high level there may be too much 'noise' so that again there is insufficient processing capacity. At the output level low arousal and corresponding relaxation may lead to too flabby a response, but too much arousal and tenseness with associated tremor may also lead to insufficient precision in response. Broadly the more difficult the task the greater the optimum arousal level, but this statement cannot be pressed too far towards precision because the epithet 'difficult' when applied to tasks is ambiguous and multi-dimensional.

It seems that warm-blooded organisms are designed to function at different levels of activity depending on the demands of the current situation. This is not restricted to the nervous system, it is basically controlled by the endocrine system and the musculature is also involved, for example, by tuning into the 'fight or flight' mode when difficulties or dangers are perceived. For man as an operator in technological systems or for man within advanced societies generally this is not functionally appropriate since it is not usually adaptive to generate excessive physical activity. An increase in heart rate, blood flow and muscle tension may well impede his performance unless he happens to be an athlete or a manual worker.

There are considerable individual differences, one of the few useful personality dimensions is introversion/extraversion. These reaction types were originally defined by Jung (1933) in terms of the direction of psychic energy which may be inward (introversion) or outward (extraversion). In arousal terms the introvert in spite of his passive and reflective appearance is naturally at a higher level of arousal than the excitable and adventurous extrovert. The explanation for this apparent paradox is that the extrovert needs and therefore seeks more environmental stimulation than does the introvert.

Between the natural endowment and the immediate demand dependent aspects there are natural rhythms more or less in phase with the time of day and therefore called circadian rhythms. There is an approximate sinusoidal change over the twenty-four hours for somatic, behavioural and introspective parameters, normally with a peak at about 4 p.m. and a trough at 4 a.m. This is disturbed and can shift for a person working at night or a traveller across time zones. There are quite large individual differences in the ease with which the cycle can shift, in some people it shifts readily in a day or two, in others it may take very much longer. There is some evidence that introverts are more active in the mornings and extroverts in the afternoon and evening, the extroverts as it were take longer to 'warm up' after sleep.

Sleep itself is a manifestation of circadian rhythm and of arousal. Arousal level also varies during sleep, most dramatically in REM (rapid eye movement) sleep which occurs very approximately at hourly intervals but more frequently towards the end of the night's sleep. Sleep requirements change with age, declining from birth to adolescence and then settling to about eight hours per night until senescence when there are frequent short sleeps (naps) during the day and more interrupted sleep during the night. Why sleep is necessary and the somatic mechanisms which control it remain unknown. So also, of course, do the reasons for the quite large individual differences.

4.1.3 Stress

Stress refers to the situation where a human operator is subjected to a load which affects his behaviour. This description might be taken to refer to the fundamental concept of adaptation or to the simple stimulus–response paradigm on which psychologists of the behaviourist school base their understanding. However the term is used at a conceptual level intermediate between these two extremes, it is intended to describe the behavioural state rather than the behaviour itself, and thus to form a descriptive background to that set of performance phenomena where there are indications of distress. There is ambiguity as to whether the term refers to the imposed load or the reaction to it. Clinically, e.g. Selye (1976), stress described the 'general adaptation syndrome' (GAS), the generalised response to stress situations with the term 'stressor' used to indicate the situation itself. Psychologically, e.g. Singleton *et al.* (1971), stress is used to indicate the imposed load and strain the reaction to it, this corresponds to engineering usage for the phenomenon in mechanics. Physiologists may use either as in heat stress indices which can be based on weighted measures of the climatic environment, or sweat rates or subjective opinions.

Heat stress is a nice illustration of the general position that single environmental measures are not directly related to single response measures. The reaction to ambient heat, as measured introspectively, by performance changes or by bodily changes is not uniquely related to temperature but to empirically determined combinations of temperature, radiant temperature, humidity, windspeed, clothing, posture, training, physical activity, sex, age, attitude, etc. Nevertheless there is no mystery, the physical laws of heat exchange and energy conservation are not violated, it is simply a question of teasing out all the relevant parameters.

The situation in relation to informational load is less straightforward. There are no physical laws which define and constrain the effects on the central nervous system of stress in the form of information input and processing although there have been attempts for example to pursue a psychological refractory period by analogy with the physiological refractory period (see next chapter). There is a very extensive literature on mental load (see next section), but it is limited in usefulness by the difficulty of separating physical, informational and emotional aspects.

The emotional aspects of stress vary from performance decrement attributed to the impression of lack of achievement, to the great array of psychosomatic illnesses. As in other fields there are problems of combining short-term and long-term aspects under the same topic label. Short-term disturbances originating in self-awareness are usually attributed to arousal changes already discussed. Long-term disturbances in the form of stress diseases are currently a popular area of interest both in practice and in theory. All theories of the aetiology of stress diseases acknowledge the dominance of the intervening personality between the stressors and their consequence. One man's disabling stress is another man's stimulating environment, but even so it may be that a person apparently enjoying the stress is the more likely to succumb to stress disease. For example, the so-called coronary-provoking Type A behaviour pattern identified by Friedman and Rosenman is one of high alertness, eagerness to compete, desire for recognition and pursuit of deadlines. Type B is the converse, see for example Cooper and Payne (1980). Stress research often reveals strange paradoxes in relationships between apparently stressful situations and the measured responses. For example, Bourne (1969) studied helicopter ambulance crews engaged in the very dangerous task of evacuating combat casualties during the Vietnam war. He showed that endocrine activity measured by a urinary steroid did not differ significantly between flying days and non-flying days, and moreover this chronic mean level was lower than that of equivalent soldiers at a training camp in the U.S.A. Interviews with the subjects supported the conclusion that their knowledge of the value of their work counterbalanced the threat of death and mutilation. The danger was coped with by a generalised emotional repression as indicated by the low steroid secretion.

A broader approach to the assessment of stress is to identify life changes by interview and to rank these changes in terms of degree of stress by expressed opinion (Gunderson and Rahe, 1974). Life change events can be divided into four categories: family, personal, work and financial. Life change units (LCUs) are assigned by degree of seriousness, e.g. death of spouse is the maximum 100 units, a minor violation of the law is 11 units. All the life changes in a given period (from 1 week to 3 years) can be added in terms of LCUs and the total used as a predictor of illness. The correlations obtained are positive, and not high, but they are often significant in statistical terms. One interesting aspect is that the LCU scale is very similar for people in different countries and different cultures from Mexico to Sweden.

There are also 'coping theories' of stress, e.g. Lazarus (1967), which emphasise the importance of the subject's personal awareness of the situation he is in. These add another important level to the parameters of stress which can now be structured at three levels (Table 4.1). The first level is the imposed load itself, the second is the somatic reaction to this load and the third is the individual observing, as it were, how the game is developing, with himself as the main player. The individual compares the demands of the situation with his own abilities to cope with such demands. If the latter exceeds the former then all is well. It can be said that there is no strain in spite of the obvious pressure of stress, or even that the stress and its effects are clear but the individual is positively enjoying using his resources to cope successfully. This explains why individuals with particular skills deliberately expose themselves to high demand situations where their special skills are required, e.g. managers and athletes (Singleton 1979).

4.1.4   Vigilance

Vigilance refers to performance in tasks where there are irregular inputs, often from cues which are difficult to detect and the output is trivial (in the form of pressing a button or making a vocal response). It was originally used by neurologists to describe the optimised arousal state of the alert organism, but was taken over by psychologists to describe new tasks which emerged in World War II. These tasks involved detecting distant enemy units by their reflection of radio pulses. These reflections were recorded either on screens (Radar) or by changes in auditory signals (Asdic and Sonar). The early studies of this problem were also called 'pipology' which nicely described the task of discriminating small changes in brief visual or auditory signals (Williams 1949).

The difficulties arise from a combination of a situation which encourages low arousal and a sensory discrimination which is near threshold. Low arousal is endemic because nothing much happens, the signals which are usually present are entirely regular and therefore monotonous to the point of being hypnotic and there is no counterbalancing physical activity. The signal to be detected is only just above the level of natural noise in the form of screen clutter or the analogous spurious random variations in the auditory signals.

Not surprisingly, performance as measured by either success in detection or speed of response deteriorates after ten or twenty minutes depending on the

Table 4.1. *Levels of 'stress'*

Level 1. Stressors or Stress	The imposed load from the environment and from information inputs (Table 4.4.)
Level 2. Strain	The reaction to the load as measured by somatic and performance measures (Table 4.3.)
Level 3. Coping response	The reaction of the individual following his audit of imposed demand, his somatic reaction to the demand and his review of his inventory of personal resources to cope with these demands

task. Performance is improved, i.e. maintained at a reasonable level for a longer period, by careful design of the environment and by any measure which maintains or improves arousal. Some of the classic research in this field was done by Mackworth (1950), who showed that performance would be improved or maintained by shorter working periods, by interruptions which increased alertness, by knowledge of results and by taking an amphetamine. The laboratory tasks he used were a pointer requiring 100 steps to complete a circle with steps at one second intervals, and, in other experiments, an auditory ping every three seconds. The signals to be detected were respectively a double step of the pointer and echoes to particular pings. This sort of task is straightforward to set up and the performance measures of misses, latency and 'false positives' are straightforward to record. A very large literature on this topic has been generated over the past thirty years (Broadbent, 1971; Davies and Parasuraman, 1982).

The latter describe six theories of vigilance as shown in Table 4.2. When summarised in this way it becomes clear that attempts to explain the phenomenon are distinctly tautological. Terms such as filtering, arousal, adaptation, habituation and so on are used in various orders and combinations to account for the observed performance in a great variety of experimental tasks which are broadly similar, but which differ in detail. Such bald summaries do not do justice to the painstaking collection of data and refined argument about exactly what happened and why, but the practical consequences are not commensurate with the academic effort invested (Davies and Parasuraman list more than 800 references). There has been rather more success in describing what happens (as opposed to explaining it) by the use of signal detection theory (p. 199).

There is undoubtedly a practical problem which can be described in 'allocation of function' terms. Compared with machines the human operator is much

Table 4.2. *Theories of vigilance*

(summarised from Davies and Parasuraman, 1982)

Inhibition theory	This is based on conditioning theory. The response to a detected signal is a conditioned response, which is extinguished gradually by inhibition because it is not reinforced
Expectancy theory	The operator is assumed to predict signals on the basis of his preceding experience, and to expect fewer signals as the task progresses. He responds accordingly in terms of his observations and his actions
Filter theory	When an operator attends to the same display for long periods his performance is increasingly subject to 'internal blinks' – momentary losses of attention
Arousal theory	Arousal deteriorates during prolonged attention to a single display because the brain becomes less responsive or because the operator loses motivation
Habituation theory	A variation of arousal theory with emphasis on the natural adaptation to a repetitive situation
Motivation theory	A variation of arousal theory which suggests that the operator loses his willingness to respond rather than his ability to do so

inferior at prolonged performance in monotonous information input situations, but on the other hand when alert he can be much superior at detecting weak signals in noisy backgrounds. This is particularly so when the significant signal can be quite variable and cannot be specified precisely. Thus there is often no alternative to the human operator in military watch-keeping situations, in industrial inspection tasks, and in monitoring what happens in large control systems.

However, once it is recognised that there is a problem of performance decrement in time of less than an hour, then all the established ameliorative techniques of design for interfaces, work-spaces, environments and working time can be applied. Training also can have some effects. There are quite large individual differences which are not understood, and the potentiality for selection is limited to using the specific working situation as the selection vehicle.

4.1.5 Circadian rhythms

Human activity varies roughly sinusoidally over the 24-hour day. This can be detected by three kinds of measures: somatic, performance and opinions (see below). By psychological standards these measures correlate quite well but there can be disorientation in special circumstances (e.g. when under the influence of drugs), and there are also some variable phase differences between the measures. Usually the physiological changes lead slightly on the psychological changes.

The endogenous clock which must control these effects is not understood. Similar effects occur in all multi-celled animals, and there are some effects even in single-celled organisms, but there may be many different kinds of clocks and a particular animal can have more than one. The clock is synchronised by zeitgebers (time givers) which are usually related to the sun, e.g. changes in light or temperature. If there are no zeitgebers, e.g. in sensory deprivation experiments, the rhythm may drift by an hour or two away from the exact 24-hour cycle (McFarland 1983).

Returning to human performance, there is for almost everyone a well-established daily pattern of sleeping, working and leisure interspersed with other regular events such as eating. Any disturbance of this periodicity will naturally be a source of stress. This happens on shift work and when flying long distances across time zones.

As with other arousal phenomena circadian rhythms can be detected by somatic changes, changes in performance and changes in feeling (Colquhoun, 1971).

4.2   Knowledge
4.2.1   *Human state*
There are close interactions between bodily and mental states and it is not possible to obtain a comprehensive picture of either without taking measures of both. This requires contributions from different academic disciplines (Singleton *et al.*, 1971).

The main disciplines are psychology and physiology, although anatomy is quite important. Pharmacology is increasingly relevant as the use of drugs becomes more common for remedial, pleasure and stimulation purposes. There is not, as yet, a problem of any great consequence in European industry in that drugs are not systematically used as aids to work, and there is little evidence of the effects on work of their leisure use. The exceptions are alcohol and tobacco which do have effects on absenteeism and illness, although again the evidence is sparse because it is difficult to obtain; alcohol and tobacco are often contributing causes rather than single causes. Anatomy is important in principle in that there are observable changes in posture, muscle tension and sometimes tremor with changing work demands, but these are not easy to record numerically.

Table 4.3. *Measures of strain*

			Frequency band (per s)
Physiological	Physical	Temperature Respiration Blood pressure	
	Electrical	Heart rate (E.C.G.) Muscle activity (E.M.G.) Brain activity (E.E.G.) Skin resistance (G.S.R.)	1 100 10 0.1
	Chemical	Blood content Saliva content Urine content	
Psychological	Indirect	Blink rate Flicker fusion Pressure exerted	0.3 50
	Performance	Rate of responses Responsiveness Error frequency	2 2
	Opinions	Tests Questionnaires Debriefing	

These are immediate measures, there are also long-term measures obtainable from the epidemiology of stress-related diseases

Physiological changes can be detected by various physical, chemical and electrical means (Table 4.3). If the environmental temperature is high or there is heavy physical work the body temperature rises and there is a change in respiration rate and volume. There can be local peripheral changes in temperature and more uniform but much smaller changes in core temperature. Respiration changes for many other kinds of stress and so also does blood pressure. Blood pressure is now quite easy to measure, but there are surprisingly few studies where this has been done, so that the interpretation of particular changes is not clear. Heart rate changes in two main ways: there can be a change of rate and a change in rhythm (sinus arrythmia) – recording is by electrocardiography. There can be changes in muscle activity which indicate tremor in the limbs or increased tension particularly in the neck muscles – these are recorded by electromyography. Changes in electrical activity in the brain are complex; variations in amplitude, frequency spectrum and occurrence of spindles, but for an experienced interpreter these are the most consistent indications of arousal level from alertness to various depths of sleep, recording is by electroencephalography. The galvanic skin response is different from other electrical activities in being a change of resistance rather than the generation of an electrical potential. It is recorded from the skin and is probably due to a change in rate of sweating. It is regarded as a measure of autonomic nervous system activity. It will be noted from Table 4.3 that these electrical effects are at quite different average frequencies from the slowly changing skin resistance to the very high frequency electrical activity in muscles. In stress situations there are activities of the endocrine system in parallel with those of the autonomic and central nervous systems. The endocrine system consists of a set of glands distributed through the body, it works by the release of hormones into the blood stream. Some by-products eventually appear in the urine. Endocrine activity can thus be detected by chemical analyses of blood or urine and possibly also by saliva analysis, although this is rarely used. For further details see Levi (1975).

Psychological measures also can be divided into three kinds: indirect, performance and opinions. Blink rate has been used as a measure of arousal in that a person tends to blink less frequently when there is intensity of focus on a specific issue, not necessarily purely visual. On the other hand frequency of blinking increases with awareness and anticipation of stress (Gregory, 1966). The technique has not been developed partly because recording is not easy and partly because the results are equivocal. The measurement of flicker fusion frequency, originally studied as a general indicator of fatigue (Rey, 1971), has been revived in relation to the use of VDU screens where awareness of flicker is one of the detrimental effects (Meyer *et al.*, 1984). Again this is not merely an indicator of visual fatigue because the retina is functionally very close to the brain. In line with observed muscle tension, attempts have been made, not very successfully, to measure strain by asking the subject to continuously grip a device while carrying out some other task in the hope that the strength of grip either involuntarily or voluntarily would correlate with effort of other kinds. Performance and opinion measures are the same as those described elsewhere in this book. One general point about test measures is that interrupting some other performance and asking the subject to complete a task such as reaction-time or visual checking never seems to work, a subject can always increase his effort for a short interval and the interval itself provides a spurious rest period. Performance measures intrinsic to a task are much more likely to be valid than artificially imposed additional tasks.

Starting from stress as distinct from strain the main stressors found in current industry are listed in Table 4.4. They are subdivided into physical, psychological and organisational. As in other applications of behavioural science it transpires that, although the underlying phenomena are not completely understood scientifically, a considerable practical contribution can be made from a general awareness of the problems that are likely to occur and what can be done about them. It will be noted that some general organisational stressors are listed. These can be dominant and are not always easily detectable even from discussion with workers in the particular situation. It is quite common to find that the series of complaints which initiate an investigation are ostensibly about some physical variable such as noise, but it emerges from the detailed investigation that the underlying cause of discontent is traceable to organisational features such as high work-load, poor supervision or remote management. If remedial measures are taken at the organisational level it is remarkable how the complaints about the physical stressors disappear. This is not to suggest that no action is required in relation to physical stressors, their effects may be in long-term damage which workers of high morale will not be unduly concerned about. Fortunately these long-term effects are relatively well understood and are predictable on the basis of physical measurements rather than opinions.

Most of what is known refers to single stressors and unfortunately in practice they occur in combinations specific only to particular work situations. The remedy is to reduce each one as much as is feasible in technical and economic terms. It may be true that in the laboratory heat is de-arousing and noise is arousing, but this does not seem sufficient justification to try to use such stressors to counteract each other in practice.

4.2.2   *Mental load*

The analogy of mental load with physical load has no scientific justification although introspectively most people would agree that working hard has common features and consequences whether the work is manual or intellectual or a combination. This may be a general reflection of the cultural mores that work is paid employment viewed with some ambivalence whatever the nature of the job because of the element of compulsion. The difficulties of measuring the effects of work load are compounded by the interaction with non-work activities.

Mental load is normally considered to be a stressor and the effects may be detectable in any of the strain measures listed in Table 4.3. In a conference devoted to a most comprehensive review of mental work-load Moray (1979) separated contributors under five topics: experimental psychology, control engineering, mathematical models, physiological psychology and applied psy-

Table 4.4. *Industrial stressors and their remedies*

Stressor	Indicators	Effects	Remedies
Physical work	Oxygen consumption Heart Rate	Fatigue	Engineered support
Poor posture	Observable	Neck/back strains	Work-space design
Protective clothing	Manifest	Discomfort Decreased mobility Decreased sensory inputs	Clothing design
Atmospheric	No outside air Long air ducts Ionic counts Infra sound	Mild indisposition Low arousal	Environment design
Radiation	Measurable	Long-term	Screen source Protective clothing
Vibration	Measurable	Fatigue	Design
Noise	Measurable	Diverts attention Interferes with communication	Design
Heat/Cold	Measurable	Diverts attention	Environmental design

Psychological				
Circadian rhythm disturbances	Shift patterns	Fatigue	Discussion
Information underload	Low inputs/outputs	Low arousal	Work design
Information overload	High inputs/outputs	Over arousal Distraction	C.R. Design Training
Personal threat	Serious incidents	Over arousal Panic	Training

Organisational			
Inappropriate staffing	Observable inefficiency	Errors and omissions	Management
Management style	Absenteeism Accident rate	Low morale	Discussion

chology. There was general agreement that it is almost impossible to separate mental work-load from physical work-load or to separate cognitive and emotional aspects of mental load. It was also agreed that work-load is essentially a multi-disciplinary problem. Many authors attempted to list kinds of load and kinds of human activity in response to load, but although these are academically ingenious and interesting the resultant impression is that the interactions are as important as the categories which themselves overlap. In short, research on work-load demonstrates once again that human reactions are holistic and defeat reductionist attempts to separate independent aspects.

Another way of stating the basic problem is that the skilled human operator can, and does, function at many levels, and he can always economise by shedding detail and moving to a different level, perhaps utilising a qualitatively different model. How far he gets away with this in terms of maintaining his performance effectiveness is a function of his experience, the kind of work he is doing, the tolerance or back-up from hardware, software and other workers and sometimes just of chance.

All this is very serious for the practitioner in this field because, for his customers, many of these problems seem simple but essential for effective system design. Questions such as:

- how many operators are needed for this work?
- are these operators overloaded or underloaded?
- are there undesirable safety and reliability aspects due to the particular operator load either for the operator or for the system?
- what are reasonable working hours and rest-pauses?

The questions get more difficult as technology changes work, for several reasons:

- answers are most easily provided for predominantly physical work and physical stressors. The energy available and needed for such work can be calculated with precision, so also can be length of exposure to a given climatic stress (Singleton 1982). However technology has greatly reduced this kind of work and predominantly mental work is now the norm. For this latter there are very few descriptors at the numerical level.
- recommendations often have to be based on precedent, but when the changes are radical the validity of precedent diminishes. Previous experience is also a dubious guide, as explained by the Parkinson aphorism, "work expands to fill the time available".
- higher technology means more expensive systems with greater energy

levels and greater outputs per man – getting the manning level or work-load allocation wrong is correspondingly more serious.

– increased community wealth and standard of living from high technology means greater costs per worker hour. There is also a requirement to keep expensive systems in action, and the cost of keeping one extra worker permanently available is now very large, i.e. four or five workers on a rotating system. Thus there is less freedom to err on the side of lavish worker resource.

However there are a number of redeeming features:

– the fact that these questions and aspects can be formally posed and understood by the decision-makers is a considerable step towards the solution.

– greater expertise in the form of education and training is such that operators can make their own contribution to assessment of workload from direct experience. The days of managerially allocating 'pairs of hands' are long past.

– there is usually a minimum of two for high demand tasks because one can fail for many reasons, the crew of two is often also the optimum because of the plethora of machine support.

– reductionist methods such as Role, Job and Task Analysis can make a contribution in formalising the extrapolation from previous tasks, e.g. the aspects which remain the same and those that have changed can be identified accurately.

– expertise in the advantages and limitations of specific stress and strain measurement techniques has accumulated, and although there is no universal technique the use of particular procedures can make a contribution to overall decisions.

– the problem can sometimes be evaded by reformulation in other terms. For example, starting from allocation of function methodology and synthesising appropriate tasks in an iterative fashion using liberal injections of previous technical and operational experience.

In summary, there is no overall method of either assessing work-load or predicting required human resource. These remain as management decisions, but with important contributions on different facets from various specialists in the human sciences. Accepting that such decisions are not definitive, it is sometimes appropriate to set up continuous monitoring systems from direct ones such as records of errors and failures (Rasmussen and Rouse, 1980), to indirect ones such as epidemiological monitoring of the incidence of occupational diseases (Kurppa, 1984).

4.3 Principles, methods and procedures

4.3.1 Experiments and trials

An experiment is literally a trial, but scientifically the term is usually restricted to a specially designed situation from which measures are taken. In a trial the situation has already been designed for some other reason, but again measures are taken. Experiments usually take place in a laboratory and trials in the field but there can be field experiments and laboratory trials. An experiment has one or more independent variables which are deliberately manipulated by the experimenter, these are distinguished from the dependent variables which are measured. In a trial, if there are independent variables they occur naturally and are not under the control of the experimenter.

Both experiments and trials are fundamentally important in ergonomics or human factors because they are ultimately the basis for the claim that these subjects have a scientific background. There are three kinds of experiments:

- the pursuit of understanding expressed in the form of theory. This is how academic experimental psychologists and physiologists spend their time. The results are tested using sampling statistics to check the probability that the obtained results could have occurred by chance. It is important to note that the size of the difference is only one of several variables which strengthen the opinion that the result is significant in this sense (others are the number of subjects and the variability between and within subjects). Thus a significant result is not necessarily one of any operational consequence.

- the *ad hoc* experiment in which experimental design procedures are used to try to answer a specific question, e.g. whether one design is 'better' than another. These are called evaluation experiments, or, in the *post hoc* case, validation experiments. Here again sampling statistics may be used but the size of the difference obtained and the proportion of subjects for which the finding is valid are more important criteria. Operational significance can be quite different from statistical significance.

- the simulation in which a man–machine system is created and driven artificially (normally by software) rather than by interaction with a real environment. Here there is greater confidence in extrapolating from the experimental data to reality because the system matches reality at least in some respects. This is quite different from other kinds of experiments which depend on the designer's insight in extracting the essence of a situation or task to be used in his experiment.

The point about experiments is that the best model of man is man, the best predictor of human performance is other human performance. Experimentalists would be on safer ground if there were no individual differences. This would eliminate the need to be careful in identifying the validity of a particular subject group, and indeed it would not be necessary to use more than one subject. This is reasonably tenable for some experiments, e.g. a check of a hypothesis about colour vision might only need one subject who has normal colour vision. However, physiologists and engineers are prone to the use of small numbers of subjects and findings can become accepted in the literature without the cautionary qualification that the original data came from one or two subjects – often the experimenter himself and one of his colleagues. Psychologists usually use larger subject groups, but unfortunately there is not a complete set of rules on how to select subjects and how many to use. The criterion of getting a significant result is a misleading one. Too many experiments use fit young males, partly because of the predominantly military origin of the discipline, and partly because this is the population which university-based experimenters can most easily get at. It is thus not known whether the result would be the same for females, for older or younger people, for less intelligent people or for more experienced people. A good experimental report should contain profiles of the subjects or groups of subjects, their ages, sex, relevant experience, and preferably also some test data about intelligence and personality. This is rarely done. More recently questions have arisen about differences between races and cultures. International travel and trade in equipment and systems has increased enormously and care is now needed to ensure that principles and designs are appropriate for much larger populations (Chapanis, 1975).

In general, the report of an experiment should contain all the information necessary for any other scientist who wishes to replicate the experiment. Most important experiments have been repeated with slight variations in other laboratories and it is the consistency of results across these situations which increases confidence in the validity of the findings. Science and the scientific community is dependent on this kind of collective activity, although in psychology it is often carried too far and, for a period of a decade or two when a topic is fashionable, similar experiments are repeated *ad nauseam*, and the literature is filled with operationally and theoretically trivial data and findings.

In addition to differences between subjects there are differences within subjects. Each person learns, suffers from fatigue, is subject to mood and motivation changes. There are differential transfer effects between tasks, for example the commonly used experimental design where half the subjects do task *A* followed by task *B*, and the other half does task *B* followed by task *A*, assumes, when scores *A* and *B* are compared, that the transfer effect from *A* to *B* is the same as that from *B* to *A*. Although in most cases when *A* and *B* are similar (and if they are not there would not be much point in mounting an elaborate comparison) this is probably a reasonable assumption, but, for example, the more *A* and *B* differ in difficulty the more likely it is that transfer effects will be asymmetrical.

With multivariate experimental designs the situation is even more confusing and although these can yield an estimate of interactions using analysis of variance, this is different from transfer effects.

Transfer in the different sense of extrapolation from an experimental situation to a real situation is also fraught with difficulties. From academic experiments there is usually intervening modelling in the form of a principle or theory. The experimental data are used to check an hypothesis and it is the validated hypothesis which provides knowledge applicable to real situations. Unfortunately, almost all behavioural sciences principles and theories have limits in terms of the kinds of people or the kinds of task to which they apply, and it may need many experiments or much experience to clarify what these limits are. In the case of evaluation experiments it is unlikely that the numerical data will transfer directly, but the trends revealed by the data are better than nothing. Such data and trends can be used as contributing evidence within overall multi-disciplinary design decisions which are ultimately a management rather than a scientific responsibility.

Numbers obtained from behavioural science experiments are themselves not always quite so definitive as they are in physical science experiments. The physical sciences invariably have metrics based on *ratio scales*: there is a zero and the scale is equal interval, all statistical test methods are admissible. There are many standard textbooks describing such statistical procedures, e.g. McNemar, (1955). A ratio scale is unusual with behavioural data. At best, it will fit an *interval scale* which is linear, but the zero point is not known, e.g. the difference between 2 and 4 is the same as the difference between 4 and 6, but it cannot be assumed that 4 indicates a value twice as large as 2, parametric tests can still be used. Much behavioural data can only safely be considered as indicating order or *ranking*, and in this case only non-parametric statistical tests can be used, but these are still quite 'powerful' (that is, they are reasonably sensitive in detecting differences between sets of data) (Siegel, 1956). The weakest kind of data is classified as within a *nominal scale*, this is where numbers have been used simply as labels and no arithmetic is admissible (Table 4.5).

Because of the inherent variability within and between subjects a set of numbers can be presented as a frequency distribution. Much data often

Table 4.5. *Scales and statistical tests*

Scale	Characteristics	Appropriate Statistics	Examples of Tests
Ratio	Equal intervals Equal ratios	All, particularly parametric which have highest power	't' test Analysis of variance
Interval	Equal intervals only		
Ordinal	Numbers indicating order only	Non-parametric only	Khi squared Mann–Whitney
Nominal	Numbers as labels	None	None

appears to be 'normally' distributed in the characteristic bell shape of a Gaussian curve, this will happen if there are many factors randomly affecting a measure. This distribution is well behaved in that measures of central tendency – the mean, the mode and the median – are all the same, and the variance – the measure of scatter – has useful additive properties, e.g. analysis of variance is legitimate. The distribution may be skewed, e.g. for time measures there is a limit at the lower end but not at the upper end, or may even be multimodal. In these cases even the arithmetic mean or average may not be a useful measure.

There are computer programs which will generate every conceivable statistical analysis method, but it is dangerously simple to pour the data into such a package and accept the result which emerges. There is no substitute for 'eye-balling' data in a variety of simple forms such as graphs and distributions. Statistical testing is a confirmatory measure, if the difference is not detectable in some form of graph it should not emerge from a test. Correspondingly the art of experimentation is in creating a situation which fits the question, and in utilising subjects so that reliability and validity are defensible.

In trials as distinct from experiments even more problems of motivation arise. In experiments, particularly with naive subjects it is usually reasonable to assume a uniform and moderate level of positive cooperation even though, in contrast to real situations, making mistakes is of no great consequence, and there is no great incentive to try hard in terms of speed or quality. In the case of trials it is usually necessary to use experienced subjects and their motivation is much more complicated. It can easily swing from extreme negative ('I like only what I'm used to'), to extreme positive ('He's trying to help me so I'll try to help him'). The attitude of managers and other leaders can dominate the degree of cooperation, so also can any suspicions about the future of the job with these new systems. There are no general remedies for problems, each situation has to be dealt with on its merits. Some problems of selecting and using human subjects are discussed in detail in Chapanis (1959).

4.3.2 Job design

A job is an activity which takes up the working time of one person. A task may be sufficiently large to make up several jobs, and a job may consist of a variety of tasks.

Jobs must necessarily recognise that human operators come in indivisible units (persons), and these individuals have economic and social expectations in terms of reasons for undertaking particular jobs – pay, location, interests, expertise and interaction with others. Thus, although tasks can be derived from system design principles, job design is based on less definitive criteria, such as the existence of a current labour force, the potentiality for recruitment in accessible labour markets, the need for continuity of employment, the organisational requirements for stability but also change in terms of training, promotion prospects, adaptation to special needs such as safety, domestic and disability limitations and adaptation also to unpredicted, often unpredictable swings in market demands for products.

Balancing the four sets of constraints – from technical system design, organisation system design, the labour market and the market for the output (Fig. 4.1) – is a management responsibility, but there can be a useful contribution from the Human Factors specialist in his role as an expert on people in systems.

In the past twenty years there have been two main features of the industrial scene provoking innovative attention to job design. The basic influence is technological development with a consequential shifting of workers from energy dominated jobs to information dominated jobs. The second influence, following from the first, is the rising standard of living which changes worker expectations of what is tolerable and desirable, and because the cost of labour has risen both absolutely and relatively in relation to other operational costs, management has to consider the use of working time and individual worker output much more seriously. This in turn promotes and supports the interests of research workers in this subject (Fig. 4.2).

The discipline which took over the title job design and changed it from a broad industrial problem to the application of specific methods and values was socio-technical systems. Although it was accepted that the history of job design lay in the classical socio-economic approach and in work study of the 'scientific management' tradition, the new approach was very much worker

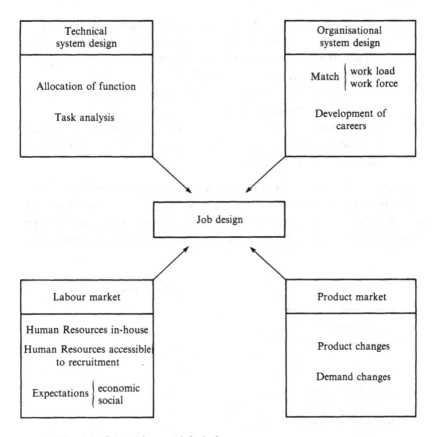

Fig. 4.1. Constraints on job design.

satisfaction and worker welfare centred rather than economics centred (Davis and Taylor, 1972; Warr and Wall 1975). The aims and concepts around which studies were constructed were quality of working life (Davis and Cherns, 1975), personal goals (Warr, 1976), worker participation (Wall and Lischeron, 1977) and job satisfaction (Sell and Shipley, 1979).

There was some economic justification in that around 1970 most advanced countries were experiencing labour problems, particularly in mass production industries. There were two main symptoms – increasing tendencies to strike and generate other difficulties in worker/management relationships, and the reluctance of the indigenous population to accept such jobs, with a consequent need to import foreign labour. There was also an element of paternalism in the imposition of an ideology – the remedy was available and was to be imposed on shop-floor workers. The method consisted of changing jobs along the following lines:

- work restructuring, with emphasis on reducing machine-pacing and process driven demands by cushioning the effects of production lines, introducing job enlargement and job rotation, and organising tasks around groups rather than individuals
- job enrichment by extending individual responsibilities, providing feedback on performance and opportunities for learning
- greater well-being by providing increased opportunities for intercommunication and social interaction, for promotion and generally for making work more 'meaningful'

In advanced countries there was considerable cooperation from industry and from governments willing to finance research and development. After more than ten years' practical experience there is some disappointment that the movement has not proved to be a universal panacea for job design problems

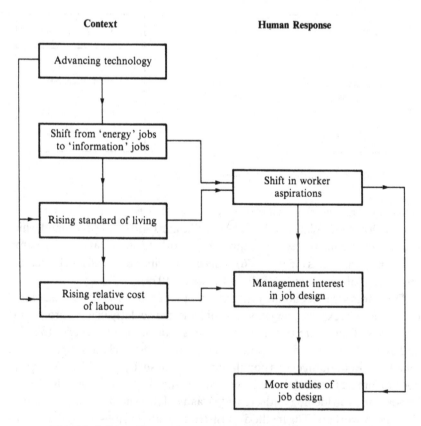

Fig. 4.2. Origin of increasing interest in job design.

(Duncan *et al.*, 1980). The following are among the negative aspects which have been noted:

- there can be suspicion from workers and trade unions that these procedures are a substitute for increasing pay
- the changes in job design can make the jobs of supervisors and managers more difficult
- industrial workers, particularly those who are part-time and casual, do not necessarily share the values and interests of research workers
- the effects as an incentive are ambiguous. Good in the sense of reducing work interruption, but not necessarily so good in promoting effort at work

Nevertheless the general principle of 'humanising' work is increasingly accepted, it is built into the labour law in some countries, e.g. Germany, and is practised in the newest technologies in others, e.g. Hellesoy, 1985. It started as an idealistic movement and ideals are never fully realised in the harsh industrial world, but it has taken a place as one of the vast range of part approaches to the complex business of making work effective.

4.4 Applications
4.4.1 Design for operation
There are some aspects of design for jobs and tasks which are general and others which are specific. An operator orientated approach can be divided into these two parts.

The general approach:
- is the working environment adequate in terms of lighting, heating and noise levels? If the worker goes to work outside a built environment are there problems of clothing design, posture and mobility?
- is the work space adequate in terms of working surfaces, working storage space, personal storage space and chair design?
- are the temporal working conditions satisfactory? e.g. hours, breaks and support facilities
- is there adequate knowledge of performance over the short-term (hours) and the long-term (years)?
- what happens along the time dimension – are there periods of underload, overload or the intermittent need for rapid response?
- is there clear guidance and support from written materials, from technical specialists and from more senior levels in the organisational hierarchy?

- is the allocation of function about right or could it be shifted at any of these levels: input (instrumentation), central processing (computing), and output (energy sources and tools)?
- are there facilities to ensure that skills are adequate and kept up to date (training and intrinsic learning)?
- is there potential for job enlargement and job enrichment?
- are the social interactions appropriate? These again are at three levels: work interaction (is the job within a series or in parallel with others), social interaction (the working community), and support (management, specialist services and subordinates).

The specific approach:
- someone has decided that expert resources should be applied to the study of this job. Who and why?
- has the problem been identified as one of productivity, quality, reliability, safety or some combination?
- is there available documentation about job and task descriptions? what do current or potential operators think about the job? (structured interviews)
- what are the views of immediate supervisors and more senior management?
- if there are direct customers, what are their views?
- what are the views of personnel specialists about matters such as availability of labour, absenteeism, and labour turnover?
- what are the views of the technical specialists who have specified the job?
- are there other services which might have relevant information such as medical and training?
- is there any morbidity data about accidents and illnesses, short-term and long-term?

The specialist studying the job will need to find a way of structuring all the evidence he has acquired. He can then make recommendations supported by documentation. This can often take the form of three reflexive task descriptions: the operation itself, the design of the operation and the task of the specialist(s) evaluating the operation.

4.4.2   Design for maintenance

As technology advances and the allocation of production functions swings away from the human operator (automation, computer control, robotics) the problems of the human maintenance operator increase in complexity and importance. Machines get more complicated and more expensive and the need to keep them operational becomes crucial. In a high technology plant human errors that might or did cause problems of system reliability are now more frequently traceable to maintenance rather than control/monitoring tasks.

There are usually two main tasks within a maintenance job: servicing/ preventative maintenance, and fault finding/repair. These are opposites in terms of task demands and appropriate man–machine function allocation. The preventative task requires adherence to routine and an entirely systematic procedure. The fault repair task requires pattern perception, e.g. in collating symptoms and wave-forms, inductive thinking to identify the fault and availability at unpredictable times. However, the two tasks have in common the need for versatility, mobility, dexterity, self-checking abilities, and the need to apply intelligence in unforeseen circumstances.

There have been attempts to automate some maintenance functions by the military but these have not proved to be satisfactory, e.g. automatic check-out equipment. Use of modularised equipment and replacement of unserviceable modules has been more successful.

Current problems are:

- the cost of continuous availability of maintenance staff
- the inherent contradiction between the requirement for flexibility and versatility and the need for consistency to promote safety and reliability
- the time pressure to get systems back on line versus the need to avoid short cuts which might generate more failures in the longer term
- the development with experience of probabilistic modes of fault finding and repair which are contradictory to the formal procedures
- difficulties of providing comprehensive supervision
- distribution of working hours and provision of 'on call' facilities
- skill problems in that comprehensive training cuts across the traditional subject separation into mechanical, hydraulic, electrical and electronic. There is also a need for continuous up-dating because of the speed of change in equipment design
- the requirement for very large libraries of routines and procedures

The systematic approach to design for maintenance is the same as that for operations with changes of emphasis in the context of the above special features.

4.4.3　*Inspection tasks*

Inspection is part of quality control. In industry the current tendency is to move away from the make–inspect separation of tasks and to try to get the makers to do as much as possible of their own quality control. Nevertheless there remain many manufacturing systems where inspection is the last task in the production process. It can be divided into two kinds: passive inspection where the inspector relies entirely on visual search, e.g. bottles moving along a conveyor belt, and active inspection in which the inspector manipulates the inspected article and may use various instruments to check the performance, e.g. television sets.

Passive inspection

This is not basically suited to the human operator in that there is an imbalance of personal activity, an accentuation of the input side mainly visual performance, and nothing much happening on the output side. The task comes within the category of vigilance described earlier, although in the industrial situation there is a very great variety of objects to be examined. The quality standard for acceptance/rejection is often vague and may be influenced by social factors such as the relationship between the inspectors and the producers. Research on the 'catch' often reveals that the performance is much worse than was assumed by the organisation (Murrell, 1965). The task design procedure is standard ergonomics:

- selection criteria, e.g. screening in terms of basic visual performance
- training with emphasis on visual cues and fault specifications
- work space design in terms of postural and thermal comfort
  display design with emphasis on lighting and contrast. Experiments are sometimes useful to check the relative effectiveness of brightness, colour, changes in transmitted light versus reflected light, figure/ground accentuation and so on
- particular attention to the study of vigilance decrement aspects and remedial measures in terms of work/rest periods, rotating tasks and general avoidance of detrimental monotony
- investigation of social interaction between producers and inspectors, e.g. is the producer at fault penalised? are the inspectors developing expected rejection rates and adjusting criteria to keep rates constant in time or consistent across producers?
- organisational aspects such as method of payment and status within the company

Drury and Fox (1975) contains extensive discussions of performance theory relevant to inspection and description of applications in steel, food, rubber, glass and electronic industries.

Active inspection

Here the inspector manually manipulates either the article to be inspected, e.g. shoes and musical instruments, or various tools and measuring devices used within the inspection process, e.g. electronic circuit boards and machine components. It may require considerable mobility and dexterity for large items, e.g. cars and other complete machines. Checklists are often used. There are less stringent problems of vigilance decrement because of the variety not only in activity but also in the sensory inputs utilised. There is often extensive reliance on auditory and tactile cues which increases with experience at the task. Design of the work-space is particularly important because a large range of support devices (lights, tools, instruments) may be used intermittently within each inspection. Ease of access and manipulation can often be improved.

4.4.4 Shift systems

Shift-work has always been necessary in some industries e.g. transport and health care. The incidence of unsocial working hours is probably increasing because of the expansion of leisure industries and capital intensive industries where equipment costs must be rapidly amortised.

There is now a great variety of shift systems intermediate between the normal five day 35–40 hour week and continuous operation over seven days and 168 hours. Maintenance staff may alternate with production staff by working either at night or at weekends. Production staff may work a double day shift system.

The problems which arise vary from the physiological/psychological aspects of circadian rhythms to social/cultural aspects of regional traditions and availability of transport and leisure activities.

The evidence about quality of work and accidents within shift systems is equivocal because it is rare that shifts are directly comparable: there may be differences in hours at work, in the kind of work done or in the kind of workers, e.g. for process controllers the predominant task on a day shift may be authorisation of specific maintenance tasks, but if the maintenance staff are on day shift only, the controller has a quite different job on the night shift. The reverse can also occur, e.g. in metal working industries where days are devoted to production and nights to maintenance.

In manufacturing and processing the problems are much reduced by increasing automation. It is now quite usual to find many large plants working steadily through the night with no human intervention except to cope with unforeseen circumstances. All the setting up and maintenance is done during the day. In service industries such as health and transport there remains the need for man-power intensive continuous operation. The most acute case is aviation, where the problems of alternating shifts are compounded by movement across time zones. The total working hours are much less than those in manufacturing.

There are quite large individual differences in tolerance of shifting rhythms of work and corresponding bodily changes including sex differences. There are also social and domestic reasons which result in many individuals preferring to work unusual hours. Although physiological circadian rhythm phenomena are clear and universal it does seem in practice that psychological, social and economic factors can override the physiological factors, at least for a proportion of the working population. A review of recent methodological and applied research on abnormal hours of work is contained in Folkard (1987).

4.4.5   Use of VDUs
Visual Display Units also known as Visual Display Terminals (VDTs) are now used by tens of thousands of workers throughout the world. There is no precedent for such a rapid and large scale change in work-spaces in such a short time – about ten years. Inevitably there have been problems. Most of them could have been avoided or at least reduced by the application of simple well-established ergonomic principles, viz.:

- consider carefully how the new aid will change the particular job
- design the layout of the work-space incorporating the keyboard and screen as a part of the total work-space, almost all VDU users have other tasks which do not include the VDU
- pay particular attention to posture in relation to keyboard operation and screen visibility
- lighting design, both natural and artificial is obviously of particular importance
- consider chair design, particularly chairs with linear and rotating movement in relation to an extended work-surface
- devise a systematic induction process which includes familiarisation, properly supportive manuals and adequate training

All this would seem to be entirely straightforward, but experience indicates that in practice these matters are very rarely dealt with properly with consequences in terms of sickness and alienation which could so easily have been avoided. For futher details see Grandjean (1986), Corlett *et al.* (1986).

Operators can be divided into categories, the casual user and the continuous user. They have quite different problems and need to be considered separately.

The casual user

This group of workers includes managers, engineers, scientists, architects and teachers. They vary in relevant skills enormously from the dedicated 'hacker' to the senior manager who has a terminal on his desk because it is fashionable. One of the basic skills they lack is in keyboard operation. There is considerable scope for training in keyboard utilisation so that it does not require attention and continuous visual guidance. The standard typing two-handed operation is not necessarily appropriate, there is a case for making it a one-handed operation so that the other hand is free to use telephones, pens and other keyboards. These operators do not normally take kindly to having to use manuals, menu systems provide a better match for their needs and inclinations.

The continuous user

This group includes typists/secretaries using word processors, data entry clerks, software writers and data handlers. They are faced by a machine interface which is fundamentally unfriendly in that the display is fixed in position, restricted in size and not easily read. The control also requires a more or less fixed body position except for hand movements and finger manipulations. Thus there are two problems which require the most detailed design attention if the interface is to be satisfactory: display characteristics including lighting, and postural aspects. The many factors to be considered are detailed in Table 4.6. The longer the working time at the interface the more marked are the effects. A normal desk/clerical job involves considerable movement both of materials on the working surface and in going elsewhere in relation to sub-tasks such as obtaining materials and filing. Desk-based computer operation is much more restrictive and consequently generates many more problems particularly in relation to the eyes and the musculature. Culture is included among the operator variables because there do seem to be national and regional differences in the frequencies and ranking of various symptoms. In some countries muscular skeletal problems dominate, e.g. repetitive strain injuries in Australia. In others various symptoms of visual strain appear to be more common, e.g. European countries. In some countries there have been temporary scares about radiation effects. Although the strain symptoms in response to the common stress may vary geographically, the symptoms of the individuals are real enough and often require medical treatment. The Trade Unions in most countries have expressed great concern and in 1984 there was an international Trade Union conference specifically on VDUs (Nedzynski, 1984). The effects on health are appraised in Bergquist (1984).

Table 4.6. *Ergonomic aspects of VDUs*

The Screen	Task Variables
Size/Resolution	
Position/Orientation	
Polarity*/Colours	Hours of work
Luminance/Contrast	
Flicker/Jitter	Work: Structure
Character – height	Organisation
width	Load
space	
line space	Training/Retraining
Type face	
Electrostatics/Radiation	
bright on dark or reverse	

The Keyboard	Operator Variables
Thickness	
Profile (slope)	Vision
Colour/Contrast/Labelling	Age
Key: size	Sex
spacing	Motivation
profile	Mood
travel	Stress reaction
operating force	Culture

The Workspace	Possible health hazards
Lighting	Muscular-skeletal effects
Noise/Heat/Radiation	Eye strain
Viewing distance	Headaches
Desk: height	Epilepsy
size	Skin rashes
shape	Effects on pregnancy
Layout: disc use and	
storage, printer	
position, paper	
storage	

In general, it seems that in the early 1980s there were indications that strange and unique problems were appearing amongst users of VDUs. With further accumulation of evidence it emerges that there are unlikely to be any unusual effects such as those suspected from radiation and electrostatic charges. Rather the problems are the classical ergonomics ones of eyestrain and muscular–skeletal disorders consequent upon inadequate application of established work design principles. The effects are mostly due to prolonged fixed posture and a small invariant visual field.

References

Bartlett. F.C. (1943). Fatigue following highly skilled work. *Proceedings of the Royal Society B*. **131**. 247–57.

Bartley, S.H. and Chute, E. (1947). *Fatigue and Impairment in Man*. New York: McGraw-Hill.

Bergquist, U.O.V. (ed.) (1984). Video display terminals and health. *Scandinavian Journal of Work, Environment and Health*. **10**. Supplement 2.

Bourne, P.G. (ed.) (1969). *The Psychology and Physiology of Stress*. New York: Academic Press.

Broadbent, D.E. (1971). *Decision and Stress*. London: Academic Press.

Chapanis, A. (1959). *Research Techniques in Human Engineering*. Baltimore: Johns Hopkins Press.

Chapanis, A. (ed.) (1975). *Ethnic Variables in Human Factors Engineering*. Baltimore: Johns Hopkins Press.

Colquhoun, W.P. (ed.) (1971). *Biological Rhythms and Human Performance*. New York: Academic Press.

Cooper, C.L. and Payne, R.L. (1980). *Current Concerns in Occupational Stress*. Chichester: Wiley.

Corlett, N., Wilson, J. and Manenica, I. (eds.) (1986). *The Ergonomics of Working Postures*. London: Taylor & Francis.

Davies, D.R. and Parasuraman, R. (1982). *The Psychology of Vigilance*. London: Academic Press.

Davis, D.R. (1948). *Pilot Error*. Air Ministry Publication 3139 A. London: H.M.S.O.

Davis, L.E. and Cherns, A.B. (eds.) (1975). *The Quality of Working Life* (2 vols.) New York: The Free Press.

Davis, L.E. and Taylor, J.C. (eds.) (1972). *Design of Jobs*. Harmondsworth: Penguin.

Drury, C.G. and Fox, J.G. (eds.) (1975). *Human Reliability in Quality Control*. London: Taylor & Francis.

Duncan, K.D., Gruneberg, M.M. and Wallis, D. (eds.) (1980). *Changes in Working Life*. Chichester: Wiley.

Floyd, W.F. and Welford, A.T. (1953). *Symposium on Fatigue*. London: Lewis.

Folkard, S. (ed.) (1987). Irregular and abnormal hours of work. *Special Issue of Ergonomics*. **30.9**.

Grandjean, E. (1986). *Ergonomics in Computerised Offices*. London: Taylor & Francis.

Gregory, R.L. (1966). *Eye and Brain*. London: Weidenfeld & Nicolson.

Gunderson, E.K.E. and Rahe, R.H. (eds.) (1974). *Life Stress and Illness*. Springfield Ill: Thomas.

Hellesoy, O.H. (ed.) (1985). *Work Environment, Stratfjord Field*. Bergen: Universitets Jorlaget.

Jung, C.A. (1933). *Psychological Types*. New York: Harcourt.

Kurppa, K. (ed.) (1984). International Symposium on research on work-related diseases. *Special Issue of the Scandinavian Journal of Work, Environment and Health*. **10.6**.

Lazarus, R.S. (1967). Cognitive and personality factors underlying threat and coping. In Appley, M.H. and Trumbull, R. (eds.) *Psychological Stress*. New York: Appleton Century Crofts.

Levi, L. (ed.) (1975). *Emotions, their Parameters and Measurement*. New York: Raven Press.

Lloyd, P. and Mayes, A. (eds.) (1984). *Introduction to Psychology*. London: Fontana.

McFarland, D.J. (1983). Clock-driven behaviour. In Harre, R. and Lamb, R. (eds.). *The Encyclopaedic Dictionary of Psychology*. Oxford: Blackwell.

Mackworth, N.H. (1950). Researches on the measurement of human performance. *M.R.C. Special Report No. 268*. London: H.M.S.O.

McNemar, Q. (1955). *Psychological Statistics*. New York: Wiley.

Meyer, J.J., Barroquet, A., Rey, P. and Pittard, J. (1984). Two new visual tests to define the visual requirements of VDU operators. In Grandjean, E. (ed.) *Ergonomics and Health in Modern Offices*. London: Taylor & Francis.

Moray, N. (ed.) (1979). *Mental Workload*. New York: Plenum.

Muscio, B. (1920). *Lectures on Industrial Psychology*. London: Routledge.

Murrell, K.F.H. (1965). *Ergonomics*. London: Chapman and Hall.

Nedzynski, S. (Chairman) (1984). *International Trade Union Guidelines on Visual Display Units*. Geneva: International Confederation of Free Trade Unions.

Rasmussen, J. and Rouse, W.B. (1980). *Human Detection and Diagnosis of System Failures*. New York: Plenum.

Rey, P. (1971). The interpretation of changes in optical fusion frequency. In Singleton, W.T., Fox, J.G. and Whitfield, D. (eds.) *Measurement of Man at Work*. London: Taylor & Francis.

Sell, R.G. and Shipley, P. (eds.) (1979). *Satisfaction in Work Design*. London: Taylor & Francis.

Selye, H. (1976). *Stress in Health and Disease*. Reading, Mass.: Butterworth.

Siegel, S. (1956). *Non-parametric Statistics for the Behavioural Sciences*. New York: McGraw-Hill.

Singleton, W.T. (1953). Deterioration in performance on a short-term perceptual motor task. In Floyd, W.F. and Welford, A.T. (eds.) *Symposium on Fatigue*. London: Lewis.

Singleton, W.T. (ed.) (1979). *Study of Real Skills Vol. 2. Compliance and Excellence*. Lancaster: M.T. Press.

Singleton, W.T. (ed.) (1982). *The Body at Work*. Cambridge University Press.

Singleton, W.T., Fox, J.G. and Whitfield, D. (eds.) (1971). *Measurement of Man at Work*. London: Taylor & Francis.

Taylor, A. and Sluckin, W. (eds.) (1982). *Introducing Psychology*. Harmondsworth: Penguin.

Wall, T.D. and Lischeron, J.A. (1977). *Worker Participation*. London: McGraw-Hill.

Warr, P.B. (ed.) (1976). *Personal Goals and Work Design*. London: Wiley.

Warr. P.B. and Wall T.D. (1975). *Work and Well-being*. Harmondsworth: Penguin.

Williams, S.B. (1949). Visibility on radar scopes. In Lindsley, D.B. (ed.) *Human Factors in Undersea Warfare*. Washington: National Research Council.

5 Information processing

5.1 Concepts

5.1.1 Information acceptance

The processes on the input side of the human operator are, in serial order: sensation, perception and cognition. These are functional terms not neatly separated and not unambiguously related to physiologically identifiable mechanisms. Even the order is complicated by interaction and feedback processes.

Sensation

The sense organs are separately identifiable in that they contain specialised transducers: cells which are particularly reactive to light, pressure, chemicals or temperature. This separation is not the same as the classical five senses in that it merges the auditory system with the somaesthetic system within pressure detectors, and taste and smell within chemical detectors. The somaesthetic system provides experience of pressure discontinuities at the surface and in the movement of the body, it detects movement about joints (the kinaesthetic system), angular and linear acceleration (the vestibular system) and skin pressure (the tactile system) (Fig. 5.1). Its importance is underestimated because, by contrast with the distant senses, it functions with minimal conscious awareness. Taste is not important at work except for specialised tasks related to catering. In addition to its close relationship with taste, smell is useful in fault detection of high temperatures and leaks. Essentially the work of the human operator is guided by three main sensing devices: vision, hearing and somaesthesia. Sensation implies a generalised awareness of changes in light, sound or bodily position and posture. Thus the brain is involved as well as the specialised sense organs.

Vision incorporates several different functions: highly selective discrimination, brightness, colour and movement detection. Because the maximum acuity is restricted to a small central area, it works not so much by receiving a large static picture but rather by continuous scanning, stabbing around in the visual environment, guided partly by the movement detection facility which is more peripheral within the visual field. Each eye is supported by large muscles and an almost perfect control system so that it can be repositioned quickly and precisely. The visual functional area that can be scanned is enlarged by the close integration of eye and head movements. Thus vision is well adapted to cope with spatial arrays either in the natural world or in designed displays from consoles to large walls of instrumentation. For this purpose light can be regarded as travelling in straight lines at infinite speed and thus the data received is in the here–now with the proviso that there is no blockage intervening between the eye and the event.

Hearing is sensitive to the frequency and amplitude of oscillatory pressure changes in air, which, when they are translated into sensation, correspond roughly although not exactly to pitch and loudness respectively (Stevens, 1951). The term sound is used indiscriminately to describe the physical variables and the correlated sensations, this leads to confusion on matters of measurement. The term noise is used loosely but generally means sound which is of no interest. Auditory sensation just about includes rhythm and melody which are complex patterns predominantly tempo and pitch dependent respectively. The speed of sound is detectable although not usually important, but it is important that the ears are not directional. By contrast with light, sound coming from any direction is equally well detected, and it can travel round obstacles. The direction also is approximately detectable.

Eyes and ears are nicely complementary in that the former detect patterns in

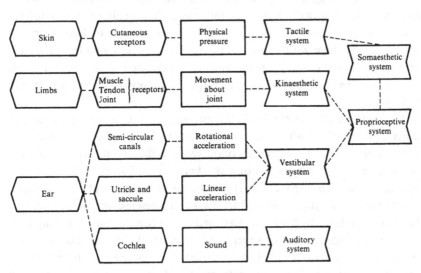

Fig. 5.1. Motion and vibration detection. (Modified from Singleton, 1972b).

space and the latter detect patterns in time. Ears work in all directions and can thus guide the unidirectional eyes towards events.

Both eyes and ears depend on the somaesthetic sense which provides knowledge that the body exists, and where it is in a general orientation sense. It also provides the stable platform on which the other sensory mechanisms are sited. This is much more complicated and more important than it may appear at first consideration. For example, an eye alone could not distinguish between movement of the environment and the movement of the eye. Any object in space, including the human body, has six degrees of freedom, three orthogonal linear directions and three rotational. The body also has relative movements within itself, the limbs and the head can move in relation to the trunk and there are movements internal to these subsystems – altogether there are almost two hundred joints. All these movements have to be generated and monitored by an elaborate control system and this control system can only function on the basis of data from sensors. The sensors for movement about a joint and for linear and angular acceleration are all within the somaesthetic system. In considering this control system and the integration of data from all sensors we are entering perception as distinct from sensation.

Vision and hearing mechanisms are described in detail in the previous volume *The Body at Work*.

Perception

Roughly speaking perception is the attachment of meaning to sensation. Meaning has two features: an indication that a unitary event has happened and the significance of that event for the individual. Thus there are general and idiosyncratic aspects. The significance also could be subdivided into knowledge of it and knowledge of what to do about it, although all these are no more than bench-marks in a continuous process intervening between inputs and outputs.

The first phase of perception is the integration of data coming in through different channels. Reality is attached to data by the recognition that there is correlation between the responses of the sensors. If doubt remains an attempt is made to resolve it by consulting another person. There is a simultaneous process of selection in that all kinds of things are happening out there, and only some of them warrant attention. Incidentally the designer of displays creates a fundamental difficulty for the human operator in concentrating so completely on the visual channel, visual perception is an artefact of the designed environment. For this reason the observer in an artificial visual environment is never entirely sure that he is dealing with reality. He cannot obtain intersensory confirmation.

Having detected an event the operator then has to decide what it means to him and to do this he must bring in memory functions. The event is related to similar events in the past using also his recollections of what he did about them with what degree of success on previous occasions. Thus the potentiality for action emerges and there is a final choice of the most appropriate response, including none as one option.

A sequence of received events, with or without overt responses, builds up into the operator's internal model or picture of the external world (Chapter 2). The key features of this model building process are worthy of reiteration:

- it is based on multisensory activity – a platform created by the somaesthetic sense from which the two distant senses, vision and hearing, can operate. In a perceptual context this is called the haptic system (Gibson, 1968)
- it is highly selective in creating events from the mass of activity going on in the environment
- it is dependent on previous learning from early childhood acquisition of how to relate intersensory data to the immediately preceding events – the environment is assumed, mostly correctly, to be continuous and regular in space and time
- there is a strong contextual element – the model in use matches the current reality although it can be switched (reformulated) if there is evidence of mismatch. The exceptions are 'day-dreaming' and intensive thinking
- meaning varies from the generalised to the specific, the latter implies a particular operator with his particular skills and current task

There is a further complication in the mix of natural and symbolic vehicles for data. The symbolic presentations, from icons to alphanumerics and graphics, have specialised meaning either separately or in combinations. The attachment of this kind of meaning again depends on extensive learning in educational, training and experiential settings. In relation to designed displays in particular Garner (1962) divides meaning into structure and signification, only the former can be measured.

Where the perceptual process ends and effector processes take over and whether there are also intermediate processes of thinking and decision-making is a matter of semantic debate. If perception is concerned with adding meaning and meaning is defined as knowing what to do next, then the remaining scope is for effectors only. There can be mental activities which are not closely related to immediate stimulation and these can be described as cognitive processes. The difficulty arises because these are all functional descriptions of parts of a holistic mental activity. Mental processes are so integrated as to make any separation into functions arbitrary and not susceptible to precise definition of boundaries.

Cognition

Cognition is the whole business of thinking and knowing, decision-making and problem-solving, hopefully rational and unencumbered by emotional overtones. The separation from perception along one dimension and conation along an entirely different dimension is not fundamentally sustainable but it is convenient and superficially tidy. It makes for more ready comparison with what goes on in computers (Newell and Simon, 1972), and also relates to other disciplines such as psycholinguistics (Vygotsky, 1962). Cognition research was triggered by the development of these newer disciplines and by the application of control and communication theories to psychology, which generated the analogies of the human operator as a servomechanism and an information processing device. Cognition begins when data becomes information, that is the evidence relates to some task which concerns the particular operator at the time. How this information is treated in terms of preliminary storage and how it is thereafter integrated, circulated, manipulated and combined with information already stored from previous experience is the stuff of cognitive psychology.

One of the early seminal books in this area (Neisser, 1967) focussed on visual and auditory processes whilst recognising that more central processes of concept formation, remembering and the like, are equally important if less understood. Although Bartlett's (1932) book on remembering is often quoted as one of the forerunners of cognitive psychology, it is not usually noted that much of this book is not about individual activity, it is about communication between people and about issues of cultural differences.

The current emphasis by psychologists on individual cognition is unfortunate for two reasons. Firstly, these processes are not directly observable and thus anything we know about them can only come from either introspection or communication between people. Secondly, high level cognitive activity in technological situations is a group activity at least as much dependent on communication between minds and between minds and technical aids as it is on activity within the mind of an individual. The *raison d'être* of information technology is the support for cognition.

Introspection is always confused by rationalisation, communication is structured by languages and pictures, and although these must relate to individual thinking quite how remains a matter for study and speculation. In a technological world what matters is not how the individual thinks, it is how the group supported by technical aids thinks. It might be argued that we must understand individual thinking before we can understand how to collectivise it and support it, but it seems more likely that we will derive understanding of how the individual must function from productive experience of how to facilitate those functions.

5.1.2 *Information transmission*

Information acceptance has been described above using psychological concepts. By contrast, useful concepts relating to information transmission have been developed mostly by mathematicians and engineers specialising in communication. These concepts have some relevance to animals as well as to machines and *cybernetics* was suggested by Wiener (1948) as the title of a new topic dealing with control and communications and providing cross-fertilisation between physical scientists and biological scientists. So far the traffic in ideas has been mostly from the former to the latter but the exploration of artificial intelligence for example, (see below), may enable the biologists to provide concepts which will help the computer specialists.

Signal detection theory

Signal detection theory is derived from stochastic analysis originally developed to describe radar performance. In the behavioural context it assumes that signals and noise as represented in the mind can be expressed as probability density functions which for convenience of calculation are assumed to be normally distributed and of equal variance (Davies and Parasuraman, 1982; Wickens 1984). With this assumption they are bound to overlap, and the extent of overlap will determine the proportion of errors. These errors are divisible into two categories: misses and false positives corresponding to the traditional distinction between omission and commission errors (Fig. 5.2). The greater the separation of the distributions (measured in the standard symbology by d') the lower the proportion of errors. The observer can, in principle, adjust his decision criterion and change the proportion of misses to false alarms. By doing so he changes another parameter (known in the standard symbology as β). β and d' can be calculated from raw data in the two-by-two outcomes table with signal present and noise only present along one axis, and presence or absence of response along the other axis. In spite of all the assumptions it has been demonstrated that this model matches human performance in the laboratory. It is intuitively appropriate in emphasising that there is a trade-off between the dilemma, in a situation of incomplete evidence, of failing to act when one should and acting when one shouldn't. For example, acquitting a prisoner who is actually guilty versus convicting a prisoner who is actually innocent.

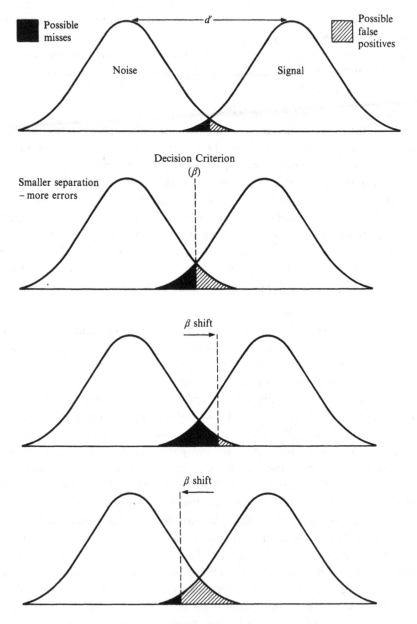

Fig. 5.2. Decision criterion in relation to signal and noise distribution of the evidence as represented in the mind.

Information theory

General communication theory has been the concern of electrical engineers since telegraphy was invented. There have been several different attempts to define information. The one that appealed to psychologists was that developed by Shannon, partly because Weaver was on hand to provide a verbal and behaviourally oriented interpretation of the set of mathematical theorems enunciated by Shannon (Shannon and Weaver, 1949).

Information is defined in terms of its contribution to reduction of uncertainty as to what has happened in the context of what might have happened. For example, if there are four unilluminated bulbs and one of them lights it presents twice as much information as the situation where one of two available bulbs is illuminated, assuming that the observer has no reason to suppose that any one light coming on is no more and no less probable than any other. These numbers indicate that a logarithmic scale is used. Logarithms to the base 2 are normally used so that if there are two equally probable alternative possible events, an actual event conveys one bit of information.

Thus, information per event $H = \log_2 (N)$, where N is the number of equally probable events. If the probability is $p = 1/N$ this can be written $H = -\log_2(p)$. If the probabilities are not equal then there is some structure or redundancy in a series of events and the general equation for the entropy of an information source is $H = -\Sigma p \cdot \log p$. This is called the Shannon–Wiener equation.

The theory can be extended to cover cases of continuous information. Noise can also be incorporated, but since the statistical structure of a signal plus noise is more complex than that of a signal alone, noise actually adds information. This unwanted information content is called the equivocation of a transmission. Correspondingly an operator will add information in the form of more noise when he responds to a signal, this is called ambiguity. Thus the ambiguity must be extracted before a signal can be identified knowing the response and the operator must filter out the equivocation to isolate the signal.

Other aspects of the theory which are not intuitively obvious are that a greater amount of information does not necessarily correspond to a larger stack of data. The amount transmitted or shared between the source and the destination depends on what has been pre-arranged or what is expected. For example, two heavy manuals of data might be arranged to be equally probable in terms of presentation. In this case only one bit of information is needed to transmit either manual, no matter how large they are or how they differ in size. The less likely an event is to happen the more information it conveys if it does happen. Information is not related to meaning. For example if the question is asked, 'Is it raining at the moment?' or 'Will you marry me?' the answer 'yes' in each case might contain one bit of information but the meanings in terms of range and extent of consequences are rather different.

In common with all rigorously defined concepts, information is invaluable in clarifying ideas and discussions. It is useful in behavioural science because the human operator does behave like an information channel or source of limited capacity. Publications on the application of information theory to psychology began to appear with increasing frequency from 1950 onwards. It was applied to a large range of phenomena which can be included in the information processing category (Table 5.1). The results in terms of changing independent variables and consistency across experimental studies indicate excellent 'goodness of fit' except for higher level cognitive processes. Since meaning is not involved, Shannon-type theory is not applicable to conative processes. An overall view of concepts of information (Shannon, Gabor and Fisher) and their relationship to meaning is provided in Cherry (1966) and MacKay (1969).

Transfer theory

The rapid development of automatic control devices in the post-war period led to the formation of a new profession within electrical engineering – the control engineer as distinct from the power engineer. It was appreciated that the human controller in aircraft and later in process systems behaved, in many respects, like an automatic control device. The human controller can be regarded as one kind of mechanism within the system control loops. Incorporation of the human operator is variously known as manual control, tracking and human dynamics. The controller, human or mechanistic, is regarded as a black box which can accept certain inputs and, in response, can generate certain outputs. The description of the dynamic relationships between inputs and outputs is called a transfer function or describing function. From the generalised control viewpoint this approach is advantageous in that the human operator is just another part of a loop within a control network, all of which is described in the same terms. From the behavioural science viewpoint the human operator transfer function is a succinct and unambiguous description of human behaviour in this situation. For further details see Kelley (1968), Bernotat and Gartner (1972), Sheridan and Johannsen (1976). As described in this way the human operator is functioning in a highly skilled mode but at a cognitively low level. He is a 'good' controller and an adaptive one in that he can change his dynamic characteristics to match peculiarities in the hardware/ software parts of any dynamic man–machine system.

The dynamic aspects described are essentially short-term in taking account of timing and amplification, not long-term in that effects due to learning,

Table 5.1. *Psychological measurement using information theory*
(after Crossman, 1969)

Topic	Task	Results
Absolute judgement	Position of a pointer on a line Angle of inclination	Channel capacity 3.2 bits/judgement 4.5 bits/judgement
Immediate memory	Reproduction of lists of digits or letters	Capacity about 30 bits
Choice responses	Reaction time with varying number of choices	Changes with learning and with display/ control compatibility. 3–25 bits/s
Motor control	Alternate tapping on targets of different width different distances apart	Channel capacity 10 bits/s
Perception	Reproduction of figures and text. Discrimination of auditory signals	Operator can detect and 'use' redundancy if it is relatively simple. Behaves like a channel with a capacity limit
Control processes	Detection of multi-dimensional patterns including rejection of irrelevancies	Complex redundancy of this kind takes time to unravel. Not describable in information terms
Stimulus/response processes	Tracking	Throughput of continuous positional information 2–5 bits/s. Doubles if 'preview' is accessible
Language	Social communication	Operator can use redundancy to reduce effects of noise

fatigue and switches of strategy are normally excluded. Details of some of the short-term behavioural characteristics are given below. It is possible to derive a measure of channel capacity different from the informational measure in terms of the operator's *bandwidth*, measured by the frequency range over which he can respond appropriately. If the human operator (or any other analogue control device) responds only over a range between A and $A + W$ cycles per second then not more than $2W$ independent signal values per second can be transmitted. This is the channel capacity neglecting noise. If there is noise and the signal to noise ratio is known the consequent restriction on channel capacity is readily calculated. There have been many experiments over a wide variety of situations to determine the human operator dynamic characteristics. These involve spectral analysis or 'mimicking'. This latter is a particularly elegant method in that an automatic device parallels and converges on the way the human operator behaves, its characteristics are easily read after it has matched the way the human operator is performing.

Dynamic behaviour of subsystems such as the human eye, grasping a moving object using eye–hand coordination and arm–hand pursuit movements can also be described as transfer functions.

The approach can be extended to cover situation monitoring, in particular monitoring of instrument displays. Smallwood (1966) devised an instrument scanning model which assumes that all instruments are equally important, there is a constant attention shift time, readout time is dependent on required precision and a reading is stored instantaneously. The operator guides the scanning by an internal model and after any one reading, switches to the next one which is identified as the one most likely to have changed appreciably. Carbonell (1966) used a queuing theory model in which the operator, in dealing with a queue of instruments waiting to be read, decides which one should be dealt with next by minimising the risk of keeping the others waiting. The process is complex but can be simulated by assuming that the signals are generated by a random walk process. The greater the task load the more erratic the sampling becomes, this agrees with the observed behaviour of pilots. Baron and Kleinman (1969), after reviewing previous studies, devised a combined control and data selection model with an elaborate data reconstructor using a mathematical model developed for navigational systems – a Kalman filter which essentially weights contributory evidence from different sources. Observational noise and a perceptual delay are also incorporated.

It will be appreciated that the mathematics associated with these modes of behaviour is complex but still does not match the complexity of observed behaviour. Another difficulty is that the basic behavioural data needed to feed into the models, such as cost/value functions are not available with any precision. Nevertheless the ingenuity of the modellers and their insights into how to cope with the interactions of many parameters are impressive. Reviews of this field are provided in Sheridan and Ferrell (1974) and Rouse (1977).

5.2 Knowledge
5.2.1 Data acquisition

Almost all presented data is intended for acceptance through one or other or both of the distant senses: vision and hearing. It is true that the operator receives information from the controls he uses and from movements of vehicles he manoeuvres, but although this information is important it is regarded as coincidental rather than presented.

The performance of the eyes as a dynamic system is formidable, up to 100 000 fixation points are attainable within a roughly circular region of about 100° about the visual axis. The torque/inertia ratio is about 436 radians/s and a new steady state position can be achieved in about 5 milliseconds. Thus the eye has no trouble in tracking moving objects, the torque/inertia ratio of an aircraft is about 4 (Fogel, 1963). The accommodation process (refocussing) is much slower and the change of 'set' to receive new information is slower still so that the overall scanning speed between data sources is about 200 milliseconds.

The auditory channel has about the same energy threshold level and range and the same capacity as the visual channel. Reaction times (the interval between the presentation of a stimulus and the initiation of a response) are slightly faster if the stimulus is presented to the ears rather than the eyes. Under the most favourable conditions, auditory reaction time is about 160 milliseconds and visual reaction time about 180 milliseconds. Such times are rarely of practical importance because the operator can usually anticipate when something is going to happen, if he cannot this itself is an indication that the design of the information presentation should be reconsidered. The relative advantage of the sensory channels are shown qualitatively in Table 5.2.

5.2.2 Information transmission

In situations involving selective action, e.g. key pressing, the human operator can transmit between 5 and 10 bits per second. The lower level is more appropriate if some symbolic interpretation such as reading or listening to alphanumerics is required. There is also a limit on what can be received from a given presentation of about 2 bits per item (Garner, 1962). This can be at least doubled by providing 'perceptual anchors' such as orthogonal axes which structure a display, or by using a correlated multi-sensory presentation. In a situation where there is a stream of independent stimuli a 'psychological

Table 5.2. *Relative advantages of the sensory channels*
(from Singleton, 1969)

	Kinaesthetic (motion and force sensing)	Auditory (hearing)	Visual (seeing)
Reception	Requires no attention	Requires no directional search	Requires attention and location
Speed	Fastest	Fast	Slowest
Order	Not registered independently	Most easily retained	Easily lost
Urgency	Almost impossible to incorporate	Most easily incorporated	Difficult to incorporate
Noise	Not affected by visual noise	Not affected by visual or kinaesthetic noise	Not affected by auditory noise
Accepted symbolism	None	Melodious Linguistic	Pictorial Linguistic
Mobility	Little flexibility of position	Most flexible	Some flexibility
Suitability	Response feed-back information	Dominantly time information	Dominantly space information
		For rhythmical data	For stored data
	For immediate check on actions	For warning signals	For routine multi-channel checking

refractory period' (Welford, 1968) can be detected of about 500 milliseconds during which no response is initiated, the time seems to be occupied by checking the response to the previous stimulus. Table 5.1. contains other data. These results were obtained from untrained subjects in artificial laboratory conditions. They are not directly transferable to the normal work situation where experienced operators are dealing with complex arrays of interrelated presentations and response options. Nevertheless these numbers, which are all in the domain of tenths of seconds, confirm that the human operator is very slow and of very limited capacity compared with the performance of electronically based sub-systems.

The total sensory capacity is about 10^9 bits/second which is clearly in a different domain from the output rate of 10 bits/second. This confirms the qualitative impression that the human operator can accumulate a lot of evidence to update a complex model of the real situation and use it to arrive at highly selected strategies which appear as simple outputs.

The receptor systems are faster than the effector systems and this provides the beginnings of anticipation, the important human faculty to predict what is going to happen. As Kelley (1968) points out, evidence about the past and even the present is important only in its contribution to predicting the future. The human operator can use the structure of events and processes to extrapolate into the future by assuming that the regularities will continue, this is called 'perceptual anticipation' (Poulton, 1974). An even more elaborate predictive facility is to consciously order the events which have to be dealt with either in a queue or by tagging into categories such as urgent/pending/can wait. More generally the operator can cognitively predict what is going to happen from his knowledge and experience of the world and how it works, this applies to economic, social and political events as well as to changes in the physical world. The need to react quickly should always be questioned, it is an indication that either information or skills do not match the complexity of the situation.

There are two laws which have been derived using information theory. *Hick's Law* states that choice reaction time is a linear function of the logarithm of the number of choices. This follows if there is a limited channel capacity and the operator is working at the limit in attempting to make accurate responses as rapidly as possible. Hick (1952) also pointed out that since an error implies that less information has been transmitted it is possible to specify a speed/accuracy trade-off in numerical terms, again assuming a fixed operational channel capacity. He demonstrated that reaction time data and errors fit this formulation reasonably well. Hyman (1953) was able to show that the principle applies when events are not equally probable. Fitts (1954) devised an index of difficulty for movements, $\log (2A/W)$ where A is the amplitude of movements and W is the width of the target at the end of the movement. *Fitts' Law* states that movement time is a linear function of this index of difficulty. Again this follows from the concept of a channel of limited informational capacity and its validity has been demonstrated by experimental data.

Returning to more precise descriptions of more limited phenomena, relevant transfer functions have been proposed by Tustin and McRuer and Krendel. Tustin's equation is:

$$G(s) = e^{-ts}(As + B + \frac{C}{s}).$$

This indicates that the response in continuous manual control is subject to an exponential lag. A, B and C are separate gain constants indicating that the operator is responding to derivatives as well as to the amplitude of stimulus at a given instant.

McRuer and Krendel's equation is:

$$G(s) = \frac{Ke^{-ts}(T_L s + 1)}{(T_N s + 1)(T_I s + 1)}$$

This incorporates an exponential lag and also a neuromuscular time lag T_N of about 0.1 s, a lead time constant T_L of about 1.0 s, and a lag time constant T_I of about 10 s.

Looking at the situation in this way promotes the suggestion that, since the operator can utilise derivative information, it might usefully be built into the displays or the controls (see below). For a more extended description of manual control and decision-making see Wickens (1984).

5.2.3 Decision-making

The human process of making a choice between alternatives in the context of incomplete information about the situation and the alternatives remains obscure. Certainly nothing is known which can be expressed quantitatively. Chapters 2 and 6 contain general discussions of how the skilled operator functions generally and under risk conditions. These ideas are useful in contributing to current issues of computer support for decisions but even with a high demand for such knowledge from designers in the information technology field progress remains slow.

5.3 Principles, methods and procedures

5.3.1 Displays

A display is a part of a man–environment or man–machine interface which conveys information to the human operator. Information by definition relates to the operator's purposes and tasks. He is moving through a multidimensional space, either physical or functional or both, and at any instant he will have some uncertainty about his ends and his means or both (Singleton, 1972a). Information reduces this uncertainty. What is actually presented is data and it is from these data that information can be extracted, the art of presentation is to facilitate the process of extraction.

The operator is designed to cope and is accustomed to coping with a natural world saturated with data most of which is irrelevant to his purposes and tasks. His problem is selectivity, and he can either direct his attention to or have it called by a display. Calling his attention is particularly significant in relation to alarms which are discussed separately below. If as is normally the case he is volunteering his attention this may be task-based (set) or more specifically item-based (search). Visual search is active and spatial (scanning) and auditory search is passive and temporal (awaiting signals). The term attention also covers the parallel or succeeding function of identifying signals in noise. Noise in this sense can be either visual or auditory, it describes the background of similar activity above which the signal must rise before it can be detected. Thus the signal to noise ratio is the first criterion of the utility of a display. The psychological equivalent of this is the figure/ground relationship. These ratios are not easily quantified but the qualitative principle of enhancing the signal at the expense of the noise provides a general design guideline. Contrast is a key parameter. Other relevant considerations in the visual case are brightness, size and familiar shapes for signals, and glare, clutter and fuzziness for noise. Auditory signal/noise ratios are extremely complex, the reduction of masking depends on the complex interaction of frequency, intensity and tonal variables, particularly when speech is involved. For details see Morgan *et al.*, (1963).

The Gestalt principles of symmetry, regularity, completeness and in general wholeness and economy apply. By following these principles it is possible to improve on nature and design artificial displays which are much better structured than are natural displays. They match the needs of the operator by doing part of the extraction process for him. For example, Fig. 5.3 shows a map of Birmingham as it is in a topographical matching sense and as it is in essence from the point of view of a motorist navigating within the city. As a display this second 'cognitive map' will appeal to any driver because it corresponds to the image which a driver very familiar with Birmingham keeps in mind. The noise has been reduced compared with the 'true' map. The same strategy of simplifying and structuring whilst maintaining the relevant data was used in the design of the well-known London underground map.

As in other kinds of information channels, noise may be generated at the source or at the destination. The relationship of internal noise (neural noise) in the human operator with noise associated with the presentation is not clear, as Welford (1984) points out, if the sum of squares of variances applies then if one or other is relatively high the lower one will be of little significance. Neural noise is thought to increase with age.

Whatever the mode of presentation the key to good display design is structure. This will partly match and partly determine how the operator is thinking, the objective is compatibility. The presented information should be compatible with an operator's needs and with the real world, particularly if he is using the world directly to gain part of his information. Ideally he should effectively look through the presentation, using it as a window on the world.

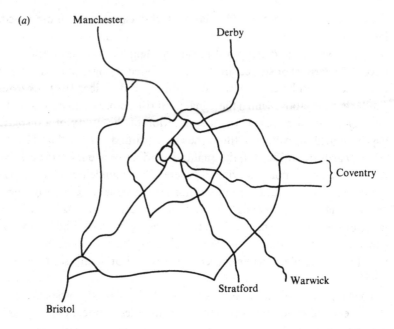

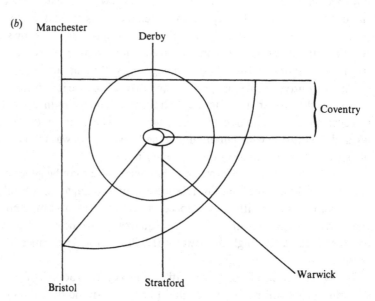

Fig. 5.3. The map of Birmingham changed from topographical accuracy to cognitive matching.

The test of perfect design is that the compatibility is such as to allow him to do this without conscious awareness that there is a display intervening between him and reality. This does not imply that it should pictorially resemble reality, a numerical presentation which meets his requirements will be translated without conscious effort into information relevant to the task. Easterby (1984) analyses the reception process into the sequence: detection, discrimination, identification, recognition and comprehension. This sequence incorporates sensation and perception. He notes that detection, discrimination and identification are all processes which involve categorisation. Related tasks are searching, sorting, scanning and skimming. Related display characteristics are legibility, conspicuity (signal/noise ratio), readability and meaningfulness. This approach of identifying relevant parameters is qualitative rather than quantitative, but it nevertheless helps to ensure that a designer moves through his choice process with appropriate awareness. Note that the three main dimensions along which these parameters can be distributed are processes, tasks and display attributes.

There are two separate problems of display design: the psychophysics and the coding. The psychophysics problem is to match the data to the characteristics of the sensors and their position. This covers legibility, conspicuity and readability. The coding problem is to match the data to the perceptual and cognitive functions of the operator, in short to make it as meaningful as possible. Learning is highly relevant to coding but not very much to psychophysics. The optimal match to central processes may change as skills develop. In particular the display which is more easily used at first sight may not suit the highly skilled operator, e.g. an experienced process operator may prefer lists of parameter values to an elaborately structured mimic diagram which would be more intelligible to an outsider.

A list of kinds of diplays is shown in Table 5.3. These might be visual or auditory and if visual they might be dials or screen presentations. The design of scales and pointers is well understood and is reported in all ergonomics manuals. The design of screen formats (see below) is becoming increasingly important because such formats are replacing dials in many workspaces including flight-decks and process control rooms. The replacement is not complete, partly because of reliability questions and partly because dials individually and collectively do have advantages. Reliability is better for dials because they can be 'hard-wired' directly to sensors, there is no intervening data processor to go wrong. In fact the main distinction is between hard-wired presentations and data processor driven presentations which are usually but not necessarily on screens. Broadly the dial set is better from psychophysical aspects, it is more easily scanned and read. Definition on screens is still

Table 5.3. *Kinds of display and distinctions between displays*

Real/Artificial	The environment naturally provides data, e.g. the view through a windscreen. This is a real display by contrast with an artificial display which depends on designed instrumentation, e.g. the car dashboard
Static/Dynamic	The data on a static display does not change, e.g. a legend plate, whereas the presentation on a dynamic display changes in time, e.g. a pressure gauge
Pictorial	A topologically matching presentation, e.g. a dot moving on a map
Qualitative	Indicates a change of state but not numerically, e.g. an oil pressure warning light
Quantitative	Presents a number or a set of numbers either digitally or in analogue fashion
Hybrid	Any combination of the above three kinds, e.g. an Air Traffic Control display has all three: a map, alarm signals and numbers indicating heights and identities
Analogue	Data is presented in terms of the length of a bar or a point on a scale
Digital	Data is presented directly as a number or a set of numbers
Mixed A/D	e.g. numbers on bars or counters within scales
Storage	Contains data about the past as well as the present usually with the purpose of extrapolating to the future, e.g. a moving chart containing a trace
Predictor	Contains data about the future or evidence which facilitates prediction of the future
Quickened	Contains some weighted derivative information, e.g. a mixture of displacement and rate of change of displacement
Unburdened	Contains weighted integrative information
Command	Tells the operator what to do rather than what the state of the system is

relatively poor, there are more problems of surface reflection and screen size is very limited so that multiple screens are often needed. Dials and lights more easily lend themselves to fitting into large-scale arrays visible from a considerable distance and often incorporating associated switches. It is more difficult to hold group discussions around a screen. The various aspects of this trade-off or optimal allocation are summarised in Table 5.4. The design decisions to be considered in any display design are summarised in Table 5.5.

Table 5.4. *Relative advantages of hard-wired and computer-driven displays*

Hard-wired	Computer-driven
Dials, charts and lights	*Usually presented on CRT screens*
More readable	Less readable
The most reliable including robustness in cases of fire or seismic disturbance	Susceptible to data processing faults
Can be directly associated with controls	Can be associated with controls using touch screens but not easily
Can be built into mimic diagrams	Cannot easily be associated with large mimic diagrams, but can present small scale mimic diagrams
Can be built into large arrays well suited to rapid visual scanning and associated control manipulations	Area of presented data relatively small, clumsy in multiple arrays
Matches needs of group discussion, e.g. complex diagnosis	Unsuitable support for group activity Feasible for two people, each with his own console and common software
Relatively static format with only measures changing	Suitable for hierarchies of formats, easy to provide guidance such as overlap and zoom facilities and windows (displays within displays) Formats can be dynamic, either with detailed measures changing or with readings only changing within fixed frameworks
Alarm facilities appropriate for attention gaining but not for alarm series (order and timing not easily indicated)	Less attention gaining alarm facilities. Good for alarm lists which automatically indicate relative timing of alarms
Structural changes difficult (eased by using modular surfaces)	Highly flexible for structural change
Generally low versatility	High versatility

Although the discriminatory abilities of the sense organs might indicate otherwise it is not desirable to use more than five colours or five tones which the operator has to identify unambiguously. Correspondingly spatial identification within a uniform array is only accurate for a line of not more than five uniform switches or dials.

There are display stereotypes, that is habits which operators transfer to an

Table 5.5. *Display design checklist*
(from Singleton, 1969)

Dimension	General problem	Possible objectives	Parameters, techniques and principles
Necessity	Does the user's need justify the provision?	Is it worth the expense and complication?	Cost effectiveness studies
		Can the operator manage as well or better without it?	Justification other than on grounds of information: – tradition – apparent quality – styling
		What happens if it malfunctions?	Critical incident studies Possibilities: – presents no information – presents false information
Sufficiency	What data may the operator need which has not been provided?	Would more data be useful: – as routine? – to set up or change the system? – in case of malfunction? – about past state? – present state? – future state?	Man-machine allocation of function Task analysis use of: – storage displays – quickened displays – predictor displays
Legibility	Can an operator with average senses see or hear what is required easily?	Is unnecessary activity required to extract the data?	Activity may: – take longer time – involve more concentration, effort – involve change of: – posture – position

Table 5.5. (*cont.*)

Dimension	General problem	Possible objectives	Parameters, techniques and principles

		Is the presentation about the right strength?	Visual parameters:
			– position
			– size
			– orientation
			– illumination
			– pointer–size
			     – shape
			     – contrast
			– lettering–size
			     – style
			     – excess
			scale–division
			     – graduation
			     – clutter
			Auditory parameters:
			– amplitude
			– frequency
			– attack
			– clarity

		Is the signal/noise ratio high enough?	Lighting parameters: – contrast – shadows – glare – reflections Sound parameters: – background noise
		Is it clear where the data are available?	
		Is it clear what the presented data are about?	Connections with real events: – physical – symbolic – legends
		Have unnecessary data been eliminated?	
		Is the accuracy appropriate in terms of: – instrumentation? – perception?	Error summation studies

Table 5.5. (*cont.*)

Dimension	General problem	Possible objectives	Parameters, techniques and principles
Compatibility	Does the display conform: – to the real world?	Is the operator using real/artificial displays? If so: – does movement of indicators correspond to real movements? – is the pattern of display items similar to real things or data sources?	
	– to other display items?	Have the most appropriate grouping principles been followed?	Possible grouping principles: – sequence of scanning – priority – frequency of use – similarity or identity of function
		Have the most appropriate additional grouping cues been used?	Possible grouping cues: – colour – shape – size – position – scale style – pointer style
		Are different dials, pointers consistent when appropriate?	
	– with previous habits and skills?	Will the operator require special training?	Skills analysis
		Is there likely to be a discontinuity with earlier operator experience?	Population stereotypes

Table 5.5. (*cont.*)

Dimension	General problem	Possible objectives	Parameters, techniques and principles
	– with required decisions and actions?	Does the presentation encourage the operator to:	
		– think about the right problem in the right way?	Encoding to match perceptual models
		– select the right action and move in the right direction?	Control/display relationships

unfamiliar display in terms of how it is expected to function. Broadly a displacement from left to right, from down to up or clockwise is assumed to be an increase in whatever parameter is being indicated. Contravention of this stereotype will result in a gross increase in errors.

Displays are normally thought of as reflecting the system state. They may also be designed to present alternative actions and their consequences, or at an even higher level they can present policies and objectives.

5.3.2 *Controls*

A control is a part of a man–machine interface which accepts information from the human operator. Controls have an associated display element in that they must be identified and located by the operator before he can utilise them. Identification can be by position, size, shape, colour and label or any mix of these.

Associated with electrical systems there are three main types: the switch, the selector and the knob. Switches may be push-button or toggle, a selector may have up to about ten different positions, knobs are intended for continuous variables. For mechanical systems keys, cranks, levers, wheels and pedals are used.

Most controls are intended for hand operations but the feet also are used in transport vehicles, cranes, earth-moving machines and a few production machines. These are pedals except for a few specialist machines such as those in the garment trades where a wheel or disc is rotated with considerable delicacy. Pedals have two main advantages: they relieve the hands for other operations, and the operator can use much greater forces. There is a corresponding disadvantage in restriction of posture and a consequent need for even more careful design of seats. When no part of the weight can be supported on the feet and the force exerted on pedals reacts on the back-rest the design of seats is critical. The weight of the feet is significant and controls should be designed to support this weight.

Almost all controls are of the displacement type where the movement is intended to indicate the required change in the machine/environmental state. Pressure controls could be designed in which the force or torque indicates the command but they are rare. For mechanical reasons many controls have an integration of pressure into the displacement. These aspects are dealt with in detail in ergonomics manuals.

Corresponding to display design problems of psychophysics and coding there are control design problems of anatomy and dynamics. The order of a control describes the relationship between the control movement and the consequent movement of the controlled system. A zero order control causes a displacement corresponding to the displacement of the control itself, but there can be different levels of amplification measured as the control gain. A first order displacement causes a change in the velocity of the controlled member. Second order are acceleration controls and third order are jerk controls. Higher order controls than this are too difficult to use for any purpose. The kinds of control are summarised in Table 5.6.

Controls also have stereotypes in terms of operator expectations analogous to display stereotypes. That is, displacement left to right or clockwise is expected to result in an increase in the controlled variable. Down to up and backward to forward are ambiguous without experience of the particular control. Toggle switches are peculiar in the U.K. compared with most other countries in that 'up' indicates 'off' rather than 'on'.

5.3.3   *Interface design*

A man–machine interface is conceptually a plane across which information is exchanged between a human operator and mechanisms or the environment. It contains display and control elements which should be regarded as links between the man and his surroundings rather than as parts of the machine.

Obviously displays and controls should be positioned for readability and operability respectively. The less obvious determinants of position are to do with how the interface maps on to mechanisms and how it maps on to the operator. Criteria for the operator include frequency of use, relative importance and urgency. Criteria reflecting the mechanism may be based on topo-

Table 5.6. *Kinds of control*

Switches	Can be push-button or toggle. Toggle switches require more positive operation and indicate state by position. Push-buttons more readily operated accidentally unless protection is provided, require associated light to indicate state. N.B. the indication that a switch has been operated is not the same as the indication that the system-state has been changed
Selectors	Used for step changes between up to ten different states
Knobs	Used for continuous variables
Keys	Can function mechanically or electrically or mixed. For continuous use, e.g. keyboards, detailed design of surface, pressure change with displacement and coded identification (mainly by position) requires detailed attention
Cranks and levers	Used when mechanical advantage is required, becoming less common as power-assistance becomes easier to provide
Wheels	Good for precise positioning because of agonist/antagonist relationship of two hands (or feet). Range of feasible hand positions
Pedals	Have implications for detailed seat design
Displacement	Change of system-state is a function of distance or angle through which control moves. Opposing and restoring forces need design consideration, e.g. springs, viscous damping
Pressure	Control does not move but change of system-state reflects force applied
Displacement	Zero order control where controlled system follows control movement directly, possibly with amplification i.e. gain factor more or less than unity
Velocity	First order control where controlled system velocity changes with displacement of control
Acceleration	Second order control where controlled system acceleration changes with displacement of control
Jerk	Third order control where controlled system third derivative changes with displacement of control
Rate-aided	Mixed displacement and velocity control, used for example in gunnery. Other mixes of orders can be designed but are rarely used because of training time required. Can occur for mechanical reasons e.g. car 'accelerator' is a mix of all four orders

graphical matching or more conceptual aspects such as the flow of materials, power or information. Such mimics rely not only on positioning but also on lines or shapes or differently coloured areas to indicate relationships.

Relationships between particular displays and controls can also be indicated by position, similarity of colour or shape, or by connecting lines on the panel. Controls may be collected together and separated from displays if there are space restrictions on operator movement or if there is high urgency in operation. For most systems except vehicles there is advantage in allowing the operator mobility, it suits him physiologically and provides much greater space to meet other design criteria. When the interface is attached to a specific machine the identity of displays and controls is less ambiguous, although their interrelationships may be more obscure and there may be more readability and postural problems.

There are display/control stereotypes particularly in parallelism of relative movements. The relationship between a control which moves backwards and forwards and a display which moves up and down is highly ambiguous and best avoided in any console design. Contravention of stereotypes can lead to longer response times, greater errors and rates of error, longer training times and more rapid fatigue onset.

Formal evaluations of interfaces either by performance comparison or by attempts to measure operator loads are extremely elaborate, difficult and expensive. It is more appropriate to rely on concept validity following from sound design principles.

5.3.4 Centralised control systems

Technological developments have generated the need and created the possibility of controlling more and more complex systems from a central point. The need arises because the systems are tightly coupled, what happens in one place has effects speedily in many other places within the system. There may or may not be urgency in the need for response from central control. On the one hand malfunctions will be expensive or dangerous or both, on the other hand there is always some distributed control which will take care of unwanted events which are 'within the design basis'. The key central control function is monitoring with a view to coordination of activities and occasionally changing state. The distributed control systems will usually involve operational human activities as well as automatic loops and the information gathering system may contain more human operators. At the centre is one key operator, but he is not alone, he is the senior member of a team or crew, and he has specialist advisers on tap.

The analysis and description of these systems can be a formidable task

Table 5.7. *Common and distinctive features of different information systems*

	Military	Commercial	Industrial
Data sensing	Devices need guidance	Entered via keyboards	Routine scanning and processing
Decision-maker	Military officer	Financial analyst	Engineer
Information coding	Spatial	Lists	Levels and flows
Operator aids	Maps	Elementary	Time trends
Priority indicators	Orders	Trading conditions	Alarm systems
Opposition	Intelligent aggression	Intelligent competition	Benign

(Table 5.7). For example, in a military system a whole battle area might be monitored with interacting land, air, surface sea and undersea elements, although currently land/air and sea/air (surface and below surface) are usually still treated separately. In a nuclear power station (Singleton, 1985) there are between 10 000 and 20 000 separate inputs from sensing devices and perhaps 30 VDUs, with additional hard-wired consoles monitored by three or four operators in one room, but with many other subsidiary manned control rooms. A multidimensional hierarchy of diagrams is required supported by extensive lists. The number of parameters is such that long lists are often the only way of providing comprehensive descriptions of parts of the potential information presentation.

Not surprisingly a key problem is to ensure that everything relevant has been thought of and recorded. Even with small systems such as numerically controlled machine tools or desk-top computers with a range of software packages, the flexibility of the potential systems is such as to tempt the designer to provide more facilities than the user can readily comprehend. Hence the importance of procedure manuals.

In bigger systems the starting point will be Role Analysis to clarify who is responsible to whom for what. That has to be determined before any further steps can be taken in designing interfaces, procedures or training. Roles may differ in different modes of system operation if, as is commonly the case, there are two operators, one senior to the other. Each will probably have his separate tasks, there may be some joint tasks, the work of the junior one will be monitored by the senior one, and there may also be some reverse monitoring.

The tasks in each of these four categories need to be described. The operators may have access to the same suite of VDU formats or some may be accessible only to one of the operators. They will probably share an interest in the hard-wired displays but each may have his own set of controls. They will probably share the same procedures library, for some tasks the procedure may be separated into two different parts, one for each operator. It is quite difficult to prepare and present documentation which indicates how these two operators are intended to interact and how they relate to common consoles and to their separate consoles. The system also needs to be designed to accommodate a trainee who forms a third party in these complex interactions. It is usually necessary to have an on-line training phase intermediate between the training school and assuming the responsibility for the junior key role within the pair.

System malfunctions and human errors

There are two related problems: the minimisation of error rates and the minimising of the effects of errors on system performance. Errors can be reduced by the standard Human Factors aspects of good design and focussed by an understanding of how errors occur. There are certain common phenomena in diagnostic errors:

- an operator may persist in pursuing an inappropriate hypothesis formed too hastily, but once formed it directs the search for evidence, supportive data are accepted and non-supportive data are rejected. This is known as mind-set. It is assumed to be less likely if the diagnostic process is shared between operators and more particularly if there is an independent monitor of events situated elsewhere, e.g. a Technical Support Centre
- there can be confusion between malfunction in the plant and malfunction in the information system reporting plant activity. This can usually be checked by the use of the built-in redundancy in the instrumentation
- there can be misunderstanding between operators, either between those in the control centres or between the control room staff and operators in the plant. The remedy is more formalised procedures for such interactions
- serious incidents invariably contain several independent hiatuses which have occurred simultaneously by chance. Such incidents are impossible to predict and the only remedy is in training based on a conceptual understanding of how the whole system is intended to function. Again it is assumed that several independent minds applied to the problem can facilitate speedy and correct diagnosis

This last point verges on the second question of the negative interaction between human errors and system malfunctions. There are several identifiable aspects:

- during serious incidents caused by localised hiatuses, e.g. fires and explosions, the effects may spread to support systems as well as to the normal on-line system including the information system. Thus, some of the evidence may be misleading and some of the standard remedies described in the emergency procedures may not function but may appear to do so. If the control room operator suspects that this might be the case he will normally send a system operator to take a close direct look and report back
- safeguard systems may fail to function because they have been inadequately maintained but this is not discovered until they are needed, and even then there will be further delays because the operators are expecting the incident to be taken care of automatically
- correspondingly there may be errors in the emergency procedures which are not noticed before they are needed in a real emergency
- because the operator is the ultimate back-stop he may have to contravene procedures or override automatic safeguards when a situation has arisen which he decides has not been thought of during the design processes. If he makes a mistake in such a decision both he and the system are in serious trouble. There will be meta-procedures which guide him as to what he can or cannot do in certain generalised scenarios, normally they also involve checking between operators perhaps at several levels
- the design may include operator lock-outs but if the designers have overlooked certain contingencies there could be serious problems. Normally such lock-outs are conditional and can be finally overridden after consultation between operational staff

Human limitations
General human limitations are the core of ergonomics and are described elsewhere in this and the previous book *The Body at Work*. There are however several which specifically influence control room design:

- because hardware related sciences are so much more definitive than human sciences design is inevitably driven by technology. At best the ergonomist can make a supporting contribution and he can be overridden for valid technical or cost reasons. For example, the ergonomist may be concerned about the plethora of alarms (see below), but he may find that one minor sub-system has several apparently low priority alarms because the contractor who provided that sub-system has specifically claimed that he cannot be responsible for reliability unless certain parameters of its state of operation are permanently presented to the plant controller

– it is the nature of instrumentation, hard-wired or data processed, that the presentation to the operator can only be a two-dimensional flat display. There is a fundamental mismatch with the needs of the operator who usually has to think pictorially in four dimensions: three space and one time, and conceptually in many more. This mismatch can be reduced by all kinds of strategies such as alternative displays giving various parameters in pairs, mixed graphic – alphanumeric presentations, and use of colours and shapes to incorporate extra dimensions, but these inevitably add to the operator's decoding problems. The general solution would be a three-dimensional display which changes in real time and which can be shifted rapidly forwards or backwards in time, but this is currently beyond the resources of the instrumentation specialists

– the designer also needs aids to support his multi-dimensional thinking. These take the form of drawings, computer-aided design presentations, models, mock-ups and simulators. They are useful also to the ergonomist in checking from his specialist point of view

– a system design process consists of many parallel activities. Ergonomics can be regarded as one of these processes or as cutting across most of the others. In particular the ergonomist cannot function except in the context of decisions by others. For example, he cannot complete his evaluation of a console design unless he has a mock-up or simulation, a procedure and at least one skilled operator available

– the ergonomist is concerned with all human operators who relate to the control room, and he may have some difficulty in persuading the designers that the commissioning engineers have claims for consideration equivalent to the operating staff. There is often considerable supplementary instrumentation in the control room whilst the plant is being commissioned

– in addition to normal operations a system has to be maintained, refurbished at intervals and eventually decommissioned. All these stages in the system life can influence the effective control room design

– for a large system there will be a number of subsidiary control rooms. The linkages between these rooms and with the central room need consideration. In some cases data are fed from and through the satellite rooms to the main room, in other cases data are primarily directed to the main room and are then distributed to the satellites. This interacts with the responsibility and functional allocation between the rooms which itself may differ between normal operations and emergencies. Problems can occur unless there is definitive mutual understanding of these allocations

– the ergonomics documentation for a large system design may itself be difficult to structure. There will be several main themes: operator oriented ones such as role analysis and task analysis, system oriented ones such as functional diagrams and information flow diagrams, and interface oriented ones such as console drawings, format hierarchies and link analyses. A specific information document will be the core of one topic and a subsidiary in relation to other topics.

5.3.5 *Alarm systems*

From a Human Factors viewpoint an alarm is a claim on the operator's attention. In a typical control room situation there is a gross mismatch between the amount of data presented and the limited human information processing capacity described earlier in this chapter. Even in smaller data presentation arrays there may be particular requirements for urgent action. In all cases an alarm attempts to prioritise data to be noted.

An alarm system may be as simple as one visual or auditory signal, such as the 'Identification Friend or Foe' warning on a visually-sighted surface to air missile, or as complex as a mixed hard-wired/computer driven system containing 24 000 separate alarms as in a nuclear power station. Between the two extremes are a variety of systems as indicated in Fig. 5.4.

The design of alarm systems is necessarily a process requiring a multi-disciplinary approach and this has characteristic difficulties.Taking process control at the complex end of the design spectrum, an alarm can be considered from five points of view:

- the mechanism
- the system
- the interface
- the plant operator
- the incident investigator

Each generates a different concept of what an alarm is.

Mechanistically an alarm is the consequence of a parameter (usually temperature, pressure or voltage) which is outside the limits specified by the designer for the normal operation of the mechanism. In systems terms an alarm is a logically derived output from a pattern of functions indicating an unwanted system state. At the interface an alarm is within one of the two sets of displayed information – the system state information and the alarm information. For the plant operator an alarm is a claim on his attention. For the incident investigator the occurrence and phasing of alarms is important evidence of what happened and when.

Much of the confusion in discussions about alarm systems stems from a failure to recognise that there are these different viewpoints. Each is legitimate in its own context but to mix them without qualification is to invite the failure

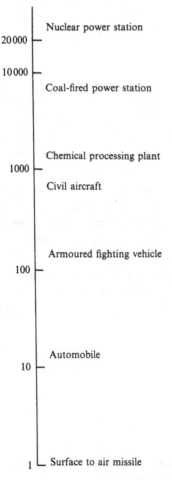

Fig. 5.4. Numbers of alarms in various systems.

of constructive debate and progress in design thinking. For this reason alarm systems are generally very poorly designed. The standard interface symptom is that during an emergency there will be alarm flooding or cascading. The operator is suddenly faced with a vast array of horns, bells and flashing lights – not a situation supportive of calm diagnostic reasoning. From the cognitive point of view a valuable source of diagnostic evidence is the sequence in which alarms appear and this evidence may be lost if too many appear too quickly. It is true that alarms are usually printed in a list in time order and perhaps with attached time stamps but again if the rate is too high the printer will lag behind real events. At one point during the Three Mile Island incident the computer printout was one and a half hours behind (Perrow, 1981).

An alarm is obviously intended to signal a departure from normal but 'normal' is usually defined in terms of the on-line performance of the system. Clearly what is alarming when the aircraft is cruising or the process plant is producing is different from what is alarming when the aircraft is taking off or landing, and the process plant is being started up or shut down. When a plant is relatively inactive but is being maintained, refuelled, refurbished, commissioned or decommissioned the control room will be full of alarm signals because the state is not normal. This stems from the failure to consider that different alarm systems may be required for different phases of plant activity. There is an unfortunate paradox in that most systems are least dangerous when in normal operation. It follows that an alarm system is, in principle, least required in the activity phase for which it is usually designed.

The design of alarms has a number of important purely technical problems, e.g. how to preserve the integrity of the source and the channel and how to avoid chattering which occurs when a parameter oscillates around the level at which the alarm is triggered. There would appear to be considerable scope for building alarm logic behind the interface which in principle could cope with suppression and prioritising, but operationally such systems have not been very successful. The difficulty seems to be that there are too many unforeseen combinations of contingencies, many of them stemming from maintenance operations in the plant. From a Human Factors viewpoint the design issues can be separated into interface problems and operator problems.

Alarm interfaces

In current technology there are available seven kinds of alarm presentation:

- auditory alarms, codable by frequency, loudness, position and quality
- annunciators arranged in matrices, codable by colour, legend and position

- alarm signals set within physical/functional diagrams occupying wall-
  space
- alarms associated with specific status displays
- alarm patterns and hierarchies on VDUs
- alarm lists on VDUs
- esoteric systems such as flashing the ambient lighting or using large
  moving readable texts

Alarm signals can of course be local to plant as well as centralised.

Auditory alarms should be used parsimoniously either as alerting signals which indicate that the operator should scan the visual presentations intensively or for various general emergencies such as fires in the plant and large-scale system failures. The ears have the great advantage of all round coverage which is an asset in claiming attention. On the other hand plant operators are not professional musicians and their discrimination of pitch, loudness, quality and location cannot be assumed to be high. The number of different auditory alarms in a control room should not be more than about five. Even this range of alarms can cause difficulties if one or more are very rare.

Visual alarms are of two kinds: hard-wired and screen based. Hard-wired can be associated with particular status displays, e.g. red lights near dials, can be specialist display elements, e.g. annunciators arranged in matrices, or can be elements within mimic diagrams. Mimic diagrams can also be presented in miniature form on screens. Screens are used also for lists. It is, of course, important that there should be consistency in the overall pattern of what is displayed for what purpose by what means.

The alarm system architecture should take account of the following questions for each signal:

- Is it intended as a warning or as a trigger for action?
- Is it intended to act as a diagnostic aid?
- Is it intended to convey numerical or verbal data as well as a qualitative claim on attention?
- What is the justifiable attention claim intensity relative to other alarms?
- Is it intended to direct the operator as well as warn him? If so, is it a direction primarily towards a plant parameter or a location?
- How does it relate to other alarms in terms of likely spatial and temporal patterns?

There are also some more general questions requiring consistent rules:

- Usually all presented alarms are recorded but should they all be transferred to a permanent data base?

- Usually alarm information is redundant in that the same information is available on status displays, but is this always necessarily the case?
- Usually each alarm has to be urgently and positively interpreted by the operator. Is this necessarily the case? In practice for many reasons an operator will accept an alarm and thereafter ignore it.
- Should there be different alarm systems for steady state operation and transient state operation?
- What are the criteria for distributing alarms between the presentation modes listed above?
- Should there be emergency procedures associated with particular alarm patterns? If so how are these identified and linked?

The alarm recipient

The human operator can cope with 5–10 bits per second, whereas the transmission capacity of high technology systems is measured in megabits. One has to be careful with this contrast because information is not stuff moving around but nevertheless there clearly is a mis-match and a need for the operator to be selective.

This selectivity can take place at many stages within information processing (Fig. 5.5). He can change the direction of his eyes, his eye focus, his attention, his level of arousal, his model of the situation and his overt activity. At the sensory level he can only look in one direction at one time. The eyes can shift position very quickly – in about 0.2 seconds – but the more central attention process is the real limit of scanning speed. This will vary with the unexpectedness of the signal (i.e. the information content) and with the coding and computation needed to extract meaning.

The rate at which visual alarms can be processed depends on what the operator has to do about them. If the action expected of him is merely to acknowledge by pressing a key he could deal with one every few seconds. At the other extreme if he has to relate the alarm to changes in a whole pattern of variables and diagnose the cause of the disturbance it could take him up to an hour to deal with one alarm. If on a continuous basis alarms are too frequent they cease to be alarms and become data presentations, if they are too rare he may not maintain an appropriate arousal level. For most purposes he can cope comfortably with one per minute but ten per minute would restrict his ability to keep track of what is happening. Thus, about five per minute would seem to be a reasonable maximum within the provisos mentioned above.

Attention, by definition, is single channel, the operator cannot attend to more than one thing at a time. Quite what is meant by 'one thing' varies with the task and the level of skill of the operator.

The model to which the operator adds new data will depend on the context, so also will any requirement to switch models. For example, he may sometimes think in terms of plant geography, where things are in relation to each other or he may think in terms of plant physics – temperatures, pressures and flows. Whatever his model he needs contextual cues as well as the alarm signal itself in order to attach any meaning. The informational content of each alarm signal is not usually considered systematically by the designer. Some of the relevant cues are shown in Fig. 5.6. Essentially the operator must be supported in his search for meaning, and although this depends in the background on training it also depends in the foreground on the place of the alarm signal within the stream of other events, either other alarms or status data.

Support for action comes from procedures, and from discussion with colleagues although cues such as colour and legend can be included in the alarm attributes.

The following are some of the specific points which need to be considered before determining an alarm architecture:

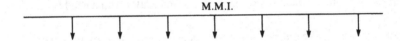

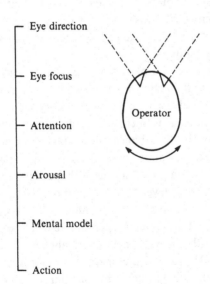

Fig. 5.5. The shifts triggered by alarms.

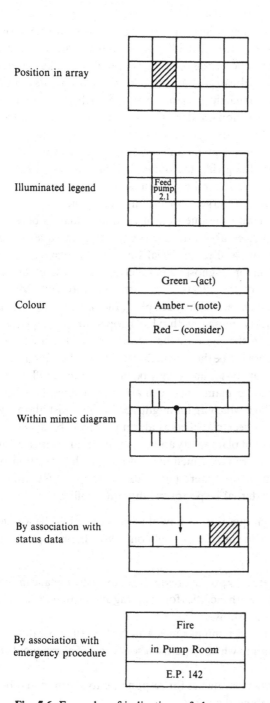

Fig. 5.6. Examples of indications of alarm context.

- It is observable that skilled operators do their own prioritising by scanning data sources and dividing their decisions into three caregories. Between the two extremes of 'do nothing' and 'take action now' they insert a third category of 'no action yet but needs watching'. There is a case for matching the alarm system to this human characteristic by having cautionary alarms (amber) as well as demand alarms The traffic light analogy could be carried a stage further by using green for an action demand and red for 'stop and think' There is a case for giving the operator a facility to instruct 'don't bother me now but remind me again later', e.g. re-present at end of shift or after a more urgent operation is complete
- In conjunction with the question of allocating alarms between the various modes listed above there is the more general question of the relative utility of parallel and serial streams of alarm data. A serial method is useful for diagnosis, a parallel method is useful for indicating the spread of the effects of a particular transient. Most high technology systems are 'tightly coupled', that is what happens at one point will quickly interact with what happens at other points
- The operator in the sense of the destination of the alarm data is usually considered to be the man in direct control of the plant. There is usually also a supervisor and it may be that he needs a different set of alarms. In complex plants there can also be a technical adviser with his own interface which again might need a specialist alarm system
- Data which has been classified as alarm worthy is by definition key information about plant safety and economy. It can be used as such in addition to its primary function of directing the attention of the operator. It might be of interest to a plant scientist, a safety engineer, a manager, an external inspector or an inquiry officer

Finally there is a design question of how the operator might be assisted by computers on his side of the interface (Singleton, 1987). In principle this could take the form of:

- storage of emergency procedures relevant to particular alarm patterns
- holding systems with facilities for scanning and browsing governed by rules and relationships
- storage with timed reminder tags attached by the operator
- expert systems into which patterns or sequences of alarms could be fed for comment
- simulations where strategies for responding to alarms could be tried without disturbing the plant.

5.3.6 Computer support
The engineered mechanism

A digital computer is a device that can store and manipulate numbers. This computation can be performed in such elaborate ways as to generate the appearance of much more complex functions but this is a convenient illusion. The illusion is fostered by processes such as the translation of continuous functions into digital sequences (this has resulted at least temporarily in the demise of the analogue computer), and by facilities for the translation of other symbols which can have 'higher level' meaning to and from numbers, for example in programming languages. In general numbers can be used to indicate categories as well as quantities and logical deductive operations can be performed within and between all the categories and data which have been predefined. However, there is no escape from human decisions on all questions of definition although for a particular task these decisions might be shared between designers, programmers and users. If there is any ambiguity about categories or data or if qualitative distinctions are attempted that ambiguity cannot be removed by the internal processes. There is an absolute requirement for precision and those internal processes are ultimately confined to addition and subtraction within numerical arrays. The restriction is helpful in practice because it is not difficult to distinguish between those functions which in principle can or cannot be allocated to a computer. A less direct consequence is that the computer does not suffer from human limitations such as vagueness, irrationality and dishonesty.

All this does not change with size, cost, maker or 'generation'. Currently computer designers are working on the fifth generation but the distinction between generations is how functions are performed rather than what they are. How functions are translated into mechanisms is important to the user mainly in that succeeding generations are more reliable and less costly than earlier ones.

On this very simple basis an elaborate information technology has been built up which is now so extensive and pervasive as to be regarded as a new industry. The industry exists and flourishes because it is helpful to the human operator in many of his roles.

The man–computer system

In common with every other man–machine system the man–computer system is effective because the machine can carry out certain functions more reliably, cheaply, quickly, accurately or conveniently than can the man. In the case of the computer these functions are computation, the execution of processes that follow logical rules and the use of extensive knowledge which can be stored as numbers.

The field is confused by jargon which is not rigorously defined mainly because human functions are often used as the frame of reference. Introducing terms such as intelligence, expert, knowledge and thinking presupposes that behavioural scientists know what these terms mean. They do not and the information technologist voluntarily and unnecessarily enters an area of mutual confusion. Correspondingly a term such as system architecture means whatever the user intends it to mean within a broad category of structures. A system architecture may consist of a functional diagram and description at any of the many possible levels or networks and lists of physical entities, or, most confusing of all, a mixture of these.

Machine intelligence or *Artificial Intelligence* arose from the use of computers as game players with the extensive processing facilities used to evaluate, on the basis of game theory, the alternatives as far as a 'look ahead horizon' which was usually only two or three moves forward, because the possibilities multiply so rapidly (the 'combinatorial explosion'). A.I. can be regarded as support for problem solving (Rich, 1983), achieving the appearance of intelligent behaviour (Winston, 1984) or as the replication of human thinking (Haugeland, 1985).

Expert systems began in the 1950s with the simulation of neural networks for processes such as perception, changed to heuristic search techniques for problem-solving in the 1960s, took up the question of knowledge representation in the 1970s, and more recently considered machine learning which involves trying to design rule bases which can evolve with use (Forsyth, 1984).

Michie (1974) suggests by analogy with human functions that an intelligent computer must contain an integrated cognitive system capable of forming an internal representation of its task environment, summarising the operationally relevant features and use the representation to form plans of action, execute them and check the action against the practical outcome thereby extending the representation. A comprehensive survey of A.I. terminology and developments is contained in Shapiro (1987).

This enthusiasm on the part of the information technologists to replicate or replace human functions is probably most useful in terms of its contribution to understanding human behaviour. In direct practical terms there would seem to be no value in expensively imitating human behaviour. There are five billion people in the world, most of them under-using their natural endowment of intelligence, they need support from not replacement by computers. The question is how best to delegate functions from man to machine, and this, as always, requires the understanding of interface design and of human advantages, limitations and requirements.

The human–computer interface

In Chapter 1 it was suggested that for machine- or process-control the interface design is not merely a matter of matching displays to the characteristics of the eyes and ears, the display should also be structured to match human perceptual characteristics and the dynamic response of controls should be matched to the timing characteristics of human performance (Fig. 5.7(*a*)). Correspondingly, for man–computer systems the match to the operator is much more than screens which suit the eyes in terms of brightness, contrast, colours, flicker and so on, and controls at the right height with appropriate key depression mechanics. The output resulting from the computation can be configured in a variety of ways and the guide to this configuration should be the task requirements as conceived by the operator. When this is done the display will match his perceptual processes. Similarly what the operator attempts to do is determined again by the task demands but also by the functional tools which are available and which are seen to be available. Thus the software specification for any generic human task can be separated into three parts: the software that operates on the data, the software that provides functional tools which the operator can use and the software driving the display (Fig. 5.7(*b*)).

The objective is to make the functional system visible or transparent, and this incorporates not only the software driving the computer but also the manual design and design of any required training. If all this is done effectively we have a usable system. The construction of a usability index (Shackel, 1984) depends on the identification of all the relevant parameters and methods of measurement for them. From the customer's point of view an integrated usability index may be sufficient for the comparison of competitive systems, but as a guide for the designer or for the user who has a particular set of tasks to deal with the separate parameters need to be listed.

The design of the human–computer information channel is a matter of enabling the user to do what he wants to do.

User requirements

What the user wants to do is specified by task descriptions (Chapter 1).

In considering the detailed needs of users it is appropriate to distinguish kinds of systems:

- general purpose systems usually on personal computers requiring intermediate level skills, e.g. word-processing, use of spread sheets
- systems intended to provide or support functions normally human-

based but absent or reduced, e.g. highly repetitive training and specialised control facilities for disabled individuals
– inquiry systems for use by the public, e.g. catalogues, time-tables
– special purpose systems requiring specific high level skills, e.g. analysis using particular statistical procedures, modelling
– computer driven control systems, e.g. process-control rooms, simulators

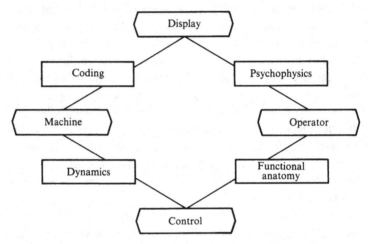

Fig. 5.7(*a*). Man–machine communication.

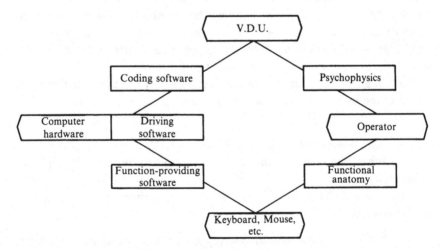

Fig. 5.7(*b*). Man–computer communication.

Clearly systems of these different kinds require separate approaches, not only to interface/facilities design but also to required support from manuals, training and assumed background skills.

For each system there is now available standard hardware and also standard software packages appropriate to many of the routines required. This is important because, although hardware and general purpose packages are inexpensive, the generation of tailor-made software remains expensive and also difficult to organise because of the shortage of skilled software writers.

Programming effort needs to be carefully targeted and task descriptions provide one set of guidelines. There are others such as the hardware and existing software advantages and limitations. As is always true in a design context, a compromise is required between the requirements of the different disciplines. This compromise can be optimised on the basis of mutual understanding which is not easy. In particular the Human Factors contribution is often underweighted because the guidelines (Task Descriptions) cannot be so easily or precisely formulated as can guidelines from other disciplines.

Two remedies can help. One is to complete a Task Analysis not only for the users but also for the designers. This helps to convince designers of the relevance and meaning of the techniques, and persuades them to think about human aspects more generally. The second remedy is to try to ensure that users have a direct voice in the design. A Task Description is a communication vehicle between the user and the designer and if direct communication also takes place this will be less systematic but it can reinforce the message of the Task Descriptions. It is still necessary to convey to designers that users are not pale copies of designers in terms of attitudes, skills or success criteria.

At a later stage in the design process this communication can be reinforced by evaluation based on user performance. Most computer companies now have Human Factors laboratories with elaborate facilities for recording performance from video cameras to multichannel records of events with time-stamps. Behind the technological facade there are all the standard human performance problems of what to record and why and how to condense the mass of readily obtainable evidence into a concise and coherent set of conclusions. It must be admitted that the contribution of the Human Factors specialist is based on experience and a general awareness of the importance of these problems rather than on a library of evaluated agreed methodology available for selective application.

Robotics

Computers can do no more than process information. In common with committees it is easy for those involved to persuade themselves that this is the key feature of all human activity. It is a key feature, but in isolation it is useless. Following a committee decision someone out there has to do something, and similarly the output of information processing has to be translated into action. If action is to be effective there must be guidance from inputs both before it and after it. Information processing has no meaning without information to process and effectors which can act on the basis of the processing. All systems must have power as well as information. This is obvious but it has to be continuously reiterated because it is so easily overlooked. There is much misguided talk about this being the information age.

Robots can translate the output of an information process into action, and can supply information to process. These functions are more difficult than information processing because power engineering is intrinsically more prone to operational difficulties and obstacles than is information engineering. This is partly because there have to be many interfaces: between the system and its environment, between information dominant processes and power dominant processes and even between mechanical moving parts.

Organisms, the prototypes of all efficient active systems, have sensors, joints and muscles as well as central nervous systems. Robots remain primitive because of the difficulty of designing the equivalents of sensors and joints. Nevertheless computer–robot systems are of fundamental general support to the human operator because they can carry out repetitive processes reliably, these processes are the basis of manufacturing industry, but they are not what people enjoy as full-time occupations. Robots are more expendable than people and thus are invaluable for highly dangerous processes.

Human factors aspects of robotics include problems of design in terms of precise allocation of function, interfaces for setting programmes and monitoring (these functions always remain with the human operator) and the difficulties and hazards of maintenance. Noro (1987) contains a review of health and safety aspects.

Conclusion

Support for the human operator can be summarised as the reduction of drudgery in computation and in other repetitive activities. In sub-systems such as word-processors they can provide much improved facilities for correcting errors and allowing changes of ideas and structures. The speed of computer computation is such as to support and even surpass human functions such as sampling and modelling system performance and reacting to threats in the military field. Storage of knowledge and data is not that much superior to paper-based methods except in ease of modifications and variety of modes of access. The obstacles to providing greater support are currently not so much within computation but in related processes such as robotics.

The conception and description of new generations of computers always seems to be essentially technology driven. It ought to be possible to start instead from the characteristics and needs of the human operator whose performance the computer is intended to support.

There are two possibilities: one is to re-think the basic architecture of the computer on more human information processing lines and the other is to reconsider the development of orthodox computing as a more matching aid to human cognitive performance.

The relevant characteristics of human performance are:

- a totally integrated process for which terms such as information acceptance, processing, storage and decision-making are artificially isolated sub-processes
- the input is highly selective and the output is essentially four-dimensional, that is, a three-dimensional spatial activity which inherently develops along the time dimension
- the development in time (learning) is a cycle of hypothesis generation, output, feedback and revision
- the internal processing is a 'push-me-pull-you' combination where output processes control inputs and input processes control outputs.
- It is mixed analogue and digital or in other terminology reactive, iconic and symbolic

The difficulties of producing a computer-based support for behavioural activity described in this way are enormous but interesting. The requirement is for imaginative information technology combined with an intuitive feel for how the human operator works.

5.4 Applications

5.4.1 Human–Computer Interface design
The U.K. organisational structure

HCI is now the preferred jargon rather than the more general man–machine interface (MMI) which was popular some years ago in the U.K. The topic received a considerable boost from the Alvey (1982) Committee (a joint committee of the Department of Trade and Industry, the Ministry of Defence and the Department of Education and Science) which decided that MMI was one of the four key aspects to the successful advance and exploitation of information technology (IT). The others were Intelligent Knowledge Based Systems (IKBS), Software Engineering (SE) and Very Large Scale Integration (VLSI). Accordingly considerable funds were provided for joint academic/industrial research in this area with an emphasis on application. The human interface was regarded as one of four topics within MMI; the others were speech processing, image processing and display technology. Not surprisingly, progress as indicated in the Annual reports (Alvey 1984–7) has been slow. This is partly because of the intrinsic difficulty of these research topics, partly because of the relative weakness of the supporting sciences, and partly because it was not appreciated, and indeed is still not appreciated, that although the problems appear to be scientifically intractable the remedial procedures and practical solutions are often very simple. For example, the creation of an effective display depends on the degree of mutual understanding between the designer and the user. The designer needs to know the objectives, skills and limitations of the user, the user needs to appreciate the facilities which the designer can and cannot provide. In short, they must communicate. Although this communication is bound to be difficult because of the different attitudes, knowledge and objectives, there are other specialists such as marketeers and ergonomists whose expertise is intended to facilitate this communication.

In considering the required direction of post-Alvey effort, the Bide (1987) Committee also placed considerable emphasis on the Human Interface (HI) and generated two lists (Table 5.8); factors understood but not often applied and factors not fully understood and not applied. It will be noted that there is no list of factors understood and applied. It is suggested above that in principle there should be a list of factors 'not understood but satisfactorily applied'. There are European programmes corresponding to the Alvey programme: ESPRIT, RACE and EUREKA. In all cases there is emphasis on the twin problems of technological advance and application. This latter is often called technological transfer. A recent Alvey Report (Morgan *at al.*, 1988) shows some signs of moving towards a more integrated approach to IKBS, SE and HI, but still treats them as separate areas of study.

Input systems

Generally these are not a problem. Inputs across interfaces with other systems e.g. process control, are fast and reliable. They usually consist of cyclical sampling systems used to update data in the computer. The main Human Factors requirement is some transparency so that monitoring and fault diagnosis are facilitated.

Inputs from human operators are basically through keyboards which are now well designed in terms of relative positions, e.g. shape and distance apart, pressure requirements and labelling. The meaning of key arrays can be changed by using menu systems where a display appears with key numbers labelled as particular functions for particular purposes. Selection within a menu can also be made by moving a cursor using keys, a mouse, a rolling ball

Table 5.8. *Human factors aspects of human computer interfaces*

(modified from Bide, 1987)

Factors understood but not often applied
Physical environment
Control design
Display design
User training
Factors not fully understood and not applied
Pattern recognition
Mental load/fatigue
Decision-making
Dialogue structure
Command standardisation
Work patterns
Organisational structures
Cultural influence
Market/User expectations

or a control lever. The mouse is currently popular. It is a hemisphere or cube which is manually moved across a surface topologically matching the screen and also contains activate buttons. Points on the screen can also be selected by light pens or by direct finger pointing (the touch screen).

One of the few apparently non-optimal features of human operator design is that the best location in relation to the body for hand–finger manipulations is not the best location for highest acuity vision. For this reason the keyboard and the mouse are easier to use than the touch screen.

Display systems

VDU screens are invariably used for this purpose. As the size and definition of screens improves, communication is facilitated in that it is possible to provide the operator with larger and better structured presentations. Colour also can be used to improve discrimination, there can be displays within displays (windows), the screen can be split into static and dynamic parts and digital data can be superimposed on schematic diagrams. Nevertheless, even so-called high definition screens do not yet approach the quality of presentation using print and diagrams on paper, or large consoles of data containing many hard-wired displays. Facilities are available for zooming and overlap of adjacent frames which partially compensate for the limited total presentation on one screen.

Format design remains an art although the appropriate questions can be listed:

- how many screens are needed
- how much data to put on a given picture
- how many levels there should be
- how the separations down the hierarchy are determined
- how to mix numerical and graphic presentations
- how to do picture joining and/or overlapping
- how to mix functional and geographical pictures
- how to mix mimics and other structures

It is not obvious how to relate screened information with other information on maps, wall diagrams, telephones and paper-based data in manuals, operating instructions and from chart recorders and printers.

At present all operators seem to devote skill and effort to collating data from different sources, recording data to match other data and generally shifting attention around the complex of available presentations.

Conclusion

The more widespread application of user-centred computer design depends on many factors, from customer demand and competition between manufacturers to availabilities of standards and techniques for acquiring and presenting relevant evidence. Williges (1987) surveys the many kinds of models available for potential use in interface design. These models are still largely underdeveloped in that they need to be applied by human factors specialists rather than directly by designers.

Knowledge of intellectual position implies clarity of concepts which in turn depends on extensive communication with others of like mind. Concept development and communication depend on agreed shared modelling of the issue under consideration.

Licklider (1982) considers the particular issue of communication between systems scientists and behavioural scientists. His paper was given in the context of discussions about cooperation and cross-fertilisation between the NATO Special Programme Panels on Systems Science and Human Factors respectively. Following a penetrating analysis of the parameters or dimensions governing effective communication, Licklider concludes that progress might be made by setting up a pilot project where success would depend on interaction between the relevant disciplines. These include systems analysis, operations research, management science, systems engineering, cybernetics, communication science, control theory, human factors engineering, ergonomics, demography, political science, computer science, information science, and the various kinds of applied psychology. The total knowledge content and practical expertise is not as formidable as the length of this list appears to indicate. All these subjects are relatively new and there is extensive overlap.

Experience with every kind of information system confirms that performance in practice is most likely to be limited by inadequate design attention to the computer input/output systems. These are often interfaces with a human operator and it is therefore necessary that system designers should have some acquaintance with the characteristics and limitations of human performance. This is itself a communication problem with which we are not successfully coping at the present time for several reasons:

- most computer system designers have a physical sciences/engineering background based on concepts and methods which are qualitatively different from those used in the behavioural sciences
- the behavioural sciences are relatively weak in theory and methods although less so in useful principles and guidelines usually called Human Factors or ergonomics
- the number of competent Human Factors specialists is very small compared with the number of Information engineers

5.4.2 Military control centres

The history of the development of military systems is nicely encapsulated in the acronyms. Originally they were Command systems, then they became Command and Control systems, C^2, then Command, Control and Communication systems, C^3, currently they are known as either Command, Control, Communication and Intelligence systems, C^3I, or Command, Control, Communication and Management systems, C^3M.

In the future they may be called networks rather than centres because many of the current problems are to do with collecting intelligence and distributing orders. The networks contain many man–machine sub-systems: some concerned with inputting data either locally or centrally, and some with action, but even the action units report back on their activities and their observations.

Thus, as in all control centres, information exchange is between people as well as between machines and people. The necessary criteria of a Command and Control centre are that there is a large data processing system used by a team of operators controlling a system which contains more human operators (Singleton, 1988), (Fig. 5.8). People are also involved in collating and interpreting the data before it is presented to the senior decision-makers. For example, a navigation centre on a ship may consist of three operators. Two are collecting data from the many sources: radar, sonar, other ships and air surveillance, and entering it into a system controlled by a more senior operator who is essentially a picture builder. The task is to create the best estimate of the position of the ship in relation to other units, some below the surface, some on the surface, some in the air. The picture includes friends and foes. It is an estimate because much of the data is uncertain. Directional data is usually better than range data, but some, put out by the enemy, may be intentionally misleading. This picture may be relayed elsewhere or may be directly observed by someone responsible for taking action. In cases of extreme urgency when the ship is being attacked the responses may be largely automatic once the targets have been identified. Target identification and location is also the problem of an artillery spotting unit which again will consist of three people. Two will be involved in guiding the sensors (which will probably be airborne with or without pilots) and accepting the data generated. There will be a third more senior man again providing a picture and indicating priorities to his subordinates. This picture or its consequences in terms of required actions will also be transmitted elsewhere.

Thus central control rooms receive some raw data and some pre-arranged pictures for which the authenticity is dependent on the skills of a hierarchy of operators within the communication system. A typical C³I centre will have

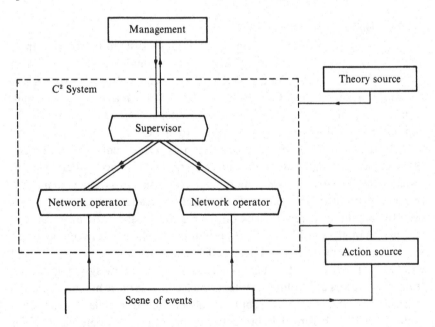

Fig. 5.8. The generic Command and Control system.

large wall maps with movable symbols, computer-driven displays of maps and text, and various kinds of hard-copy messages which have arrived via telecommunication devices. There will be a key operator trying to make sense of all this data, some unknown part of which is either spurious or intentionally misleading. The presented information is intended to reduce the uncertainty as to what is located where and in what strength. The key operator will be a senior officer supported by his staff and advised by experts in meteorology, politics and other specialities. One of his central questions is always 'what will the consequences of my decisions look like on the world television screens tomorrow?', and he is constrained by 'rules of engagement' determined by even more senior officers in consultation with their political masters.

The ergonomic design problems are:
– lack of knowledge of cognitive processes. There is an extensive literature about generalised problem-solving and decision-making, some of it related to the military context (Sage, 1981, Wohl, 1981). This provides guidelines but it is not specific enough to relate to the different cognitive processes of designers, information technologists and military personnel at different levels of authority. Senior officers coping with strategies are different from junior officers coping with action and data gathering including picture-building, and different again from non-commissioned personnel interpreting signals. Operator displays and operator aids should ideally be matched not just to human operators but to the particular kind and level of human operator. Currently this can only be attained by leaving enough flexibility to tailor design in the light of experience
– starting from the principle that an operator at any level is modelling reality and updating his model using data presentations, the question becomes how best to support this modelling activity. The process is an interactive one in that the displays should match the operator's model but equally the model will adjust to match the displays. The model and the displays must also match reality if the emergent decisions are to be effective. Reality is a geographical space containing mobile units each with its own characteristics. Superimposed on this are a set of political constraints summarised in the rules of engagement plus the important climatic variables. This conceptual framework provides a basis on which the total display array can be evaluated
– a specific difficulty about military reactions is that there is an intelligent enemy out there. A key element of skill is the facility to generate fitting responses which contain an element of surprise. This is called *flair*. It is an intuitive rather than an intellectual ability and little is known about how to support it using information presentations. The response generated may be at

the strategic or the tactical level and presumably it is a holistic response based on an overall appreciation of the situation

   – detailed design of displays within the total presentation is a matter of standard display design principles

   – the senior operator has no effector problems, he simply gives orders which others translate into output signals.

   – aids in the form of supportive dynamic models are difficult to arrange because there are too many variables. Prediction is rarely feasible, not just because of the range of error in extrapolation, but because there can be dramatic discontinuities following localised defeats and victories or weather changes

   – the picture-builders do have effector problems from the orientation of their sensors to selectivity and weighting attached to incoming signals. They can be aided by the use of software which will cope, better than can the human operator, with issues such as lines of sight when there is extensive movement in three spatial dimensions, e.g. on how to move an aerial sensor across hilly terrain in limited visibility. The problem of a mobile sensor is where it is as well as what it detects

   – the orthodox comparatively rigid military hierarchies simplify some of people interaction problems. The distinction between orders, advice and information is clearly understood

   – the remaining problems of work-space design are the same as for any other kind of work-space, these are listed in greater detail in the next section. The contrasting if complementary approaches to design which can be driven respectively by engineering technology, behaviour parameters, computer technology and task analysis are described in more detail in Singleton (1987).

5.4.3 *Process control centres*

   Control rooms for industrial plants are easier to design and operate successfully than military command and control centres for several reasons:

     – the data presented is not distorted by pre-processing dependent on human judgement

     – the system controlled is passive, there are no enemy intelligence and unpredictable reactions to be coped with

     – there are no intruding unpredictable factors such as weather changes

     – the operating life is much longer so that there is greater opportunity to develop the required specialist skills using feed-back from experience

     – human errors have, in most cases, merely economic costs. There can be costs in human lives because of energy and toxic substances released and there are occasional catastrophes, but these are rare compared with what happens routinely in military systems used in their designed context of warfare

– political overtones and problems of coping with mass-media exist but are relatively much less severe.

In relation to the last two points, nuclear plants have a special problem in that, when the stress on the operators is greatest during emergencies there are likely to be further stresses due to other agencies, some internal from senior management, and some external from mass-media wanting to know what is happening. The remedy is yet another information centre between the main control room and the inquirers.

The design problems can be separated into a number of categories corresponding to different functions. The centre is a work-space occupied by a team, an interface with the plant, a management centre and an information centre.

A team work-space

As noted in the discussion above of centralised control systems, a primary issue is the size of the team. Generally there is a core of two or three: a supervisor and one or two desk operators, but there will be other staff who are legitimately present although not on a full-time basis, such as trainees, maintenance staff and managers. Thus there is a requirement for a number of dedicated work-spaces and an additional requirement for discussion space. On the question of standing versus sitting, the usual compromise is that each full-time operator should have his own desk equipped with a battery of VDUs and telephones and with adequate space for paperwork. However, when he is manipulating plant variables he will do so from a standing position in front of large wall consoles of instrumentation containing hard-wired displays, controls and more VDUs. A large control centre can have more than 30 VDUs.

The size of the room will be determined by the location of these work-spaces, the number of VDUs and the required area of control and hard-wired presentations, and the necessary storage for documentaion.

There are two questions to be decided at a policy level, should there be windows and should there be a public gallery. There is a strong case for public galleries, not only in terms of public relations, they can be used by staff for official visitors particularly if there is telecommunication with the control room. Such a gallery provides an intermediate alternative to actually entering the control room, and room entry should be severely restricted. The case against windows is based mainly on security, although they do take up valuable wall space and the lighting level is then not entirely controllable. Internal windows overlooking large plant areas are a useful compromise. Another possibility is to have windows in the rest room but not in the control room. Security is important, the popular concept of the control room as the brain or nerve centre of the plant is a fair one. There may be more vulnerable parts of the plant but these would not be known to outsiders.

The room should also be protected from fire and disturbances such as aircraft crashes or missile attacks. Particular care is needed in the design of the heating/ventilating system. Lighting and colour design are difficult as evidenced by the fact that few existing rooms seem to demonstrate satisfactory solutions. Lighting is a necessary compromise between the incompatible requirements of screens, dials, control surfaces and documents. Furniture and floor surfaces are often neglected because they are not regarded as being within the engineering design remit. They relate to the problem of ambient noise which can be serious, not only as a general stress factor, but also as an interference with communication between team members.

A plant interface

This is the best understood function of the control centre, indeed the most common criticism is that a centre has been designed as just this, and the other functions have not been recognised as design issues. The orthodox view is even more restricted in looking only at the dynamic displays and controls. The static displays; legends, mimics and documentation are essential parts of the total information presentation. Procedures can form a whole library of volumes: there are operating instructions, maintenance instructions, suppliers handbooks on sub-systems, safety instructions and emergency instructions. The allocation between hard-wired and data-processed presentations is governed by the criterion that it should be possible to control the plant, at least on a short-term basis, without the data-processor. The division of the total plant instrumentation into categories normally follows the sequence of material, power or information flows from inputs to outputs, but it must relate also to the tasks allocated within the team. Task-related consoles should be nearest to the desk of the responsible operator, but the more tightly coupled the system is the more difficult it becomes to separate out discrete sections of the instrumentation and supporting data-processing. Problems can arise because ideally two operators may need to function in front of the same console at the same time. Recently the question has arisen as to whether or not consoles and other control room complexes including desks should be dimensioned to accommodate the female as well as the male population. The grouping of displays and controls must be considered in the context of many relevant factors, there are many quite different equally valid solutions each with its particular snags.

In addition to plant interfaces concerned with allowing the operator to monitor the system and enter the control loops, there can be a variety of operator-aid interfaces concerned with specialist problems such as safety requirements and fault diagnosis.

Given the variety of roles and tasks it becomes increasingly difficult to select the architecture of the basic interface and to provide methods for presenting all the contributing functions so that optimal design decisions can be made. Once this has been settled, the traditional problems of ease of operation and error minimisation in terms of reading displays and activating controls are relatively straightforward.

A management centre

Given the knowledge of system state which exists in the control room, it is a natural choice as the centre for controlling other activities such as maintenance. Security also can (in some cases but not all) be regarded as a main control room responsibility, because some surveillance devices intended for system monitoring can also be used as parts of security checking systems.

An information centre

The main control room is always the plant information centre. As such it may receive data from many sources including customers, e.g. in a power station the grid control communicates directly with the control room supervisor. Other sources and destinations in addition to the plant itself are the related control rooms, some of which may be off-site, for example, a media information centre or the control rooms of other plants which may share the same geographical site. The plant senior management will also need close contact with their control centre. The interface for most of these transactions is the telephone, but the design of the overall telephonic system is rarely given its proper priority, and the extensive load which arises from telephones is rarely considered in terms of its interaction with routine plant control tasks. For example, an operator may be interrupted several times whilst he is attempting to follow a complex procedure. In large control rooms this can be sufficiently serious to warrant consideration of a manned telephone switchboard within the control room. Logging or recording of exchanges by telephone is rarely taken seriously.

Communication with maintenance personnel is important for several reasons:

- the control room staff are the detectors of requirements for remedial maintenance
- when routine maintenance is undertaken the control room staff need to know because the effects will be visible on their displays. In particular, if a sub-system is shut-down temporarily the control room

staff may need to energise a back-up sub-system. Thus a procedure is required whereby permission of the control room staff must be obtained before any maintenance task is undertaken, this requires another communication sub-system with its own procedures. The control room staff must record what is happening in logs, and perhaps directly on the interface, not only for their own benefit but because the hiatus may carry over to succeeding shifts

– plant-based staff are needed by the control-room staff as scouts or messengers particularly during emergencies

Given such close interaction there is a case for specialist displays which indicate where maintenance staff are and what they are doing.

During night shifts, the control centre or its adjacent offices may contain the senior plant staff on duty. Thus they will need to be directly accessible to the outside world if responsible decisions or comments are required.

5.4.4 Aviation psychology

One of the main triggers for the development of ergonomics was the difficulties of pilots attempting to control aircraft. This kind of vehicle is potentially unstable, manifestly dangerous and demands fast reactions on the part of the controller. There is elaborate instrumentation to facilitate control in three spatial dimensions within which there are also interactions. Time is an additional and dominant variable because there are speed minima which are different in various conditions, such as cruising, taking off and landing, and consequently there is no possibility of suspending the basic function of flying to reappraise a particular situation, however complex. Since visual cues to geographic location are limited, there is further instrumentation concerned with navigation. Not withstanding all the elaborate artificial displays, the pilot still requires a view of the real world through the windscreen, and thus there are matching or compatibility problems between real and artificial displays.

In spite of all the hazards, flying – particularly commercial flying – is quite remarkably safe as measured, for example, by fatalities per passenger mile. This is a consequence of very high system reliability which in turn is a function of the meticulous care devoted to design, training, operations and maintenance, all with a proper emphasis on the importance of effective man–machine interaction.

There are three main kinds of pilot skilled in coping respectively with transport aircraft, military aircraft and light aircraft. Their tasks and problems are different in some respects but nevertheless they have many common tasks and all interact with another important operator with different tasks and skills:

the Air Traffic Controller. This partnership is not going to be removed by any foreseeable technological advances. The passenger and the public generally will insist that every aircraft contains a pilot and every flight is monitored by a human controller.

There is a potential communication problem between the two in that the pilot sees himself at the centre of his perceptual world with other aircraft around him, the A.T. Controller sees a total dynamic pattern of aircraft. This 'inside looking out' versus 'outside looking in' distinction can lead to confusion. Emotionally also there is a difference (which becomes accentuated if danger increases) in that the pilot feels very strongly his personal responsibility for the safety of passengers and crew, whilst the A.T. Controller naturally takes a more intellectual if equally responsible view of the safety of the aircraft.

It follows that the air/ground dialogue should be very carefully designed in terms of expected content, procedures and supporting information systems taking into account both cognitive and emotional aspects. Analysis of such conversation supports the view that there is a strong element of mutual reassurance as an overtone to the supposedly highly rational interchange.

In Human Factors design terms there should be continuously developing role analysis, task analysis and transactional analysis as the potentialities of new software, hardware and data networks become clearer.

The information support system has an enormous data content, and there is a need for prioritising. One manifestation of an alarm system is the automatic detection of the possibility of mid-air collision. In principle both in the air and on the ground we have a requirement for a presentation of a four-dimensional system in a hierarchical fashion. Separation into linked two-dimensional data formats requires extensive ergonomics expertise.

The pilot

Both the small aircraft cockpit and the large aircraft flight deck are confined spaces. The operator cannot move around, he has foot controls and he may be subjected to buffeting so that seat design is the first critical problem. The restricted space and the requirement for urgent action lead to the principle of wrapping the interface around the operator in a densely packaged form. Incidently, because so much of the ergonomics pioneering work was done on the pilot, there is a tendency to regard this style as ideal for all work situations and there is much misapplied ergonomics in attempting to make other work-situations look like cockpits. If, as is normally the case in industry, urgency is rare and space is not at a premium, there is much to be said for spreading the interface over a large area, this has many advantages from the reduced probability of confusing the identity of particular displays and controls to the value of a little exercise in moving around. On the flightdeck the packaging problem is now less serious with the replacement of many hard-wired displays by multi-purpose VDUs and the replacement of direct analogue type controls by 'manoeuvre demand' selective controls.

Much of the general research on various aspects of interface design was stimulated and developed in the context of flying, so that most of the principles and recommendations in ergonomics textbooks and manuals explicitly or implicitly refer to what is best for the pilot. This is also true for processes extended over time such as selection, training, simulation and fatigue. The need for rapid reactions resulted in the development of predictive displays and quickened displays (Fogel, 1963). A predictive display presents future status estimated by extrapolation from current status which is presented in parallel. It increases the required rate of information acceptance, but hopefully reduces the corresponding rate of information processing. The time interval of prediction may not be obvious and may mislead the operator. A quickened display (p. 212) again should reduce the human information processing required and can certainly reduce training time or required skill level. It will contribute to stability but reduces manoeuvrability. The information portrayed is false as an indicator of geographical system state.

In task terms the pilot is much more than an 'in the loop' controller. For recent generations of highly instrumented and automated aircraft he is a system monitor, planner and manager (Thorne and Charles, 1978). He is also the centre of an elaborate verbal communication system. He must be able to carry out several tasks apparently simultaneously, and he must resist many kinds of stress from disturbance of circadian rhythms (p. 167) to continuous awareness that an emergency may arise at any moment (Edwards, 1979). A review of the psychologists' contribution to the effective control of aircraft is contained in Roscoe (1980).

Current problems of flightdeck interface designers include the design of screen formats, design of alarm systems, access to procedures and the optimal use of computer-based aiding. As in other control centres there can be difficulties if the information coding is too elaborate and there is insufficient access to the raw data, reliance on computer control will result in a diminution of manual control skills, and provision of whole or part solutions to problems will diminish cognitive skills. Training and evaluation are better organised and controlled in the aviation industry than in any other. On the flightdeck of commercial aircraft there are management issues such as the 'authority gradient' across crew members, decisions such as when or whether to take off, and how and when to complete all the required paperwork.

In common with the air traffic controller the skill problem is to maintain a four-dimensional model of reality which is updated by visual and verbal information. A recent review of all Human Factors aspects of flying is contained in Hawkins (1987).

The air traffic controller

The density of aircraft in flight particularly near major centres of population is such that control from the ground is essential. Whitfield and Stammers (1978) point out that although safety is the primary objective there are others, in particular expediency and orderliness. Expediency in the sense of minimal interference from other aircraft results in considerable economies not only in fuel but also in passengers' time. Orderliness is important for matters such as full utilisation of airways and runways, and for ensuring that the international medley of aircraft and flight-crews conform to agreed procedures and cooperate with each other through the controller. The 'picture' which is the controller's internal model contains a developing pattern of all the aircraft in his sector, together with details of identity, their height and other attributes. This information is all presented on a screen, and at first sight such a screen appears impossible to comprehend. The controller does it on the basis of his acquired skills and because the picture develops continuously, the time dimension is important to him not only because of the potential consequences but because it provides continuity, he can perceive what is happening at any instant because it follows from what was happening previously. He positively contributes to the changing picture not only by redirecting aircraft but also by formally accepting new entries and removing exits from his sector. Unlike the pilot, almost all his output is verbal rather than motor, but his auditory interface with all the pilots he is talking to matches and reinforces the visual picture presented on the screen. He must follow highly standardised procedures, and if these are not skilfully designed they can lead to distrust and lack of respect for management. It is the nature of the job – mental load, shift work, the continuous presence of potential hazards and the need to interact with many individuals – that conflicts within the organisation seem to arise very easily. Hence the importance of a well-developed organisational structure. High technology systems still depend on the morale of practitioners which is a function of task design, training and management support. At the extreme any system is useless if the staff are on strike.

For any design changes it is even more than usually important that there should be the potentiality for smooth transition from the old to the new system. For this and other reasons the Human Factors approach to systems analyses should contain task and skills analyses of the operator, the manager, the designer and the human factors specialist.

5.4.5 Checklists and standards

A checklist normally consists of a series of questions or headings which need to be considered in the context of a particular design problem or objective, e.g. Table 5.5. They may be addressed to a designer, a human factors specialist or an evaluator such as a safety engineer. They can be advantageous for several reasons:

- much if not most of ergonomics practice amounts to little more than considering the matter in terms of the user's requirements and limitations. Once the question has been posed an answer follows. The answer is not usually unique, and does not require great expertise or very precise numerical evidence. For example, a checklist provided in Murrell (1965) asks the questions 'What are expected maintenance requirements? Has the equipment been designed to make the diagnosis of faults easy? Has the equipment been planned so that probable repairs can be carried out with minimum delay? Are all locations for regular maintenance accessible? A checklist can contain supporting guidelines and data as well as questions
- for any design there will be many related questions and even a specialist ergonomist may overlook some of them. It is not always possible to proceed systematically on the basis of concepts and principles, what is required may have emerged from previous experience. A checklist can meet these requirements. For example, in checking the 'information conditions' it is tempting to launch immediately into an analysis of displays thus overlooking the primary source of information for any worker which is contained in the instructions from his supervisor
- if a checklist can be structured in terms of theory then it provides a useful summary of the pattern of factors to be considered in relation to a particular kind of design exercise. For example, the general purpose checklist produced by the International Ergonomics Association (reproduced in Edholm, 1967) is subdivided under the main headings shown in Table 5.9. This is effectively the content of ergonomics as conceived by the IEA at the time
- the structure may alternatively be used to indicate an appropriate series of questions which are more effectively dealt with in a particular order for the particular purpose. For example, a checklist for evaluating new machine tools from the ergonomics viewpoint
- checklists are useful on education or training courses to provide

Table 5.9. *The structure of ergonomics as indicated in the IEA general purpose check-list*

(from Edholm, 1967)

Work space		
	Physical demands	
	Mental demands	
		Vision
		Hearing
		Other senses
		Dials and
		Displays
Work method		
	Physical demands	
	Mental demands	
	Flow of information	
Environment load		
Organisation of work		

students with guidance during their first attempts to conduct practical ergonomics appraisals

Standards are often structured in the same way as checklists in detailing the various aspects to be considered. However, there is a much stronger requirement to provide data about limits, or at least guidelines in relation to each parameter. Standards have been slow to develop in the ergonomics field because of the difficulty of meeting this requirement.

Pursuit of standards takes place at three levels. Large purchasing bodies such as Departments of Defence may promulgate their own standards, all advanced countries have their systems of national standards, and finally there are international standards.

Standards may relate directly to interface elements such as displays or keyboards, or may relate to general characteristics of the operator such as body size and sensory limitations. The attempt to get agreement within a committee of experts on any such topic very quickly reveals the limitations of established knowledge and the requirement for a level of precision from which many research workers in this field recoil. Thus standards are of value not only in relation to design issues, but also in generating a particular form of discipline on research thinking and a way of identifying gaps in knowledge. Committees setting standards often involve producers, users and government representatives, as well as scientists, and it is therefore not surprising that political issues and specialist pleading by pressure groups confuse and impede the development of standards. Nevertheless the process is desirable to facilitate exchange of goods and services between countries. They provide yet another avenue of communication between the intellectual and scientific approach on the one hand, and the technological and economic approach on the other.

National bodies include the French N.F., the British B.S. and the German D.I.N. Some of their standards are taken over directly for international use and vice versa, but in other cases, e.g. anthropometry, the international standard refers only to definitions and principles and it is the national standards which contain data profiles for the particular national populations.

The International Standards Organisation (ISO) is a very large institution with 2000 technical committees (TCs) and sub-committees (SCs). Many standards for specialist machines and special problems contain ergonomic data and there is in addition a committee (TC159) which specialises in ergonomics. It is intended to cover terminology, methods and data. It has six sub-committees and many more working groups. For example, SC5 on the physical environment has three working groups. Other sub-committee specific topics are guiding principles, particular ergonomics requirements, anthropometry and biomechanics (SC3), signals and controls (SC4) and work systems (SC6). In 1984, 42 countries out of a total ISO membership of 75 countries were involved in TC159, 16 as participants and 26 as observers (Metz, 1985). On the face of it this would indicate that there are 16 countries who consider that they have the expertise and the interest to cooperate in generating international ergonomic standards.

Standards in relation to information processing are more difficult to define and agree than are standards to do with corporal variables such as body size. There is another ISO committee (TC97) which specialises in personal computers and office equipment. This has included topics such as keyboards (ISO/TC97/SC18/WG7) but the personnel/computer interface topic rests with TC159.

References

Alvey, J. (1982). *A Programme for Advanced Information Technology*. London: H.M.S.O.

Alvey Programme. (1984–7). *Annual reports*. London: I.E.E.

Baron, S. and Kleinman, D.L. (1969). The human as an optimum controller and information processor. *I.E.E.E. Transactions. M.M.S.* **10.1**. 9–17.

Bartlett, F.C. (1932). *Remembering*. Cambridge University Press.

Bernotat, R.K. and Gartner, K-P. (1972). *Displays and Controls*. Section on Theory of manual control. Amsterdam: Swets and Zeitlinger.

Bide, A. (1987). *Information Technology – a Plan for Concerted Action*. London: H.M.S.O.

Carbonell, J.R. (1966). A queueing model of many instrument visual sampling. *I.E.E.E. Transactions. HFE*. 7. 157–64.

Cherry, C. (1966). *On Human Communication*. Cambridge, Mass.: M.I.T. Press.

Crossman, E.R.F.W. (1969). Information theory in psychological measurement. In Meetham, A.R. and Hudson, R.A. (eds.). *Encyclopaedia of Linguistics, Information and Control*. Oxford: Pergamon.

Davies, D.R. and Parasuraman, R. (1982). *The Psychology of Vigilance*. London: Academic Press.

Easterby, R. (1984). Tasks, processes and display design. In Easterby, R. and Zwaga H. (eds.). *Information Design*. Colchester: Wiley.

Edholm, O.G. (1967). *The Biology of Work*. London: Weidenfeld and Nicolson.

Edwards, E. (1979). The expert pilot. In Singleton, W.T. (ed.). *The Study of Real Skills. Vol. 2. Compliance and Excellence*. Lancaster: M.T. Press.

Fitts, P.M. (1954). The information capacity of the human motor system in controlling the amplitude of movement. *Journal of Experimental Psychology*. 47, 381–91.

Fogel, L.J. (1963). *Biotechnology: Concepts and Applications*. New Jersey: Prentice-Hall.

Forsyth, R. (ed.) (1984). *Expert Systems*. London: Chapman and Hall.

Garner, W.R. (1962). *Uncertainty and Structure as Psychological Concepts*. New York: Wiley.

Gibson, J.J. (1968). *The Senses considered as Perceptual Systems*. London: George Allen & Unwin.

Haugeland, J. (1985). *Artificial Intelligence*. Cambridge, Mass.: M.I.T. Press.

Hawkins, F. (1987). *Human Factors in Flight*. Brookfield: Gower.

Hick, W.E. (1952). On the rate of gain of information. *Quarterly Journal of Experimental Psychology*. 4. 11–26.

Hyman, R. (1953). Stimulus information as a determinant of reaction time. *Journal of Experimental Psychology*. 45. 188–96.

Kelley, C.R. (1968). *Manual and Automatic Control*. New York: Wiley.

Licklider, J.C.R. (1982). On communication between systems scientists and behaviour scientists. (Brussels: NATO Annex II to AC/137 – D/653)

MacKay, D.M. (1969). *Information, Mechanism and Meaning*. Cambridge, Mass.: M.I.T. Press.

Metz, B.G. (1985). From ergonomics to standards. *Ergonomics*. 28.8. 1197–204.

Michie, D. (1974). *On Machine Intelligence*. Edinburgh: University Press.

Morgan, C.T., Cook, J.S., Chapanis, A. and Lund, M.W. (1963). *Human Engineering Guide to Equipment Design*. New York: McGraw-Hill.

Morgan, D.G., Shorter, D.N. and Tainsh, M. (1988). *Towards System Thinking – a Joint Strategy for IKBS, SE and HI*. London: Information Engineering Directorate.

Murrell, K.F.H. (1965). *Ergonomics*. London: Chapman and Hall.

Neisser, E. (1967). *Cognitive Psychology*. New York: Appleton Century Crofts.

Newell, A. and Simon, H.A. (1972). *Human Problem Solving*. New Jersey: Prentice-Hall.

Noro, K. (ed.) (1987). *Occupational Health and Safety in Automation and Robotics*. London: Taylor & Francis.

Perrow, C. (1981). Normal accident at Three Mile Island. *Society*. **18.5**. 17–26.

Poulton, E.C. (1974). *Tracking Skills and Manual Control*. New York: Academic Press.

Rich, E. (1983). *Artificial Intelligence*. New York: McGraw-Hill.

Roscoe, S.N. (ed.) (1980). *Aviation Psychology*. Iowa: State University Press.

Rouse, W.B. (ed.) (1977). Applications of control theory in human factors. Special issue of *Human Factors*. **19**. Nos. 4 and 5.

Sage, A.P. (1981). Behavioural and organisational considerations in the design of information systems and processes for planning and decision support. *I.E.E.E. Transactions*. SMC **11.9**, 640–78.

Shackel, B. (1984). The concept of usability. In Bennett, J., Case, D., Sandelin, J. and Smith, M. (eds.). *Visual Display Terminals*. New Jersey: Prentice-Hall.

Shannon, C.E. and Weaver, W. (1949). *The Mathematical Theory of Communication*. Urbana: University of Illinois Press.

Shapiro, S.C. (ed.) (1987). *Encyclopaedia of Artificial Intelligence*. (2 vols.) Chichester: Wiley.

Sheridan, T.B. and Ferrell, W.R. (1974). *Information, Control and Decision Models of Human Performance*. Cambridge, Mass.: M.I.T. Press.

Sheridan, T.B. and Johannsen, G. (1976). *Monitoring Behaviour and ,Supervisory Control*. New York: Plenum.

Singleton, W.T. (1969). Display design: principles and procedures. *Ergonomics*. **12.4**, 519–31.

Singleton, W.T. (1972a). General theory of presentation of information. In Bernotat, R.K. and Gartner, K-P. (eds.). *Displays and Controls*. Amsterdam: Swets and Zeitlinger.

Singleton, W.T. (1972b). *Introduction to Ergonomics*. Geneva: World Health Organisation.

Singleton, W.T. (1985). Ergonomics and its application to Sizewell 'B' *in* Weaver, D.R. and Walker, J. (eds.). *The Pressurised Water Reactor and the United Kingdom*. Birmingham: University Press.

Singleton, W.T. (1987). Operator needs for alarm systems. In Colloquium on the application of computers to alarm detection, analysis and presentation. *Digest* 1987/103. London: I.E.E.

Singleton, W.T. (1988). Command and control requirements for nuclear plant. In Anthony, R.D. (ed.). *Human Reliability in Nuclear Power*. London: IBC Technical Services.

Smallwood, R. (1966). Internal models and the human instrument monitor. *I.E.E.E. Transactions*. HFE, 181–87.

Stevens, S.S. (1951). *Handbook of Experimental Psychology*. New York: Wiley.

Thorne, R.G. and Charles, G.W.F. (1978). The Pilot. In Singleton, W.T. (ed.). *The Study of Real Skills, Vol. 1. The Analysis of Practical Skills*. Lancaster: M.T. Press.

Vygotsky, L.S. (1962). *Thought and Language*. Chichester: Wiley.

Welford, A.T. (1968). *Fundamentals of Skill*. London: Methuen.

Welford, A.T. (1984). Theory and application in visual displays. In Easterby, R. and Zwaga, H. (eds.). *Information Design*. Chichester: Wiley.

Whitfield, D. and Stammers, R.B. (1978). The air traffic controller. In Singleton, W.T. (ed.). *The Study of Real Skills. Vol. 1. The Analysis of Practical Skills.* Lancaster: M.T. Press.

Wickens, C.D. (1984). *Engineering Psychology and Human Performance*. Columbus: Merrill.

Wiener, N. (1948). *Cybernetics*. New York: Wiley.

Williges, R.C. (1987). The use of models in human-computer interface design. *Ergonomics*. **30.3**, 491–502.

Winston, P. (1984). *Artificial Intelligence*. Reading, Mass.: Addison-Wesley.

Wohl, J.G. (1981). Force management decision requirements for Air Force tactical command and control. *I.E.E.E. Transactions*. SMC **11.9**, 618–39.

6 Risk and reliability

6.1. Concepts
6.1.1 Risk

Risk is associated with the undesired outcomes of an action or absence of an action. Every choice involves risk because the consequences are never certain and inevitably some consequences are less desirable than others. Statistically, risk can be defined as the sum of the probabilities of the separate undesirable consequences of an activity. As Rowe (1986) put it, risk is the downside of a gamble. Alternatively the pursuit of any objective can be assessed in cost: value terms and risks are associated with the costs. Risk is often defined as a compound measure of probability and magnitude of adverse effect, e.g. Lowrance (1980), but this complicates even further an already complex concept because the magnitudes of adverse effects involve value judgments which are idiosyncratic. With this kind of definition there can be no agreed measure of a specific risk.

Risk has become a social and technical rather than a personal problem because technology at any level generates hazards which are not confined to one person pursuing his private affairs. Even when using a hand-tool a worker who suffers or causes suffering might readily imply that the risk was generated not by him but by the tool design, by lack of appropriate training or by inadequate instructions. With higher technology the situation becomes still more complicated. A passenger in any vehicle is subject to appreciable risks over which he has no control once he has entered the vehicle. For some toxic chemicals and for ionizing radiation there is no sensory data which warns a person that he is at risk. A risk may be short-term in that if harm occurs it does so immediately, or may be long-term in that there can be a slight influence on life expectancy or on transmission of genes. Risks are not evenly distributed in that a plant which benefits the whole country has to be located in one place where the local residents are exposed to a greater risk following a disaster than are people elsewhere. This gives rise to the NIMBY (not in my back yard) phenomenon which can lead to violent expression of local opinion.

For reasons such as these a disjunction has appeared between the attitudes of technologists on the one hand and the lay public on the other. In a democracy the public naturally feel that they are entitled to participate in decisions which affect the risks to which they are exposed. Unfortunately they are not in a position to fully appreciate the scientific basis of the arguments that the experts use. This is not surprising because in most cases of complex technological decision-making the experts do not agree amongst themselves and this is readily detected by outsiders. Furthermore there is often a wide separation between the risks and benefits of technology, for example it is easy to insist on extreme safety measures for nuclear power generation without making a connection with the fact that such costly measures eventually appear on electricity bills which have to be paid by everyone. The politicians and other policy makers find it extremely difficult to arbitrate between the push of technology and the resistance of the public and they are not helped by the contribution of the mass media where generally there is a concentration on conflict (which is good entertainment) and a reliance on the superficial interview.

This is the background to the extensive research on risk over the past decade. See Schwing and Albers (1980), Berg and Maillie (1981), Green (1982), Cooper (1985), Oftedal and Brogger (1986), Singleton and Hovden (1987). Risk was originally seen as a technical problem involving calculation of probabilities of various untoward outcomes. Such data could be used to compare different strategies, to assess progress in reducing hazards and as part of the evidence needed to make decisions about technological innovation. Technology in this context covers a continuous spectrum from mechanical engineering at one extreme to pharmacology at the other. Centrally placed are the manufacturing processes which require elaborately engineered plant and also depend on the use of complex chemicals such as organic solvents for which the toxic effects are obscure. The field can be separated into two areas: one concerned with trauma where effects are dramatic and immediate and the other with the effects on health following the insidious exposure to toxic substances over long periods. In a class of its own, for historical reasons to do with nuclear bombs, is the effect of ionising radiation.

Avoidance of catastrophes is usually based on a target acceptable risk of about 10^{-6} per annum, per event or per unit. This is about the probability of being struck by lightning for one person in one year, a risk which is recognised by everyone as existing but not something to worry about. There is a striking absence of correlation between probabilities of harm due to particular events and expressed concern about such events. The extreme cases are road accidents with a fatality risk per year per person of $1:4000$ about which the public is remarkably apathetic, and the widespread fear of nuclear reactor accidents where the corresponding figure estimated in 1975 was 1:5 000 000 000 (NUREG, 1975). Such inconsistency has led to considerable research on factors other than risk probabilities which govern attitudes to hazards. Slovic *et al.* (1980) conducted a number of studies in which the opinions of various kinds of people were solicited. Risks of death from dramatic and sensational events, e.g. tornadoes, tend to be overestimated whilst those which are unspectacular, involve single victims and commonly are non-fatal are underestimated, e.g. vaccination. Nuclear power is unique because it is regarded as involuntary, delayed, unknown, uncontrollable, unfamiliar, potentially catastrophic, dreaded and severe. Since evidence about hazards is not definitive the interpretation tends to be biased towards supporting existing beliefs. Kahneman *et al.* (1982) demonstrate that subjective probability assessments are influenced by the recency and vividness of recalled events and that the way in which alternatives are posed can alter judgments. Brehmer (1987a) and Hale (1987) review the psychological research on risk assessment and related judgments. They conclude that behaviour is more coherent than it appears at first sight but it is multifactorial and certainly cannot be related directly to simple probability measures.

6.1.2   Safety

Safety is a legal rather than a behavioural concept. It has been institutionalised by legislation in all countries but there is no conceptual basis beyond the worthy but vague aspiration that within a well organised society people should not be allowed to harm themselves or each other. In common with other civic goals such as freedom, health and happiness, it is an ideal rather than an attainable objective and it has to be pursued indirectly. That is, there is no direct way of ensuring that a situation is entirely safe, various measures can be taken to reduce risks but there is always a residual potentiality for harm. The basic approach has to be agricultural rather than engineering. That is, safety cannot be systematically designed and constructed any more than a crop can. The conditions have to be optimised so that the crop creates itself. Correspondingly safety requires the optimising of context and conditions, in particular occupational safety is concerned with the design of the working environment and conditions of work, including training. The United Nations Organisation primarily concerned with occupational safety is the International Labour Office. The basic instrument which all member states are invited to ratify is Convention 155. Article 4.2 states that 'The aim of the policy shall be to prevent accidents and injury to health arising out of, linked with or occurring in the course of work, by minimising, so far as is reasonably practicable, the causes of hazards inherent in the working environment.' Many countries have similar statements in the preamble to national safety laws (Singleton 1987). Note the emphasis on the working environment which is regarded as the source of hazards rather than the worker himself. This current mode of thinking has emerged from the reformulation of safety laws which occurred in most advanced countries about 1970. In the 1987 Single European Act, Article 118a directs Member States to pay particular attention to the encouragement of improved health and safety at work.

The earliest attempts to cope with occupational hazards were laws to do with compensation passed at about the beginning of the twentieth century. The assumption was that an occupational injury was either the fault of the worker or the fault of the employer. In the latter case the worker was entitled to some compensation although not of course in the former case. The problem of degree and location of blame proved intractable and in any case cultures changed and it became accepted that a worker's need for compensation should not be so closely tied to who was at fault. Attempts to establish degree of disability (see p. 321) as a measure of required compensation also proved difficult.

There was a gradual swing towards prevention and laws regulating particular industries appeared, starting with the manifestly dangerous industries such as mining and construction. Inspectors were required to check that laws were obeyed and in most countries there were two kinds of law and often two kinds of inspector – those dealing with labour law (working hours, hygiene etc.) and those dealing with safety law (fire precautions, machine guarding etc.). The situation became increasingly confusing. In the U.K. for example, by 1960 there were seven different national inspectorates working from five government departments and local inspectors working for 1600 different local authorities. There were also new kinds of hazards, in particular the potentiality for occupational accidents such as explosions and chemical effluents which impinge on people other than employees.

Different countries produced characteristically different solutions but with common themes (Singleton 1983). Switzerland has a National Insurance Fund with which every employer has a contract so that liability rests with the Fund. The Fund is self-supporting and broadly the account with each employer is kept in balance so that the employer has a financial incentive to maintain a good safety record. Employees are responsible for taking reasonable care. The Fund maintains general services such as specialist safety expertise and provision of statistical norms for particular industries. In the U.S.A. the administrative and research aspects are separated in two federal bodies, respectively the Occupational Safety and Health Administration (OSHA) and the National

Institute for Occupational Safety and Health (NIOSH). The situation is monitored by a third body, the Bureau of Labor Statistics (BLS). The responsibility for safety is with employers and not with employees. In the U.K. the Robens Committee (1972) recommended radical changes including the rationalisation of the inspectorates under one body. These were implemented in the Health and Safety at Work etc. Act (1974) which created the Health and Safety Executive (HSE) and the Health and Safety Commission (HSC). The latter is a committee which determines policy. The key innovation is the concept of duties on employers, employees, persons in control of premises, any person who designs, manufactures, imports or supplies any article for use at work and the general public. All are required to take appropriate safety responsibility for their own activities. They are supported by an inspectorate which is responsible for advice and guidance as well as for policing. Germany and the Scandinavian countries also have legislation based on the working environment and have much stronger research efforts than does the U.K. (see 'Accidents' below). These latter countries are moving towards a closer integration of safety with other objectives such as quality of working life.

The common characteristics of national safety systems in advanced market economy countries are shown in Table 6.1. They function well enough as legislative and administrative institutions but, perhaps because of the sheer size of the activity at a national level, they tend to demonstrate what generously might be called continuity but ungenerously might be called inertia. There is always a very elaborate system of committees, and innovative decisions get lost in the hierarchies. They demonstrate the standard symptoms of large bureaucracies.

The fundamental difficulty is that safety is an artificial and operationally negative concept. Artificial in that behaving safely is merely a subset of acting effectively, or skilfully. Negative in that the whole approach has been to prevent certain kinds of undesirable activity rather than to facilitate desirable activity. These deficits are becoming more apparent as the engineering approach to safety gradually gives way to the behavioural approach. These are complementary in that the engineering approach concentrates on a safe environment and the behavioural approach concentrates on a safe operator (see below). Historically the effort and resources have gone into the engineering approach and because the point of diminishing returns has been reached there is renewed interest in the behavioural approach. In studying safe behaviour the question automatically arises as to how or why this is separable from effective behaviour more generally.

Occupational Safety, like risk, is separable into two problem areas, sudden trauma due to energy in the wrong place at the wrong time (McFarland and

Table 6.1. *Common characteristics of national safety systems*
(after Singleton, 1987)

---

1. A reliance on a hierarchy of acts, standards and codes of practice with increasing specificity and ease of modification going down the hierarchy.

2. An inspectorate as the basic means of ensuring compliance but with problems of how to distinguish between national and local inspection responsibilities (for what and to whom), whether to specialise in functions, e.g. electrician, or industries, e.g. furniture making, and the criteria by which to arrange inspections (random, regular, data-guided, following emergencies, by request, etc.).

3. Problems of how to separate but simultaneously maintain contact between the three essential functions of administration, research and inspection.

4. Difficulties in collecting, collating and interpreting accident statistics.

5. Proliferation of committees.

6. The problem of how to measure the cost-effectiveness of the organisation.

7. Determination of policy changes influenced by new risks in new technologies, newly identified risks in older technologies, and changes in socially acceptable risks.

8. Determination of research priorities by risk levels, numbers exposed, seriousness of consequences, feasibility and public/mass media pressure.

Moore, 1971), which is a useful definition of an accident, and harm due to long term exposure to toxic substances and environments. The toxicity problem is serious and of increasing importance, but it comes within the discipline of industrial hygiene/occupational medicine rather than Human Factors. This chapter is concerned with coping with the collision with harmful mechanical energy, although some of the concepts and methods are applicable also to toxic problems. For detailed treatment of toxic matters see ILO (1983) and Oftedal and Brogger (1986).

6.1.3 Accidents

The most succinct definition is due to Cherns (1970); 'an accident is an error with sad consequences'. As Cherns points out this leaves aside 'Acts of God' but this is constructive in that, by definition, nothing can be done about 'Acts of God' but we can do something about erroneous acts of man, namely errors. This introduces the first problem of accident statistics in that 'Acts of God' are included and their total represents the best that can be achieved in terms of accident reduction. It is a common mistake to assume that a reasonable safety target is zero accidents. The 'sad consequences' qualifying clause highlights the second problem of accident statistics, there will have been many similar errors with no consequences, obviously these are not recorded as accidents but their aetiology is identical. In short, accident data are a chance subset of the scientifically interesting data which would be the total errors.

However these objections did not impede the classical accident studies of Greenwood and Woods (1919) who compared the actual distribution of accidents to individuals in various proportions (e.g. in one sample 447 had none, 132 had one, 42 had two etc.) with the distributions expected according to three hypotheses: chance, unequal liability and bias (one accident leads to another). The best fit was unequal liability which supports the 'accident proneness' hypothesis; see also Cresswell and Froggatt (1963). Conceptually accident proneness is ambiguous in that it is not clear whether some persons are more likely to have accidents all the time or some are liable to particular kinds of accidents, or different people are differentially prone to have accidents at different times.

Operationally it has not proved possible to identify accident proneness by tests or by other means, so that it is not an avenue for reducing accidents. On the other hand there is evidence from road accidents to indicate that 'a man drives as he lives' (McFarland *et al.* 1955). As McFarland (1970) points out young males are the predominant 'accident-prone' group, alcohol is involved in about half of fatal road accidents and persons having repeated accidents are frequently found to have emotional problems and poor social adjustment.

Another general difficulty about accident statistics is that the tendency to report can confuse any requirement for comparisons between different situations. For example, it is doubtful if a highly safety conscious industry such as coal mining where reporting is meticulous can be compared with an industry such as construction which treats safety and accident reporting much more casually. In their direct observation of more than 2000 accidents in four different types of industrial workshop Powell *et al.* (1971) noted that the two workshops which had associated, fully staffed surgeries recorded 55% and 70% of the observed accidents, but for the two where there was no fully staffed surgery recorded accidents were about 5% of those discovered by the investigators. For injuries 'leading to three days of lost time' the shops with surgeries recorded almost all of them, but the shops without surgeries accurately recorded only about half of them, the other half were recorded as 'sickness' or 'uncertificated absence'. The Robens Committee (*op. cit.*) found that in the U.K. in 1970 there were 473 000 reported accidents causing absence from work of more than three days, but there were 822 000 new claims for industrial injury benefit.

In reporting or utilising statistics the precise population covered and the definition of terms used should be carefully considered. For example, should accidents to truck drivers and commercial travellers be included in occupational accidents or transport accidents or both? If both then confusion is likely if total accidents are calculated by addition. Industrial accidents may or may not include accidents travelling to and from work. This is crucial because in France for example there are twice as many fatal accidents while commuting compared with those while actually at work (ANPAT 1983).

Statistics are a poor basis for the study of accidents also because there is a causal chain in which a number of parameters intrude between the danger and the harm as shown in Fig. 6.1.

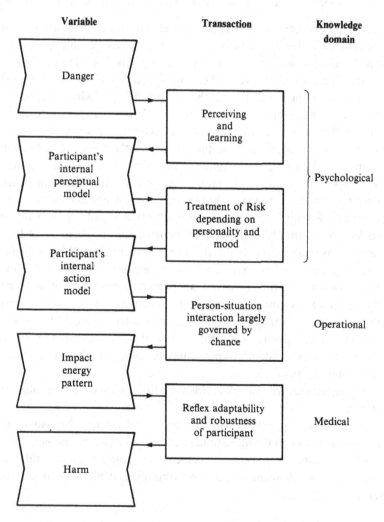

Fig. 6.1. The remote relationship between danger and harm.

Attempts to detect the causes of accidents invariably conclude that there is a pattern of events any or all of which can be identified as contributing factors. Lagerlof (1975) divided approaches to accident research into three categories:

- behavioural models such as accident proneness, psychodynamics (see next section) and choice or risk taking
- epidemiological models which attempt to relate to particular kinds of accident the attributes of the victims, the agents causing the injury and the surroundings
- systems models which attempt to trace the interactions of events and agents in the event networks which have an accident as the output

As in many other fields where human behaviour is an integral part, research is academically frustrating because there are so many possible approaches and so many disciplines each of which makes a partial contribution to the total picture. Operationally however there are often considerable dividends in terms of reduced accidents even though the understanding of what is happening and why is far from complete. Singleton (1984) reviewed European accident studies since 1970, the point of the beginning of extensive new investment in many countries, and concluded that they were mostly based on collection and collation of data from real situations with the result that there is increased awareness of the industrial situation but not very much theoretical advance. 'Most current theories are of the "system" type which can explain anything but predict nothing". This may be a fair reflection of reality in that any specific accident is essentially unpredictable even though accident rates for given populations remain very similar from year to year. Given this detailed unpredictability it may well be that the search for causation theories is misconceived and the best that can be achieved is a process-control type monitoring with adjustment of relevant parameters, some mechanism based, some behaviourally based as trends and discontinuities are detected. This could cope also with the sociocultural phenomenon that public attitudes change and for reasons which are not easily identified particular accident problems generate more or less public concern.

The reasons for treating all accident statistics with care are summarised in Table 6.2.

Given that safety and accidents are conceptually intractable issues, there is a case for retreating to the more fundamental underlying phenomenon which is that these matters arise because people make mistakes. The consideration of human error would seem to be one contribution that behavioural scientists can make.

Table 6.2. *Reasons for treating accident statistics with care*

---

1. 'Acts of God' are included: low probability events which actually happened but which are entirely unforeseeable; some are natural, e.g. earthquake, some are man-made, e.g. two farm-workers were killed by a military aircraft which crashed in the field in which they happened to be working.

2. Accidents are a random selection from critical incidents, the total of the latter is interesting but unknown.

3. 'Tendency to report' confounds comparisons.

4. Totals also depend on precise description of how an accident is defined, what are included and excluded and the population at risk (usually unknown). This also negates comparisons across studies.

5. Changes in method of reporting, sources and destinations of reports can radically affect totals.

6. The usual criterion of resultant harm is only remotely related to the initiating situation (see Fig. 6.1.)

7. There are understandable but unavoidable biases in reporting by participants and observers.

8. Recorders, analysts and research workers also have biases which are difficult to compensate for.

6.1.4 Human error

An error is a deviation from an optimal path towards an objective (Singleton 1973). A path may be definable in physical space, e.g. the path of an aircraft or may be in the more conceptual space envisaged by Lewin (1936) in which an individual is considered as moving through a life space, e.g. an educational self-development process. Such paths are not infinitely narrow and there is always some tolerance. The boundaries may be set by law or by design, e.g. a motorway lane or may be set by the person pursuing the objective, e.g. the climber. Paradoxically the higher the level of skill the wider the tolerance, excessive precision is the prerogative of the novice. It might appear more definitive to describe errors in terms of consequential damage, but this is not feasible because the relationship between any error and its consequences are a matter of chance, e.g. if I drive out into a main road without checking the traffic this is an error but there are no consequences unless there happens to be another car at precisely the right point to collide with mine.

For these reasons there can be no standard procedure for measuring or even detecting human errors. Whether or not an error has been committed depends on the objective the person is pursuing and whether he transgresses the path he has chosen or has had chosen for him. There may be many paths towards a particular objective and which one is chosen depends on many factors such as diagnosis, instructions, available resources including skill level and acceptable risks.

Explanations as to why errors occur vary from the psychodynamic to the informational (Singleton, 1973). Freud (1949) explained apparently irrational and damaging behaviour in terms of a death instinct associated with the id and supervised by the ego and superego. From this point of view a person can, if internal supervision is inadequate, deliberately and pleasurably damage himself or other people. It is clear from road behaviour in particular (Storr 1968, Parry 1968) that the car does provide an excuse for and a means of personal aggression. Human errors and consequent accidents are not necessarily unintentional. The cognitive approach to errors is to locate potential points of error within information processing. Kidd (1962) suggests that there can be:

- failure to detect
- failure to identify
- failure to weight the evidence correctly
- failure to select the correct action
- failure to act

He lists the possible causal factors for each of these and in this way provides a systematic check list of design features relevant to error reduction, e.g. failure to detect a signal may be due to input overload or underload or to adverse noise conditions. This approach is essentially a pragmatic one, it takes the origin of errors to a more detailed level but it does not explain why they occur.

A wider cognitive view is the proposition that errors occur because the mental model is an inadequate match to reality (Davis 1958, Singleton 1975). This suggests more directly the potentiality for reducing errors by training, instructions, information presentation and feedback. It also follows from the concept of action as hypothesis testing to update mental models (p. 85) that there should be potential for error correction as well as for error avoidance. Human performance is much improved if it is feasible to detect errors and correct them within continuous performance. This is more than the provision of adequate feedback, human performance is fundamentally tentative and explorative, errors are an intrinsic feature and a situation which does not tolerate them is unforgiving and unnatural. Taylor (1963) pointed out that all human engineering and virtually all psychological studies depend on measures extracted from man–machine systems rather than from man – 'the behaviour of a creature cannot be measured except through its effect on something else'. It follows that it is always the performance of the system which is being measured and the relative dominance of the man and the machine as reflected in the measured performance varies from one extreme to the other for specific situations. Rasmussen (1987) correspondingly regards human errors as man–machine mismatch situations and, from the human operator viewpoint, as experiments in an unkind environment. Reason (1987) sees mistakes as consequences of biases in planning resulting from the limited capacity of working memory, and the selective processes in obtaining data from the long-term (schematic) memory. He distinguishes between mistakes which occur in the planning phase and slips which occur in the execution phase.

In high technology systems effects often result from the behaviour of a team or crew rather than an individual. Even at the informational level this can cause complications in that there can be communication failures within the group. On the other hand there is a greater probability that at least one person in the group will have the correct hypotheses (Brehmer 1987b). Group activities are complicated by the authority issue (p. 142) and by the many other issues of group dynamics.

As in other aspects of complex behaviour the approach to understanding human errors has not been able to escape from a reductionist approach. Errors are analysed in terms of the information processing sequence, the hierarchy of skill levels, the separation of cognitive processes (memory, inference etc.), cause–effect relationships and action–reason relationships. Taylor (1981) suggests that the basic doctrine of the mechanism is in decline and uses *hermeneutics* to describe an alternative approach which he favours. This is the search for meaning which can be shared between people, but it is not easy in relation to accidents which are meaningless events. The human skill approach (Chapter 2) is holistic and teleological rather than reductionist and mechanistic and it is closely related to system theory (Singleton 1981). There still seems to be considerable potential here both for understanding and as a source of methods and procedures (see below). The problem is to describe human transactions with the environment sufficiently definitively so as to generate descriptions of human error and appropriate remedies.

6.1.5 Reliability

The practical reason for the research and development described in this chapter is the pursuit of reliable system performance. A reliable system is one that performs according to the design intent or within the design basis to use current jargon. However, designers and consequently designs are never perfect and inevitably unanticipated events will occur. This is serious in high technology systems because there is much energy around and if it transgresses the designed boundaries then there can be extensive damage, a high recovery cost and injuries to people. The aim then is to make systems as reliable as possible and to do this it helps to be able to predict system reliability, preferably at the design stage. Such evidence can be used as part of decisions or choices within system designs for particular purposes.

It is obvious that the reliability of any system depends on the engineered mechanisms and on the performance of the human operators within the system; those who set it up, those who operate it and those who maintain it. Investigations of many system failures, e.g. aircraft crashes, result in figures of anything from 50% to 80% ascribed to human error. These are for relatively direct human system input, if designers and supporting technologists are included then 100% can be assigned to human error, e.g. a valve that fails in a process system is ultimately the responsibility of those who selected the materials and the mechanism to operate in those conditions.

The human operator has both a positive and a negative impact on reliability. Positive in that he is the ultimate backstop in the attempt to correct unforeseen failures and negative in that his operational errors make a large contribution to system unreliability.

When one of the early American astronauts was asked to describe his feelings as he waited for lift-off he said that it suddenly occurred to him that his life depended on the reliability of hundreds of sub-systems, each of which had been designed and produced by the contractor who submitted the lowest tender. Extreme reliability is expensive and it is bad design to make a component or sub-system more reliable than is necessary in terms of the expected system life. Good design is not merely effective, it is also cost-effective. Hence the pursuit of the precise quantification of reliability so that cost-effective design decisions are aided.

There are considerable difficulties in generating numerical data even for hardware mechanisms. The standard curve of reliability is neither linear nor monotonic. There is usually an early erratic phase when poorly constructed or assembled components fail before the standard wear and tear asymptotic curve takes over. Hence the importance of a system commissioning phase when early failures can be detected and corrected. Another difficulty is that reliability data are inherently probabilistic. Thus, accurate data will provide information about populations but not about individual cases. It can be used to predict the required numbers of spares to be stored but not to indicate where or when a specific failure will occur.

Human failure rates were first subjected to systematic reliability approaches because of the problem of big systems and in particular the aerospace programme. In these vehicles a serious failure is catastrophic because the option of shutting the system down is not available and facilities for on-line repair are extremely limited.

Two approaches to the production of equipment were developed. The first was one of exhortation: a combination of training and propaganda aimed at trying to make sure that everyone involved was as careful as possible in completing their particular part of the production. These were called *zero defect programmes*, the art was one of varying the approach to the workers using all the available communication techniques: feedback, lectures, films, posters etc., so as to keep the message alive and avoid the development of adaptation, boredom or resistance. The second approach was to assume that errors are unavoidable but to provide ways of calculating their probable level for particular kinds of operations. This was called *reliability analysis* (see below). It will be noted that zero defect programmes operate early and within the system development operation cycle, whilst reliability analysis is an off-line support technique usually carried out either at the design stage or on the basis of operational experience. The cost of correcting defects increases markedly as the system development proceeds (De Greene 1970).

Estimation of the probability of failure of large-scale systems such as aircraft or industrial plant requires, in principle, the integration of data about machines, people and their interaction. This is impossible in the present state of the art. The fundamental problem (p. 133) is that engineered mechanisms and human operators are qualitatively different. The complementary nature of machine and man characteristics would suggest that man–machine systems ought to be more reliable than any separate failure rate data could suggest. This is probably the case but the case is not quantifiable.

Learning occurs within both design and operation. Tye (1980) points out that aircraft systems have learning curves in that the rate of notifiable accidents diminishes with accumulated flying hours (hours measured in millions) and that successive generations of aircraft start at lower points on the accident rate scale. Jacobs and Hutchinson (1973) demonstrate that road vehicle fatality rates diminish as the density of vehicles increases, that is as experience increases.

6.1.6 Disasters

Avoiding large-scale system failures is taken very seriously by scientific and technological communities because there can be loss of life and the cost is high. In addition such failures are usually spectacular so that they get intensive treatment in the mass-media which, at least temporarily, affects public and policy-making opinions and damages the reputation of the technology and its sponsors. Such incidents are normally followed by inquiries, sometimes several independent inquiries, so that what happened is well documented. The scale of the inquiries and other consequences is not related to the degree of damage to people. For example, the best known and explored disaster is the Three Mile Island incident in 1979, e.g. Rubinstein and Mason (1979), Perrow (1981). This caused no loss of life directly, but what happened and why was explored in tremendous detail by a variety of investigative bodies. The consequences for the organisation of nuclear power generation and the design of stations have been on a world scale. There were some direct operator errors implicated but there were also some mechanism failures. This is typical of disasters in that there are usually four independent unwanted events due to mechanisms, operators and management which happen to conflate to generate a situation which gets out of control. It follows that such situations are rare but unavoidable in that they cannot be predicted by either designers or management. NUREG (1975) estimated that world wide there is about one event per year which causes of the order of 100 fatalities, and about one every ten years which causes of the order of 1000 fatalities. This is true both for natural disasters such as tornadoes and earthquakes and for man-made disasters such as dam failures and aircraft crashes.

Bignell *et al.* (1977) examine in detail seven catastrophes: a level crossing crash, a landslip, a fire, a building collapse, a bridge failure, a ship sinking and an air crash. They present a consistent picture of design errors, planning oversights and communication failures. No outright villainy is uncovered, but there is considerable incompetence which is detectable with hindsight. Reports on more recent incidents such as the Bhopal chemical plant and the Chernobyl nuclear reactor confirm that the complete cause is never what one person does at one time. The event always has a history: political, technological and managerial, and with hindsight it is possible to trace how contributing events converge on the final trigger of the disaster. The disaster itself is another chain of events facilitated by system complexity and tight coupling (Perrow 1984). Most high technology systems are tightly coupled in that events quickly spread through the system by interactive effects and by lack of slack in the system which would leave room for adaptation and blocking of undesirable sequential effects.

Since the harm often spreads into the system environment there is scope for the consideration of ameliorative measures of containment and rescue facilities. These also need to be considered with care because the proposed remedy may have its own dangers. Rescuers are themselves at risk and can also add to the risks of those to be rescued.

For any large chemical or nuclear plant the first line of defence is a containment building. This is designed to contain the effects of the 'maximum credible accident' (Flowers 1976). Incredible things do happen and beyond the plant there will be some mobile and some permanent instrumentation centres which record the direction and extent of the 'toxic plume'. As a last resort there may be plans for the evacuation of the local community. Equally important is the information network which provides facilities for some remote advice and control, for ensuring that all authorities with local responsibilities are kept informed and for briefing the mass-media who have a part to play in information circulation.

Because there are many official and unofficial organisations which get involved following a disaster (police, fire services, health services, voluntary organisations, public spectators etc.), the key strategy is to ensure that there is central authority which can monitor the situation and keep the total rescue system under control. Following harrowing disasters there will be, in addition to the immediate casualties, longer-term effects emerging as neuroses and psychosomatic disorders. Those most active after the event may be least affected (Hedge 1987).

The broad strategy of *defence in depth* is now practised in relation to high technology systems. Serious events always involve a combination of circumstances. Typically:

- a system transient arising from one or more hiccups in the hardware, software or materials used in the process
- a design instrumentation inadequacy resulting in data or feedback which happens to be misleading in the situation which arises
- an error in construction or maintenance which remains undetected for months or even years because there was no check until the particular serious event was analysed
- one or more human errors in control following wrong diagnosis of what is happening

This description emphasises again the simple fact that such situations are entirely unpredictable and thus the reasonable strategy is to erect a series of obstacles to resist such an 'invasion'. Defence in depth can be made available along at least three avenues:

- detection of unwanted circumstances
- strategies for avoidance of disaster
- strategies for coping with disaster

Each of these in turn has its own array and series of defences.

6.2 Knowledge

6.2.1 *Accident data sources*

In most advanced countries data are collected at several levels:

- the overall situation is monitored by a government sponsored body such as the Health and Safety Executive in the U.K. or the Bureau of Labor Statistics in the U.S.A. Usually there is an annual report, e.g. the *Rapport Annuel de la Caisse Nationale Suisse d'occurance en cas d'accidents*, from Lucerne, and the Unfallanalyse from *Zentralstelle fur Unfallverhutung und Arbeitsmedezin* at Sankt Augustin (Hoffman, 1987). These contain data about a particular year supported by trends from previous years and highlights of any particularly undesirable situations which seem to be arising in particular trades, industries, kinds of machine or process
- there are national voluntary institutes concerned with prevention which again monitor the overall situation and produce their own reports, e.g. the Royal Society for Prevention of Accidents (ROSPA) in the U.K. and the National Safety Council (NSC) in the U.S.A.
- industry or occupation based bodies such as trade associations, trade unions, industry institutes and insurance companies collect data for their own purposes
- universities and other research institutions undertake specific studies in relation to particular interests and hypotheses
- the world situation is monitored by the International Labour Office in Geneva which produces a unique collection of data annually – the *Year Book of Labour Statistics*

For reasons already enumerated (Table 6.2) such data are not as easy to interpret as they appear at first sight. Data from different sources are almost never directly comparable, there are invariably differences in definition of terms and in the reason for inquiry or reporting which negate comparisons.

Deaths are less ambiguous than injuries or diseases, but even here there can be differences in, for example, the maximum time lapse between injury and death for which the accident is describable as fatal. Fatalities do not necessarily present the same relative pictures as injuries. For example, the ratio of injuries to fatalities is about 0.5 for aircraft accidents, 25 for rail accidents and 50 for road accidents (Tye 1977).

The situation is not improved by the tendency to increase the size of data networks and stores, the weakness is invariably in the original recording of the accident or injury. Different users of data have different requirements: policy makers, planners, managers, safety specialists, designers, trainers, ergonomists, psychologists, sociologists, epidemiologists, statisticians and lawyers ask different questions. In the interests of ready computerisation the original data are often recorded on a standard form. The questions posed on the form will suit the particular specialist who designed it and not the others who have their own legitimate specific interests. There is much to be said for the original account of an accident to be in clear prose guided by a checklist agreed by a multi-disciplinary team and supplemented by various numerical evidence such as date, time of day and ages of those involved.

6.2.2 Accident data interpretation

Here again there is wide scope for ambiguity. For example, which is the most dangerous job, the one which injures the most people or the one where the probability of injury to a person is highest? Has an industry worsened or improved its safety record if the accident rate per unit of product increases? This can happen when the number of accidents stays about the same but the number of workers involved has decreased following improved productivity.

Is an injury to an operator more, less or equally serious compared with one to a member of the public? In a ruthless war an officer will consider that losing one of his men is much more regrettable than losing a passer-by, particularly if he is in enemy territory. In civil life the opposite is usually accepted, e.g. in any transport system the crew is expected to assume greater risks than are the passengers. From the point of view of resultant distress the two should be equivalents.

On the whole, accident analysts try to avoid value judgments partly because this is scientific tradition and partly because they are always debatable. This is no problem for those in universities but it is not so easy for sponsored investigators who are expected to provide an answer, not another set of questions. For example, it is very difficult to decide how much should be invested in reducing a particular hazard. The law is no great help because it always includes phrases such as 'as far as is practicable' for which the test seems to be technical feasibility, or 'as far as is reasonably practicable' which incorporates technical and economic feasibility.

In considering any presentation of evidence it is salutary to consider basic questions such as: who says so? how does he know? who analysed these data? who collected it in the first place? what are their likely biases? what other biases are likely in the observers, participants and reporters of the original events?

6.2.3 Accident data

Following all these cautionary statements it might seem unwise to present any data. However, broad data particularly about fatalities also provide a picture of the accident situation and a basis for the assessment of

Table 6.3. *Deaths in Great Britain (1985)*

(ROSPA data)

		Proportions of total deaths
Deaths from ill health	633 000	97%
Accidents	15 000	2%
(Road accidents	6000	1%)
Suicide	5000	1%
(Falls	5000	1%)
Deaths from all causes	655 000	100%

priorities for expenditure, action and research. All the data are for Great Britain unless otherwise stated.

Every year about 15 000 people are killed in accidents including about 1000 children aged under 15 years. About 6000 are killed in the home, about 6000 on the road and about 600 at work. More than 400 people are drowned of which about 70 are engaged in sporting activity, excluding drowning about 100 are killed in sport. Hospital casualty departments deal with about 6 million accident cases each year, about 2 million due to home accidents, about 1 million due to accidents in sport, and about 1 million due to road accidents (see ROSPA reports).

The sub-division of fatalities is shown in Table 6.3. About 97% of deaths are 'normal', only about 3% are 'with boots on'. Of the latter 2% are accidents and 1% are suicides. Of the accidents about half are due to road transport and the other half due to falls, that is each of these accounts for about 1% of total deaths. These rounded off percentages produce some distortion, e.g. accidents are three times, not twice, as frequent as suicides, but they do present a picture which can be remembered and which does not change from year to year.

The rough equivalence in total numbers of road accidents and falls obscures the important fact that falls are a problem for older people, whereas road accidents spread across the age range as shown in Fig. 6.2. Within the fatal road accidents about 2000 pedestrians, about 2000 car users and about 1000 motor cyclists were killed. There are, of course, many more car users than motorcyclists, the risk of fatality using two-wheeled transport is more than double that for four-wheeled. Given also that four-wheelers do many more miles, the death rate per mile on motor-cycles is more than twenty times greater than that in cars. However, the death rate for car users per mile is ten times greater than for trains (ROSPA data).

The accident incidence rate at work is shown in Fig. 6.3. Not surprisingly, mining and quarrying is the most dangerous category, and professional and scientific work the least dangerous (by a factor of 10) by this measure. The differences, e.g. between mining and construction, should not be accepted too precisely because of differences in tendency to report and differences in difficulties of estimating numbers exposed. In agriculture more accidents

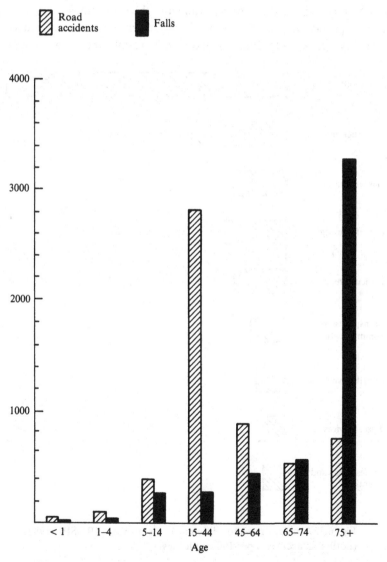

Fig. 6.2. Distributions of fatal road accidents and falls by age group.

happen to employers than to employees, but accidents to employers in industry are negligible, on the other hand the age range in agriculture is much greater than in manufacturing. In spite of the data in Fig. 6.3 it could be argued that agriculture is more dangerous than manufacturing.

Table 6.4 shows the distribution of industrial fatalities to employees in one year. Note the validity of McFarland's concept (mentioned earlier) that an accident is caused by energy in the wrong place at the wrong time.

Trends over time are not easy to pin down because of the changing regulations which change methods of reporting and the continuous changes in all industries, particularly the reduction of man-power and the increase in available energy per worker. Fig. 6.4 shows the steadily reducing number of

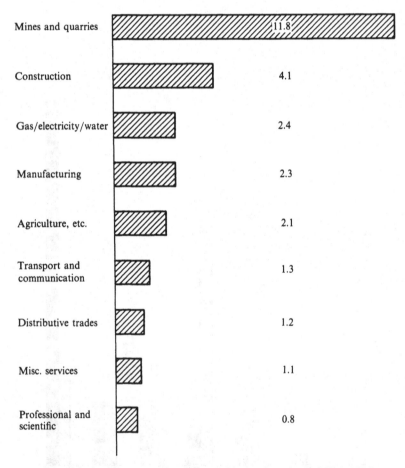

Fig. 6.3. Accident rates for different kinds of work. (ROSPA 1982) (notifiable accidents per 100 employees)

fatalities per year in the coal industry (Singleton 1982). This graph has not been updated because of the distortion due to a one-year miners' strike about 1984. Over the period shown the mining man-power was reduced to about one third of its 1950 level and the output was halved, but nevertheless the safety record is one of which the industry can be proud. A less dramatic downward trend has occurred in agriculture as shown in Fig. 6.5, again the workforce has been going down but total output has probably been increasing. During 1981–5 the number and rate of fatal injuries to employees remained broadly constant (Goddard 1988).

Table 6.4. *Employee fatalities in*
industry in one year, 1986/87

(H.S.E. data)

Caught by moving object including machinery and vehicles	153
Fall from height	81
Contact with electricity	22
Drowning and asphyxiation	17
Contact with harmful substance	10
Explosion and fire	9
Fall on same level	6
Others including unclassified	44
Total	342

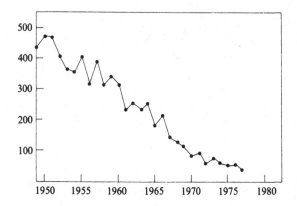

Fig. 6.4. Fatal accidents per year in the British coal industry. (N.C.B. data).

The increased concern about casualties due to accidents has many origins including the increased wealth which makes greater expenditure on safety more feasible, and the growing expectation that death is a phenomenon associated only with old age (Singleton 1984). Fig. 6.6 shows the dramatic change in distribution of deaths in each year of age during this century, and Fig. 6.7 demonstrates that the adult of today has more than a 50% chance of living past the age of 70 years.

6.3 Principles, methods and procedures

Although it is intellectually congenial to remain within the intricacies of theory and statistics there is a practical objective which is to increase safety. As in any other technological subject the principles and methods emerge from a consideration of the relationship between what happens in practice to relevant basic theory. In this case the theories are about human behaviour and the practice is the accidents which actually occur.

The links between the two are provided by knowledge about human errors and methods of studying accidents (Fig. 6.8). Note that there are transactions in both directions. The whole process is synergistic, not only does behavioural science contribute to accident reduction, the study of accidents contributes also to a knowledge of human behaviour as revealed through errors.

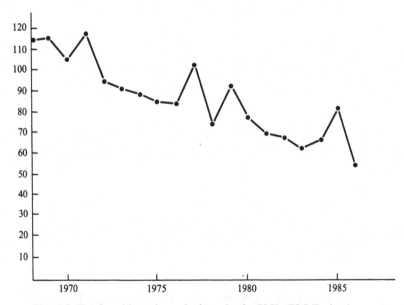

Fig. 6.5. Fatal accidents in agriculture in the U.K. (H.S.E. data).

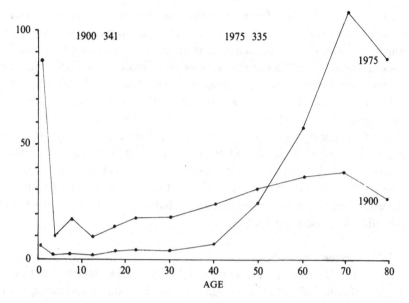

Fig. 6.6. Male deaths in each year of age in the U.K. (C.S.O. data) (thousands).

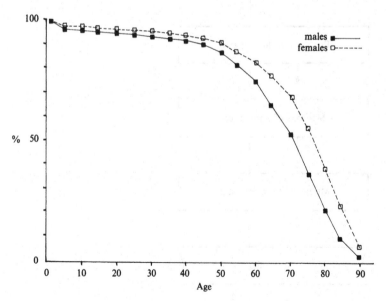

Fig. 6.7. The U.K. life-graph for the 1950 cohort (C.S.O data).

In laboratory studies of human performance errors are often regarded as a tiresome irrelevance clouding the data. Correspondingly the safety engineer sometimes looks upon human behaviour as an untidy complication best removed or at least reduced as far as possible by more automation. The thesis of this chapter is that both these attitudes are misguided and that neither type of investigator can make progress without treating human error as of intrinsic importance in the academic and the practical contribution to safety.

The theoretical picture is of a complex purposive adaptive organism engaged in transactions involving energy and information exchanges with a complex stochastic physical environment. The practical picture is of accidents which occur specifically by chance but within various overall populations there is potentiality for prediction in probabilistic terms and also for the reduction of these probabilities.

6.3.1 Accident reduction

This is straightforward in principle in that there are only four possible sources of remedial measures: design, procedures, training and management.

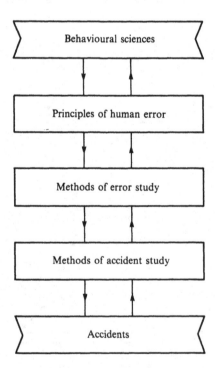

Fig. 6.8. Accident study methodology.

Design

Design for safety is a subset of design for effective operation but is often considered separately for legal reasons.

In the U.K., as described above, designers, makers and suppliers have specific safety responsibilities. As a consequence the safety inspectorate is able to adopt a passive and questioning role. The initiative is deliberately left with the producer who has to prove that what he does, did or proposes to do is reasonably safe. If not, he faces the sanctions of warnings, being refused a licence to continue and ultimately being prosecuted. Many of the issues are technical in a physical science/engineering sense but there is increasing attention to Human Factors. For big systems the proof that behavioural aspects have been considered must be demonstrated by a systematic ergonomics programme. Whether a design or product is safe is checked in two ways: does it meet the relevant safe criteria and was an agreed systematic programme followed to pursue the appropriate level of safety (NUREG CR1270, 1980). All this requires specialists.

The design procedures followed are the same as those described in Chapters 1 and 5 with some differences of emphasis. It may be that there are various engineered mechanisms which have been added specifically to increase safety. These can vary from automatic control loops (which are assumed to be more reliable than manual control) to interlocks which prevent the operator following unsafe sequences. On simpler systems such as single machines specific hazards may have been established by previous experience including accidents, e.g. the power take-off shaft on tractors which catches clothing. Providing guards and screens obviously can be beneficial, but too often such aids are added as an afterthought to an already complicated design. These may interfere with ease of operation, this is deleterious not only from the productivity viewpoint but also because the operator is tempted to remove or outflank them.

Such guarding is not a purely engineering task, it is to do with the man–machine interface which should involve consideration of what the operator is doing as well as what the mechanism is doing. For example, it is still common for the operator's task to be one of feeding the machine and removing the products. The traditional way of ensuring safety is to have a guard which switches power off if out of place, it must be moved to insert materials and then replaced before the machine performs its task. The guard is removed again to take out the product. This is clumsy and tedious from the operator's viewpoint and unnecessarily slow from the management viewpoint. A more effective solution is to have two working jigs connected so that each replaces the other inside the machine. It is then possible to unload and load one while the machine is working on the other. The operator's hands are never inside the machine and he works in parallel with it rather than alternately with it. Such design does not require great insight, it follows immediately if the designer can be persuaded to consider simultaneously the related functions of the man and the machine.

A more behavioural approach to design safety is to ensure that there is potentiality to correct errors. For example, it is often desirable to separate the choice of an action from the trigger which transmits the command to the system. The operator thereby has the opportunity to check his choice before the action commences, e.g. on machine tool consoles the operator selects the speed or direction of movement and checks his selection before he presses the initiate button.

Procedures

These overlap with both design and training within the total accident reduction strategy.

Sometimes a procedure can be enforced by an interlock design and sometimes it can be guided by an interface design either actively or passively. An active guide would take the form of a series of display items, e.g. illuminated controls which can indicate what should be done next. A passive guide takes the form of the physical layout of interfaces in a way corresponding to frequently required sequences of operations. It can be argued that if procedures are as common and fixed as this implies then as a matter of function allocation the machine should be programmed to complete tasks automatically. There are counter arguments such as the need for flexibility in particular circumstances and the benefits of contact and awareness ('feel' for the system) which the operator gains by carrying out procedures.

Training clearly has a considerable part to play in ensuring that procedures are followed either by ensuring that the location and use of procedures is formally established or by ensuring that drills are practised to the point such that they are followed without thought.

In big systems such as process control and aviation the following of written procedures is mandatory. Enforcement may be at the legal level, the company level or the crew level. Operators are aware that should there be an accident and it is clear that they did not follow established procedure they will have to justify their actions with very good reasons. There are procedures not only for routines but also for emergencies which have been recognised on the basis of design and operational experience. The quality of procedures is highly variable. Unfortunately procedures which are provided for rare emergencies may be the least valid ones because there has not been the opportunity to modify them by experience. Such modification is not easy except in cases of obvious omissions and self-contradiction. Apparent inadequacy or inappropriateness is not easily judged by operators. In highly safety conscious industries such as nuclear power there are procedures for modifications of procedures with categories of those which can be modified at site level, those which require company or area confirmation, those which must be referred back to designers and those which must be approved by independent safety authorities.

For smaller systems there are usually procedures for setting up, shutting down and maintenance which hopefully take account of safety factors. These are usually very badly designed because the designer from his position of complete familiarity is not sensitive to the problems which puzzle the user. The remedy is simple but rarely followed, procedures should always be checked with an appropriate population of users. This is not necessarily expensive, a trial with one typical user is much better than no trial. Some of the many aspects of procedure design are described in Vandenberg (1967) and Bohr (1984).

The problems are accentuated if the users are the general public who cannot be assumed to have any technical awareness. Reliance on procedures or training is doubtful, design provides the most effective protection, this is true also for some industries where competent management supervision and systematic training are difficult to provide, e.g. agriculture and fishing. It is often most effective to present information using signs and pictorial instructions (Easterby and Zwaga, 1984).

Training

Safety training should, in principle, encompass three levels:

– procedures and drills
– diagnosis and remedial action
– attitudes and housekeeping

Design and training for a drill should ensure that the completion of each action is the trigger for the next action, and conversely that some actions are always taken before others. This much reduces the possibility that any act will be omitted, e.g. a welder will always pull his hood into place after adjusting the workpiece and before increasing the flame size because he was trained that way.

Ensuring that operators stick to rigid drills avoids the common difficulty that departures from procedures usually do not result in accidents, although an accident can happen if the departure happens to coincide with some other situation states. If there is insistence that the procedure is never varied it quickly becomes automatic and there is no temptation to try short cuts. This is particularly important when a crew is working closely together so that its actions will remain in phase, e.g. a crane operator and his loaders. Another advantage of the drill conducted without conscious intervention is that it will be more resistant to effects of fatigue and stress. This, of course, is why the drills have been used in warfare for thousands of years. Continuous training in the use of procedures is necessary in relation to emergencies for the above reason and because they are not needed routinely so that operational experience is not a substitute. In high technology systems there is a general difficulty that, in emergencies, the operator is expected to take over, but if the task is normally conducted automatically he will have little practice in the manual mode. For this reason procedures are often designed to ensure that the operator will maintain the appropriate skill level, e.g. alternate automatic and manual landings for aircraft.

Training in diagnosis is much less straightforward than procedural training. This is true at every level from hazard recognition in manufacturing systems, (Hale, 1984) to fault diagnosis in high technology systems (Duncan, 1987). Fashions change in that post-war there was a move towards training in problem solving methods rather than in basic theory, stimulated by the lower quality of military maintenance personnel (Gagne, 1962). More recently in civil systems the pendulum has swung back again because there is evidence from disasters such as Three Mile Island that if operators have a more complete understanding of the theory of what is happening they will be less likely to make fundamental errors. There is no general answer, the proportions of methods and theory within any training course must be settled for each specific job. Sometimes it is appropriate to separate roles in having scientific and technical staff on hand to advise operating staff, e.g. nuclear power stations now have 'Technical Support Centres' as well as Main Control Rooms.

Attitude training as always is the most difficult, it is essentially indirect. Creation and continuous reinforcement of what is called a 'safe climate' (Singleton, 1976) remains a mix of organisation features such as training and retraining, management attitudes, activity of safety officers and committees and feedback of data on safety trends (Table 6.5).

Management

Over the past twenty years there has been a great improvement in housekeeping within industrial plant. Disused materials and machines are removed promptly, windows and lights are kept clean, gangways are marked and nothing is allowed within them and so on. All this is bound to help to

Table 6.5. *Indications of a safe 'climate'*

'Climate' in this social sense is the climate of opinion and awareness. Although not measurable it is the dominant factor in determining safety within any premises.

1. All people actions and interactions are modulated by a general awareness that risks exist but should be minimised.
2. There are limits and boundaries, not always explicit, but rigidly followed as one expression of accepted membership of the enterprise. Some things are simply not done because they are unsafe.
3. Correspondingly there are other things which are always done such as routine checks and general tidiness.
4. When working in a team it is a disgrace if action or failure of an action puts another team member at risk.
5. There is a general pride in a safe outcome from situations where there are recognised hazards.

reduce the common kinds of accidents due to things falling on people and people falling (Fig. 6.2). There is some marginal improvement in construction sites but little or none as yet on farms.

The attention of management to safety issues was most successfully reinforced by the requirement in the Health and Safety at Work etc. Act (*op. cit.*) that every employer must have available a current written policy statement with respect to safety and health at work. The first step of an inspector visiting premises is to ask to see this statement. The need for continuous updating keeps these matters within management awareness. The appointment of safety representatives and safety committees is also mandatory as prescribed by the Secretary of State and the creation and functions of these processes also increases management awareness. Even for research studies it has been claimed that presence in the plant and discussion with management and employees make their own contribution to safety.

From Bureau of Labor Statistics analyses there is American evidence that medium sized firms (100–249 workers) are the most dangerous, presumably because in small companies everything is within the attention span of management and in large companies there are elaborate systems of safety officers, committees and procedures.

The committee approach is advantageous to management for economic as well as for humanitarian reasons, because safety and quality of work can be reinforced by the same strategies. On the other hand committees can become ritualistic and parodies of their original intentions. A safety committee can meet and go through a routine agenda to the satisfaction of members but with no consequences for anyone else.

6.3.2   *Hazard reduction*

A hazard is a potential accident. Thus hazard reduction is the intended result of all work on safety, but it is also a more specific activity based on analysis of existing situations. Hazard analysis is forward looking and complements accident analysis which is backward looking. It is more common in the newer industries, partly because they are new and therefore tend to look to the future rather than the past, and partly because they contain higher energy levels which lead to more serious but often fewer accidents. It is therefore more important to take preventative rather than remedial action. Hazard reduction can be an expert activity but it should also be practised by every manager and worker. For example, a manager sensitive to hazards would notice and take action if a particular worker had long hair or loose clothing which might get caught in a machine, a farm worker sensitive to hazards would avoid leaving heavy objects propped against a fence or building which young children might later pull over. Awareness of hazards can be increased by formal training, but more usually it depends on a knowledge of where the danger lies in a particular industry, trade or environment. Fortunately almost everyone is interested in their own work situation and is prepared to read and talk about it. Hazard reduction at this level depends on information circulation through safety committees and safety bulletins. It also depends on setting examples which will be copied.

The expert behaves in an analogous way but rather more formally. Equipped with his background knowledge of accidents which have occurred or can occur, he will observe all situations and functions from this point of view and make appropriate suggestions. The general starting point is energy in the form of electricity, heat, movement, gravity (bulk, height etc.) or toxic substances. The hazard analyst will note all sources of energy and the possibilities that it might be released unintentionally and thereby do harm.

Table 6.6 illustrates the questions a skilled observer asks himself during an inspection tour. These need to be tailored to particular kinds of premises or work-places, but it is surprising how many different hazards can be detected by a simple structured approach of this kind. Such a survey precedes a discussion with whoever is in charge to decide what, if anything, needs to be done.

Hazard reduction in high technology industry (Fig. 6.9) is a much more elaborate process starting with the original design and reinforced by training and operational feedback.

6.3.3   *Error reduction*

Attitudes to errors are always ambivalent. On the one hand we expect that a responsible person should be able to account for his actions, on the other hand we recognise that to err is human.

Table 6.6. *Hazards check-list (low technology)*

Electricity
1. Are all plugs, sockets, conduits and cables in good condition?
2. Are there cables which can be tripped over or damaged by machines?
3. Can lights or cables be touched by hands, heads, or loads being carried or transported?
4. Are there any situations where electric power is adjacent to water, e.g. taps or wet floors?
5. Are all the maintenance tasks the responsibility of properly qualified personnel?

Heat
1. Are hot surfaces either guarded or easily detected?
2. Is there any way in which a person can come into contact with flames or hot materials?
3. Are all fires suitably guarded against persons, clothing and inflammable materials?
4. Are the fire precautions appropriate?.
5. Is there any need for special clothing or tools?

Movement
1. Are all stairs in good condition and equipped with handrails?
2. Are all gangways kept completely clear?
3. Can there be collisions in doorways or junctions?
4. Where are there possibilities of foot or hand slip?
5. What about the moving materials and machines?

Gravity
1. What sorts of accidents could occur through things falling?
2. What sorts of accidents could occur through people falling?
3. Can anything roll around?
4. Is all lifting properly organised and trained for?
5. Is all seating robust and stable?

Toxic substances
1. Is all containment adequate?
2. Is there a need for protective clothing, including footwear?
3. What happens if spillage occurs?
4. For open containers, is the air movement in the right direction?
5. Are workers trained in what to do following an accident?

There are many ways of categorising errors as shown in Table 6.7. The commission/omission distinction is superficially attractive but of no great practical importance in terms of either aetiology or consequences. The difference between systematic errors (biases) and random (unpredictable) errors is useful in that biases can be detected and corrected for. Unfortunately human errors are usually at neither extreme, there is some consistency and some apparently chance element which adds to the difficulty of correction. The formal/substantive distinction is important in understanding why an error happened. A formal error is one in which the intention was correct but the action was inappropriate, a substantive error is one in which the intention itself was misconceived – the programme is justifiable given the objective but the defined objective does not match the requirements. The other classifications:

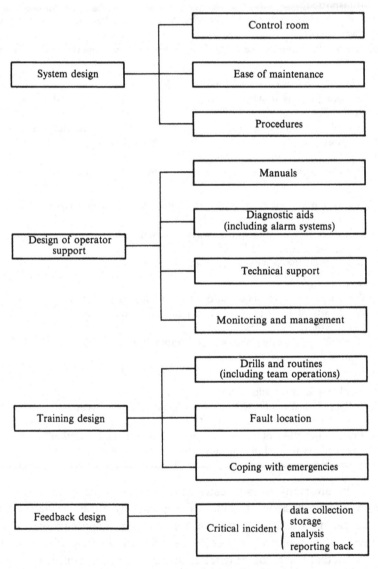

Fig. 6.9. Hazard reduction by design (high technology).

Table 6.7. *Categories of errors*

Error dichotomies
Commission   : Omission
Systematic   : Random
Formal   : Substantive
Detectable   : Undetectable
Reversible   : Irreversible
Man recoverable : Machine (recoverable (or neither)

By location within information processing
Detection failure
Incorrect identification
Incorrect weighting
Incorrect action selection
Incorrect action
   (after Kidd, 1962)

By performance
Failure of performance
Incorrect performance
Out-of-sequence performance
Non-required performance
   (Meister and Rabideau, 1965)

By responsibility
Incorrect diagnosis
Insufficient attention
Inadequate procedure
Inadequate supervision

By remedy
Design
Procedures
Training
Management

By skilled performance failure
Fair risk (chance)
Excessive risk (attitude)
Wrong risk assessment
Inadequate spatial/symbolic interpretation (cues)
Inaccurate sensori-motor performance (action)

Table 6.8. *Error reduction/correction methodology*

Error reduction
1. Reduce probability of pathological reaction.
   (Selection, Health monitoring, Group interaction)
2. Optimise arousal conditions.
   (Environmental, Informational)
3. Training, Procedures and Interface design.
   (Matching of internal modelling and information structures)
4. Consider Serial issues.
   (Feedback, Load variation, Fatigue)
5. Establish policies and attitudes.
   (Organisation and Management)

Error correction
1. Avoid convergent decision situation.
   (where urgency increases with delay)
2. Provide rapid feedback on actions and their consequences.
3. Design for error recovery feasibility.
   (e.g. separate choice decisions and initiate actions)
4. Replace continuous control by action selection.
5. Provide man–man monitoring.

---

detectable – undetectable, reversible – irreversible, recoverable by man, machine or neither all centre on the key principle that the human operator makes mistakes but is very good at correcting them given the opportunity.

Thus there are two questions, how to reduce the probability of error and how to correct or compensate for errors (Table 6.8). An error reduction methodology essentially requires the application of general ergonomic principles as described in Chapters 1, 2, 5 and in '*The safe system*' below with some specialist considerations such as avoiding situations where the longer a decision is delayed the more urgent it becomes. This can readily arise in vehicle control and in process systems, the human operator is particularly prone to error when subjected to this kind of stress. This principle underlines the strategy of aiming for forgiving systems and awareness of limits (Singleton, 1982). A forgiving system is one which has generous tolerance limits (the width of the path within which performance is tolerable as described earlier) and which also provides opportunities for recovery of errors. The concept of the forgiving system first became clear in relation to fighter aircraft, some of which are notoriously unforgiving, but it has much wider application. Awareness of limits is a related concept; machines, operators and systems have performance limits at which discontinuities occur and beyond which accidents can occur. A system is safer if the operator is made aware of all these limits by training and

Table 6.9. *Examples of detailed error classifications*

Aerospace (Altman, 1967)	
Inputs	Sensing
	Detecting
	Identifying
	Coding
	Classifying
Decisions	Estimating
	Logical manipulation
	Problem solving
Outputs	Chaining
	Omissions
	Insertions
	Misordering

Aviation (Fitts and Jones, 1947)	
Displays	*Controls*
Legibility	Substitution
Misreading	Adjustment
Reversal	Reversal
Interpretation	
Confusing instruments	Unintentional activation
Scale interpretation	
Illusions	
Forgetting	Forgetting
Inoperative instruments	Unable to reach

also by accentuation from the system, e.g. a car is safer if it is obvious when instability is developing, but is unsafe if a discontinuity such as skidding occurs without preliminary warning.

Error classification like any other behavioural classification has to be selected to fit the particular purpose. Table 6.7 also shows classifications of different types. Table 6.9 illustrates the possible detail in classification based on analyses of particular sorts of data.

In summary the general if indirect path to error reduction is systematic ergonomics, the direct path is to describe and classify errors which have occurred and consider remedies in the light of this evidence (Singleton, 1972).

6.3.4 The safe system

As already explained, a safe system is an effective system and the techniques for achieving this are summarised in Table 6.10. These techniques

Table 6.10. *Systems-based safety strategy*

Allocation of function (Man:Machine:Procedures)
Work space and interface design
Environmental design
Procedures design
Selection and training (Highly qualified personnel)
Contingency planning
Human and Hardware based monitoring
Working hours and other working conditions

Table 6.11. *Controller error minimisation*

Automatic control support
Procedural support
Machine – man monitoring
Machine based over-ride facilities
Man – machine monitoring
Manual over-ride facilities
Man – machine intercommunication
Man – man intercommunication
Arousal maintenance facilities
Fatigue avoidance facilities
Skill development facilities
Maintenance of rarely used skills

complement the more operator oriented techniques for controller error minimisation (Table 6.11).

Interest and activity in relation to this topic has increased over the past twenty years because systems have got bigger, more expensive, more tightly coupled, with faster integration and greater energy content. Not all factors mitigate against safety. The operator is now more remote from the scene of materials and energy activity which makes him safer, the greater productivity and more complete automation means that there are fewer people around to get damaged. On the other hand probability of damage to the public is greater than it used to be. The importance of reliability, basically because of increased capital investment, indirectly supports greater safety.

The importance of maintenance as a contributor to reliability and safety has also increased. A hiatus in a big system is now about as likely to have its origin

Table 6.12. *The safe organisation*

---

1. Pervading influence from leadership style at all levels of management
2. Reliance on a safety policy document which is endorsed by all managers and regularly reviewed
3. Systematic collection and dissemination of accident data
4. Comparison of company performance with national norms for the company type
5. Training of supervisors and foremen in safety sensitivity and accident recording
6. Training of operators and maintenance staff in safe procedures, e.g. lifting for manual workers
7. Use of safety committees to which workers' representatives are elected and managers attend as a primary responsibility
8. Provision of specialist safety officers when appropriate with clear terms of reference and channels of access to promote action
9. Constructive use of outside experts such as official safety inspectors and consultants for special problems
10. Integration of safety and health support services

---

in a maintenance error as in a controller error, and the maintenance operator is personally more at risk than is the controller.

Operation and maintenance can be approached with a strategy separated into the safe operator, the safe system and the safe organisation (Singleton, 1976). The organisation is itself a system, but a people dominant one, and safety in this context depends on creating a safe climate. This is expressed in the attitudes and style of workers at every level. It is directly observable as good housekeeping, but its effects are manifested and maintained in the many different ways listed in Table 6.12.

Leplat (1984) regards the analysis of accidents as a specialised form of systems analysis with an emphasis on potential or actual dysfunctions within the system. This involves analysis of series and patterns usually starting from an incident or error, working backwards towards sources and forwards towards consequences (Leplat 1982). The backward looking analysis is called a genesis study (Leplat 1977). From the fact of the incident it follows that there have been some variations from standard system performance and one object-ive of the analysis is to locate these variations. This approach is analogous to that of Kjellen (1984, 1987) who searches for deviations in system variables of many kinds: human errors, energy changes, communication failures and so on. Saari (1984, 1986) concentrates on disturbances in the flow of information and also on the use of information feedback in behaviour modification.

6.4 Applications

6.4.1 *Risk analysis*

Practice under this heading has become very popular in high energy systems such as bridges, dams, oil platforms, chemical plant and power stations. The objective is to assess risks and the relationship between various risk activities and their joint outcome. The ultimate purpose is to reduce accidents, but there are a variety of more immediate reasons for embarking on such analyses:

- as part of the evidence comparing different designs
- as safety-related feedback during a design process
- as a safety check before a design is translated into practice
- as a marketing aid demonstrating the expected safety level of a design
- to ensure compliance with safety regulations
- to conform with regulations or agreements with a safety authority or a contract sponsor

The techniques used depends on the kind of system to be analysed and the purpose of the analysis. Rowe (1986) suggests that Risk Analysis can be either top down or bottom up. A top down analysis starts with the purpose and works through a decision model to the specification of the studies required to collect relevant data. A bottom up analysis (more strictly a synthesis) starts with the elemental risk data (doses/effects of toxic substances or probabilities of mechanical failures) and relates these to the likely behaviour of the system under study by looking at all the possible pathways and defences. Andersen (1984) suggests that the first step is to define system boundaries and then proceed through the sequence:

- identification of hazards (see '*Hazard reduction*' above)
- analysis of causal events
- analysis of consequences
- estimation of risk

It is important to establish system boundaries because one key feature of risk is the interaction between the system and its environment. The environment may impact on the system, e.g. storms or aircraft crashes, and the system may leak into the environment, e.g. physical objects, toxic substances or radiation. It will be noted that the main part of these large scale risk analyses is writing scenarios of what might happen in what circumstances.

More detailed risk analyses involve generating event trees and fault trees, preferably with attached probability data. This is called *Probabilistic Risk*

Assessment (PRA). It is difficult enough for hardware systems such as fluid networks or for information systems such as alarm trees, and it becomes virtually impossible if any attempt is made to incorporate man–machine interactions. This is very serious because the human operator is in the system as an agent for the detection and correction of malfunctions. If his impact on the system cannot be quantified then risk or reliability analysis becomes of limited value on both theoretical and practical grounds.

6.4.2   *Reliability analysis*
This overlaps with risk analysis, but there is a difference of emphasis in that risk is about safety and reliability is orientated more towards efficiency and economy. It is enormously important to system operators that systems are reliable. For big systems such as aircraft or process plants it is not only potentially dangerous, it is also extremely expensive if the system does not function as planned. For smaller systems, such as cars and machine-tools, customer and user preference is strongly influenced by reliability.

Event Tree Analysis (ETA) is used to trace the consequences of particular initiating events, it is essentially a 'what if' technique. *Fault Tree Analysis* (FTA) is the reverse process which starts with events which will result in system or sub-system down-time and works backwards through component failures and human errors. In both cases attempts are made to attach probability values to particular levels in the chains. Perhaps the main value of these analyses is in identifying what could happen and thus initiating rethinking about how to avoid these chains of happenings. Particular sub-systems can be identified which must have very high reliability, if necessary by duplication or triplication, or by alternative back-up systems. It is also possible to identify 'common mode failures' which are particularly serious in causing simultaneous breakdowns on a large scale, e.g. due to loss of power supplies.

There have been many attempts to develop *Human Reliability Assessment* (HRA) techniques. The best known is the *Technique for Human Error Rate Prediction* (THERP) developed at the Sandia Laboratories (Swain and Guttman, 1983). This parallels hardware reliability analysis in starting with probability of failure for standard elements such as switch operations, and combining these along sequences to arrive at assessments of overall reliability. The numbers are qualified by various 'performance shaping factors', e.g. stress level. Nevertheless there has been much criticism by psychologists of such a mechanistic technique. There are also holistic techniques which depend on expert judgment. The essence of these techniques is how to extract more informed opinions from experts. For example, the *Success Likelihood Index Methodology* (SLIM) (Embrey, 1987) aims to orientate experts in weighting the relative importance of various performance shaping factors relevant to the performance of a particular task. Weightings can be converted into ratings and ratings can be summed to arrive by another conversion at overall probabilities of failure. This is a modern computer-based version of the classical psychophysical methods.

The intensive pursuit of simple numerical answers is a concession to the engineers who like to have concrete data, preferably in a form where it can be combined with their own data about the reliability of hardware systems. This is a serious trap for the unwary who, given a set of data, readily overlook the shaky nature of the sources and processes used to generate it.

A more defensible approach is to use established Human Factors principles to optimise the performance of a given kind of operator in a given system and thereby arrive at the best attainable level of human reliability.

6.4.3   Safety compliance

Given that in any country safety is something which the authorities have undertaken to enforce, there are two problems: what to enforce and how to enforce it.

What to enforce is difficult enough because there are economic, social and cultural influences on top of scientific and technical problems. Economic decisions are usually shifted to employers by the use of phrases such as 'as far as is reasonably practicable', but the authorities must show some awareness of cost-effectiveness, otherwise they will place their own companies at too great a comparative disadvantage to those of other countries where safety precautions are less rigid. Cost also should come into assessing where to direct the safety effort. Even the largest countries do not have infinite budgets, and if risk reduction per unit cost is much greater in one direction than in others there is sense in moving in that direction. Socially and culturally the authorities need also to take some account of movements in public opinion. For example, in most developed countries there is more investment in radiation and chemical hazards than in the more mundane, but in terms of the evidence more significant sources of damage such as lifting and falling (Singleton 1984). Technically it is extremely difficult to describe to what degree something is harmful. Sometimes the scientists make some attempt to translate their evidence into a usable form, e.g. Pochin (1986), but more usually they restrict their efforts to producing isolated bits of data and someone else, invariably a committee, has to do the translation into legislation. For these reasons and because of continuous change as experience and evidence develops advanced countries have three levels of edict:

– *Laws* generated by the national legislative bodies which are usually framed in general terms and are changed only every ten or twenty years. During the past decade the main changes have been to try to cover a greater proportion of the total working population. Earlier in the century the laws dealt only with factories but they now cover shops, offices, the hotel and catering industry, transport and public places

– *Standards* which are mandatory but are formulated by the safety and health institutions. The difficulty here, as described above, is how to translate scientific data into forms of words and numbers which can lead to consistent enforcement by inspectorates and achieve the basic objective of protecting the population without unnecessarily adding to costs. For example, for environmental agents from noise to chemicals there is the difficulty of combining maximum allowable intensities with maximum overall exposures. Formulating a new standard can take several years

– *Codes of practice* which are advisory and thus can allow much more flexibility while retaining the background presence of the law. If an employer is sued for negligence the case is that much stronger if it can be argued that a code of practice was transgressed

This graded system allows scope for the inspectorate to combine their conflicting roles of policeman and adviser. Other aspects of the functions of the inspectorate are whether to organise by industry or by trade, how to separate local and national responsibilities and how to organise the sampling process of inspection visits. Industry versus trade is difficult because it is the industry which is localised geographically and therefore easier to monitor, but increasingly specific expertise is necessary to inspect effectively. In most countries the inspectorate is organised by areas, but fortunately areas tend to have trade specialities and the inspectors specialise accordingly, e.g. in the U.K. the East Scotland office deals with distilling and brewing, and the Midlands office deals with metal working. In Switzerland the Zurich office deals with metal working and the Aarau office with the chemical industry. Normally local inspectorates deal with general labour laws. There are national branches of the inspectorate which deal with highly technical problems such as radiation levels. Arranging tours of inspection has to have some random element to reduce predictability, but, on the other hand, 'selective persecution' must be avoided. In the U.S.A. the situation is actually made more difficult because the law allows individuals to request inspections, most of the inspectorate time goes on coping with these complaints.

The three necessary service functions are administration and inspection described above and research. Research can be taken to cover everything from collection of accident data to behavioural aspects of safety. Collected data meets several different needs: feedback on overall performance from a safety and health management viewpoint, provision of specific norms from an operational management viewpoint (a manager can compare his performance with the average for the industry), and highlighting of trends and new hazards from an epidemiological viewpoint. Provision of new evidence for standards and codes of practice is an associated scientific function. There is a case for separating this total research from the administration and compliance functions, but when this is done as in the U.S.A. the communication difficulties seem to be greater.

It will be appreciated that safety compliance is man-power intensive and therefore increasingly expensive in relative terms as societies advance. How to maintain the optimum level of activity and resource is a problem for every society.

These issues and solutions have been described at some length because there has been greater progress and experience here than elsewhere. Yet the problems are characteristic of all areas where it is desirable to translate science into technology and practice including the behavioural sciences. Acquiring the knowledge is the smallest, and in many ways the easiest part of the whole business of getting it applied in practice.

6.4.4   Accident research

Accident research is susceptible to rather better management than other areas because it is a field with definable boundaries and because there has been extensive experience in the past twenty years.

The sponsor and customer of the study is usually a safety authority and it is desirable to tailor the objectives by two criteria. Firstly, the likely mechanism of implementation – is the purpose to guide policy or to fit into an established mode of information dissemination such as codes of practice? Secondly, what is the balance of importance between severity and frequency of accidents, or are cultural criteria intervening? e.g. the topic happens to be fashionable.

There is a parallel question of the type of benefit. Is it broadly to increase understanding, that is to develop theory? or is it intended to be a more direct decision aid to practitioners or policymakers?

The costs of research are not only financial, there is also time and personnel. Objectives and procedures often need to be determined by the time available before the results are required. It is irresponsible to undertake a particular project unless there are staff available with appropriate knowledge and skill to conduct the investigation.

The availability of personnel will also affect the theoretical approach: the emphasis may be from physical and engineering sciences, from behavioural sciences, from mathematics and statistics or from more specific expertise such as accident and risk theories *per se*.

There are two possible sources of data: existing records and new sources. The existing records may be in the form of accident statistics, accident reports and accident investigations. The limitations of statistics have been described already. Accident reports are frustrating for the behavioural scientist because the emphasis is usually either legal (who was responsible), medical (what was the damage) or engineering (what machinery was involved). It is rare to find a comprehensive account of what those involved were actually doing or trying to do, why they were doing it, and what were their circumstances (time at work, time of day, weather, etc.) Investigations of serious accidents are always carried out for specific purposes. These purposes, the context and the kind of people who conducted them (often dominated by lawyers) need to be appreciated so that the inevitable biases can be taken into account.

Studies undertaken within research projects can generate new evidence by interviews, observation of incidents and experiments which may be laboratory based or field based. There are special obstacles within accident studies for each of these procedures. Interviewees have been involved and their reports are inevitably biased against the attachment of any blame to themselves. Direct observation of accidents is almost impossible because of the waiting time and the ethical issue that it is not feasible to stand by and observe without attempting prevention. Correspondingly it is not feasible to generate realistic but risk free accident situations either in the field or in the laboratory.

For all these reasons accident studies tend to start with available data and to generate hypotheses from these about behaviour more generally which can be checked by specific studies, such as interviews and experiments. It also becomes clearer why there is so little theoretical material specific to accidents.

References

Altman, J.W. (1967). Classifications of human error. In De Greene, K.B. (ed.). *Systems Psychology*. New York: McGraw-Hill.

Andersen, R.S. (ed.). (1984). *Risk Analysis in Off-shore Development Projects*. Trondheim: SINTEF.

ANPAT, (1983). Commuting Accidents. (Association Nationale pour la prévention des accidents du travail). In *Encyclopaedia of Occupational Health and Safety*. Geneva: International Labour Office.

Berg, G.G. and Maillie, H.D. (eds.). (1981). *Measurement of Risks*. New York: Plenum.

Bignell, V., Peters, G. and Pym, C. (1977). *Catastrophic Failures*. Milton Keynes: Open University Press.

Bohr, E. (1984). Application of instructional design principles to nuclear power plant operating procedures manuals. In Easterby, R. and Zwaga, H. (eds.). *Information Design*. Chichester: Wiley.

Brehmer, B. (1987a). The psychology of risk. In Singleton, W.T. and Hovden, J. (eds.). *Risk and Decisions*. Chichester: Wiley.

Brehmer, B. (1987b). Development of mental models for decisions in technological systems. In Rasmussen, J., Duncan, K. and Leplat, J. (eds.). *New Technology and Human Error*. Chichester: Wiley.

Cherns, A.B. (1970). Accidents at work. In Welford, A.T., Argyle, M., Glass, D.V. and Morris, J.N. (eds.). *Society: Problems and Methods of Study*. London: Routledge and Kegan Paul.

Cooper, M.G. (ed.). (1985). *Risk: Man-made Hazards to Man*. Oxford: Clarendon Press.

Cresswell C.W. and Froggatt, P. (1963). *The Causation of Bus Driver Accidents*. Oxford University Press.

Davis, D.R. (1958). Human Errors and Transport Accidents. *Ergonomics*. **2**. 24–33.

De Greene, K.B. (1970). *Systems Psychology*. New York: McGraw-Hill.

Duncan, K.D. (1987). Fault diagnosis training for advanced continuous process operations. In Rasmussen, J., Duncan, K. and Leplat, J. (eds.). *New Technology and Human Error*. Chichester: Wiley.

Easterby, R. and Zwaga, H. (eds). (1984). *Information Design. Section 5 – Applications and Consumer/Safety Signs*. Chichester: Wiley.

Embrey, D. (1987). Human reliability assessment: the state of the art. In *Human Reliability in Nuclear Power*. London: I.B.C. Technical Services.

Fitts, P.M. and Jones, R.E. (1947). Analysis of pilot error experiments. Reprinted in Sinaiko H.W. (ed.). (1961). *Selected Papers on Human Factors in the Design and Use of Control Systems*. New York: Dover.

Flowers, B. (1976). *Nuclear Power and the Environment*. Sixth report of the Royal Commission on Environmental Pollution. London: H.M.S.O.

Freud, S. (1949). *An Outline of Psychoanalysis*. London: Hogarth Press.

Gagne, R.M. (ed.). (1962). *Psychological Principles in System Development*. New York: Holt, Rinehart & Winston.

Goddard, G. (1988). *Occupational Accident Statistics*, 1981–85. Employment Gazette, January.

Green, A.E. (ed.). (1982). *High Risk Safety Technology*. Chichester: Wiley.

Greenwood, M. and Woods, H.M. (1919). The Incidence of Industrial Accidents upon Individuals with special reference to Multiple Accidents. *Industrial Fatigue Research Board Report No. 4*. London: H.M.S.O.

Hale, A.R. (1984). Is Safety Training Worthwhile? *Journal of Occupational Accidents*. **6**. 17–33.

Hale, A.R. (1987). Subjective risk. In Singleton, W.T. and Hovden, J. (eds.). *Risk and Decisions*. Chichester: Wiley.

Health and Safety at Work etc. Act. (1974). Chapter 37. London: H.M.S.O.

Hedge, A. (1987). Major hazards and behaviour. In Singleton, W.T. and Hovden, J. (eds.). *Risk and Decisions*. Chichester: Wiley.

Hoffman, B. (1987). *Unfallanalyse. 1985*. Sankt Augustin: Berufsgenossenschaften.

I.L.O. (1983). (3rd. rev. ed.). *Encyclopaedia of Occupational Health and Safety.* 2 vols. Geneva: I.L.O.

Jacobs, G.O. and Hutchinson, P. (1973). A Study of Accident Rates in Developing Countries. *Transport Road Research Laboratory Report.* LR 546.

Kahneman, D., Slovik, P. and Tversky, A. (1982). *Judgement Under Uncertainty.* Cambridge University Press.

Kidd, J.S. (1962). Human tasks and equipment design. In Gagne, R.M. (ed.). *Psychological Principles in System Development.* New York: Holt, Rinehart & Winston.

Kjellen, U. (1984). The role of deviation in accident causation and control. In Kjellen, U. (ed.). *Occupational Accident Research.* Amsterdam: Elsevier.

Kjellen, U. (1987). Variations and the feedback control of accidents. In Rasmussen, J., Duncan, K. and Leplat, J. (eds.). *New Technology and Human Error.* Chichester: Wiley.

Lagerlof, E. (1975). Industrial safety in Sweden. In *Occupational Accident Research.* Stockholm: Work Environment Fund.

Leplat, J. (1977). Reconstruction and genesis of accidents. In *Research on Occupational Accidents.* Stockholm: Work Environment Fund.

Leplat, J. (1982). Accidents and Incidents Production: Methods of Analysis. *Journal of Occupational Accidents.* 4. 299–331.

Leplat, J. (1984). Occupational accident research and systems approach. In Kjellen, U. (ed.). *Occupational Accident Research.* Amsterdam: Elsevier.

Lewin, K. (1936). *Principles of Topological Psychology.* New York: McGraw-Hill.

Lowrance, W.W. (1980). The nature of risk. In Schwing, R.C. and Albers, W.A. (eds.). *Societal Risk Assessment.* New York: Plenum.

McFarland, R.A. (1970). *Human Factors during the Next Decade 1970–1980.* Presidential address to the Human Factors Society, San Francisco.

McFarland, R.A., Moore, R.C. and Warren, A.B. (1955). *Human Variables in Motor Vehicle Accidents.* Cambridge Mass.: Harvard School of Public Health.

McFarland, R.A. and Moore, R.C. (1971). Safety Engineering. In *Encyclopaedia Britannica.*

Meister, D. and Rabideau, G.F. (1965). *Human Factors Evaluations in System Development.* New York: Wiley.

NUREG (1975). Reactor Safety Study. *An Assessment of Accident Risks in U.S. Commercial Nuclear Power Plants.* 75.014. Washington: Nuclear Regulatory Commission.

NUREG CR1270 (1980). *Human Factors Evaluation of Control Room Design and Operation Performance at TMI 2. Vols 1–3.* Washington: Nuclear Regulatory Commission.

Oftedal, P. and Brogger, A. (eds.). (1986). *Risk and Reason: Risk Assessment in Relation to Environmental Mutagens and Carcinogens.* New York: A.R. Liss.

Parry, M.H. (1968). *Aggression on the Road.* London: Tavistock.

Perrow, C. (1981). Normal accident at Three Mile Island. *Society.* **18.5.** 17–26.

Perrow, C. (1984). *Normal Accidents: Living with High Risk Technology.* New York: Basic Books.

Pochin, E.E. (1986). Radiation and an index of harm. In Oftedal, P. and Brogger, A. (eds.). *Risk and Reason.* New York: A.R. Liss.

Powell, P., Hale, M., Martin, J. and Simon, M. (1971). *2,000 Accidents*. London: National Institute of Industrial Psychology.

Rasmussen, J. (1987). The definition of human error and a taxonomy for technical system design. In Rasmussen, J., Duncan, K. and Leplat, J. (eds.) *New Technology and Human Error*. Chichester: Wiley.

Reason, J. (1987). The psychology of mistakes: a brief review of planning failures. In Rasmussen, J., Duncan K. and Leplat, J. (eds.). *New Technology and Human Error*. Chichester: Wiley.

Robens Committee (1972). *Report on Safety and Health at Work*. London: H.M.S.O.

ROSPA. Royal Society for the Prevention of Accidents. *Accident Statistics for Great Britain*. (published annually)

Rowe, W.D. (1986). Identification of risk. In Oftedal, P. and Brogger, A. (eds.). *Risk and Reason*. New York: A.R. Liss.

Rubinstein, T. and Mason, A.E. (1979). The Accident that shouldn't have happened. *I.E.E. Spectrum*. November.

Saari, J. (1984). Accidents and disturbances in the flow of information. In Kjellen, U. (ed.). *Occupational Accident Research*. Amsterdam: Elsevier.

Saari, J. (1986). The effects of positive feed-back on housekeeping and accidents at a shipyard. *Journal of Occupational Accidents*. **8**. 237–50.

Schwing, R.C. and Albers, W.A. (eds.). (1980). *Societal Risk Assessment – How Safe is Safe Enough?* New York: Plenum.

Singleton, W.T. (1972). Techniques for determining the causes of errors. *Applied Ergonomics*. **3.3**. 126–31.

Singleton, W.T. (1973). Theoretical approaches to Human Error. The Ergonomics Society Annual Lecture. *Ergonomics*. **16.6**. 727–37.

Singleton, W.T. (1975). Skill and accidents. In *Occupational Accident Research*. Stockholm: Work Environment Fund.

Singleton, W.T. (1976). *Human Aspects of Safety*. London: Keith Shipton.

Singleton, W.T. (1981). System theory and skill theory. In Singleton, W.T. (ed.). *Management Skills*. Lancaster: M.T. Press.

Singleton, W.T. (1982). Accidents and the progress of technology. *Journal of Occupational Accidents*. **4**. 91–102.

Singleton, W.T. (1983). Occupational Safety and Health Systems: a Three-country Comparison. *International Labour Review*. **122.2**. 55–68.

Singleton, W.T. (1984). Future trends in accident research in European countries. In Kjellen, A. (ed.). *Occupational Accident Research*. Amsterdam: Elsevier.

Singleton, W.T. (1987). Risk-handling by institutions. In Singleton, W.T. and Hovden, J. (eds.). *Risk and Decisions*. Chichester: Wiley.

Singleton, W.T. and Hovden, J. (eds.). (1987). *Risk and Decisions*. Chichester: Wiley.

Slovic, P. Fischhoff, B. and Lichtenstein, S. (1980). Facts and fears: understanding perceived risk. In Schwing, R.C. and Albers, W.A. (eds.). *Societal Risk Assessment*. New York: Plenum.

Storr, A. (1968). *Human Aggression*. Harmondsworth: Penguin.

Swain, A.D. and Guttman, H.E. (1983). *Handbook of Human Reliability Analysis*. Albequerque: Sandia Laboratories.

Taylor, D.H. (1981). Hermeneutics of Accidents and Safety. Ergonomics **24.6**. 487–95. Reprinted in Rasmussen, J., Duncan, K. and Leplat, J. (eds.). (1987). *New Technology and Human Error*. Chichester: Wiley.

Taylor, F.V. (1963). Human engineering and psychology. In Koch, S. (ed.). *Psychology, a Study of Science. Vol. 5*. New York: McGraw-Hill.

Tye, W. (1977). *Basic Safety Concepts*. Paper 512 at the 15th Anglo-American Aeronautical Conference, London.

Tye, W. (1980). Design for Safety. Reported In Singleton, W.T. (1982). Accidents and the progress of technology. *Journal of Occupational Accidents*. **4**. 91–102.

Vandenberg, J.P. (1967). Improved operating procedures manuals. In Singleton, W.T., Easterby, R.S. and Whitfield, D. (eds.). *The Human Operator in Complex Systems*. London: Taylor & Francis.

7 The citizen and the environment

7.1 Concepts

This is one of the shorter chapters because, with the exception of road vehicles, the research effort is considerable but the practical application is limited and shows no signs of expanding rapidly in the near future. Nevertheless it is worthwhile to introduce the topic because at least potentially there is a considerable Human Factors contribution to the issues.

7.1.1 The technology-based society

The issue in general terms is that, throughout the world, changes in the environment, work and leisure are now based on advances in technology. If these changes are left to the physical scientists and engineers the consequences are not entirely satisfactory to the customer, the ordinary citizen. In his role as the people's representative in technology design teams the Human Factors specialist ought to take some responsibility for improving this state of affairs. There are a number of difficulties:

– the ultimate responsibility is with the politicians elected to government, but in terms of intellect, education and training, politicians are not well equipped to assimilate and weight the conflicting advice they receive, and national constitutions were designed for a different era. For example, most countries have a governmental Department of Transport, but no country has an integrated transport policy. There are too many vested interests, the interactions are too complicated, the consequences of decisions extend well beyond the life cycle of any one government – in general the problem is too big. Some impact is possible at regional and district levels, but not on a national scale. Historically it was often achieved for a single mode of transport; in the early eighteenth century Europe was covered by an extensive canal network, succeeded at the end of the century by an even more extensive railway network, each was built within a few decades which must have involved tremendous human effort and organisation. More recent and more mechanised examples are the post-war roads built in the far west of the U.S.A. by the Eisenhower government and the network of European motorways which followed the example of the prewar German autobahns. In retrospect it seems surprising that ergonomics did not emerge from any of these enterprises. With a few exceptions civil engineers are more notable for their drive than for their intellectual analysis.

– governments are currently dominated by economic advice and objectives. Economists rarely think in terms related to human problems.

– other specialists such as architects and planners have seized the opportunity to approach the issues of the built environment. Once again their thinking has not been people-based. For example, the problems of high-rise living were fairly clear even before the event to psychologists, but not to those who designed and implemented the policy. It was obvious that old people and mothers with young children were going to have difficulties in not being able to reach the open air except via lifts subject to vandalisation. However, no one foresaw that living in high buildings would result in rejection of all responsibility for spaces such as halls, lifts, stairs, corridors, not only in terms of good housekeeping but extending also to what happens to people in these spaces. The consequence is that the influence of environmental planners peaked around the '60s and '70s and has since declined because of the obvious failures. It is disheartening to professionals when it emerges that ergonomically and aesthetically satisfying total environments seem to emerge better by evolution than by formal design.

– some of the problems blamed on the technologists including the planners are not so much due to the formal approach but rather to increasing densities of population. The greater this density the more difficult, but perhaps the more necessary, it seems to be to design satisfactory living conditions. It has even been suggested, with an excessively brutal realism, that given such high population densities an appropriate solution has emerged accidently. This is to encourage these people to congregate in small groups in darkened rooms watching flickering screens. This impression is reinforced by travel through the dreary 'flatlands' surrounding most European cities in both Common Market and Comecon countries.

– as standards of living rise new problems emerge because an amenity which reaches saturation ceases to be an amenity. Governments in communist countries are aware of the problems which arise if resources and leisure are allowed to increase faster than leisure facilities become available, the consequence is increased alcoholism and other drug abuse. In all countries the automobile is a marvellous amenity providing that only a small proportion of the population have them, if everyone has them they become a curse except where population densities are low. Similarly the European hankering for rural as opposed to urban life can be satisfied if the proportion of town people in a village remains low, when the townies outnumber the indigenous villagers the area becomes commuterland and the objective is lost.

It is difficult to make and dubious to even claim to be able to make a contribution to such large problems. The approach cannot be scientific at least in the restricted sense of reliance on theory established by experiment. Field-based approaches incorporating assessment and prediction of available re-sources was in vogue in the 1970s stimulated by the Club of Rome (Forrester, 1970; Meadows, 1972; Mesarovic and Pestel, 1975; Peccei, 1977). These efforts were frustrated by the difficulty of estimating world resources of any commod-ity, e.g. new resources of oil are steadily discovered by further exploration, and by the fact that individuals and communities adapt by changing their require-ments as costs and consequences change. As a London *Times* leader of 4 May 1988 put it 'compiling statistics – from raw material as changing and resource-ful as human beings – is an inexact science. Fortunately there is hunch, suspicion and anecdote to help ministers discover what is really going on. They should make more use of them'.

For these and no doubt many other reasons there is an intuitive suspicion of 'social engineering'. It is regarded as an intrusion on individual freedom of choice, but this is inevitably a matter of degree of emphasis. In a well ordered society freedom cannot extend beyond freedom under the law. Governments cannot make things happen in the way that an engineer designs and constructs a machine, they can only create the conditions which will encourage those things to happen which they would like to happen. In addition, predictions of human behaviour are inherently probabilistic, there is bound to be slack in the system which will enable the individual to determine his own destiny and move upwards, downwards or sideways through the various economic, social and technical levels (Singleton, 1967). It can also be argued that it is rigid systems of caste, class and taxation rather than societies with planning systems which restrict the individual's freedom of manoeuvre. Planning, like every other executive activity, is only objectionable when it is incompetently and ineffi-ciently conducted. The solution would seem to be to introduce more human parameters into government and planning in evolutionary rather than revol-utionary style as experience and knowledge accumulate. There must be an extensive reliance on knowledge from practical experience rather than from academic theory, although hopefully theory will follow from the evidence of experience.

7.1.2   *The technology-based environment*

This is a less intractable issue than the societal infrastructure. The environment is dominated by technology from transport to methods of agriculture. For example, industry and domestic property is now strongly influenced in location by access to motorway networks. Even air transport requires large airports and it has only recently been appreciated that an airport radically influences a region not merely in terms of environmental variables such as noise, but more pervasively in terms of the whole pattern of the regional economy and transport system. Within airports as public places the ergonomics aspects of lighting, information presentations, design of services, reception desks and luggage movement are now dealt with satisfactorily. Correspondingly there has been a great improvement in the design of public information systems in railway stations, hospitals, shopping centres and other similar places which are unfamiliar to some of the user population. The design approach is a combination of systems analysis of traffic flows and requirements together with appropriate displays containing alphanumeric data and coding by colour and by the use of easily identified symbols. In agriculture the technology is not merely the physical sciences–engineering combination, but also the chemical–biological influence on seeds, fertilisation and pest-control. This creates many safety issues (see Chapter 6) and there are remedial procedures based on machine design, container design, labelling and presentation of instructions. The accelerating impact of technology over the past century is now such that there is very little 'natural' landscape at a more detailed level than the height contours. In Europe every panoramic view is a consequence of human will and effort, not merely in obvious features such as roads and electricity pylons but in the detail of the boundaries, the vegetation, the flow of water in rivers and the tree patterns. This impact will be even greater in the next few decades because the productivity of agriculture is now such that a considerable proportion of the land is not needed for growing food. Quite what to do with it and whether behavioural scientists can conduct studies which will influence these decisions remains to be seen.

There are not very many useful concepts which can be used even to discuss these issues, but the related terms: *territory, social distance and defensible space* are relevant. Territoriality was first noted in the behaviour of birds about fifty years ago, and once noticed it was obviously a key feature of animal behaviour. Animals, in groups, families or occasionally as individuals, often function within a geographical area for which they attempt to define the boundary and which they protect from intrusion by outsiders. There are degrees of definitive ownership, the nest or its equivalent is even more fiercely protected than the surrounding area in which hunting takes place. Outsiders recognise when they are intruding but may do so aggressively in an attempt to take over some or all of the space. The concept was developed and extended to human behaviour, perhaps rather too imaginatively, by Ardrey (1966). Territorial behaviour is instinctive and human beings hopefully have a considerable rationality superimposed on their more primitive propensities. Nevertheless the violent reactions aroused at national levels by disputes about frontiers and on a much smaller scale the ease with which arguments about office spaces or about fences between neighbours can arise suggest that this factor remains potent. Newman (1972) extended the notion to the built environment and distinguished between public space, semi-private areas and private territory. One strategy for reduction of violence and vandalism is the cultivation and extension of semi-private space which is under surveillance and for which the individual or group feels some responsibility. For example, the siting of cloakrooms in factories can usefully reflect this phenomenon. In a village the whole local area is semi-private space and special note is taken of strangers. The phenomenon of social distance relates to private space which is located with reference to the individual rather than to geography. Although there are individual differences, most people are irritated or uncomfortable if others, particularly strangers, get too close to them. Even in a city street a pedestrian regards the space immediately in front of him as his into which others ought not to intrude, the same is true for motorists.

There are interactions between bonds and boundaries defined socially (groups), and those defined geographically (environments). Horizontal distance is different from vertical distance within built environments – hence the social problems of high-rise buildings. Within offices 'them and us' differences arise in relation to those across the corridor or those on the other side of the lifts, stairs and toilets. Toilets and canteens are spaces shared by different groups, this is perhaps why joint staff committees are often accused of spending so much of their time discussing 'tea, towels and toilets'.

Canter (1975) divides the environment into the thermal, the acoustic, the luminous and the spatial, and separates the issues of buildings, cities and natural environments. The separation of relevant parameters is an important aspect of conceptualisation, otherwise the questions are too general to have answers. Not surprisingly, the physical variables are the easiest to analyse and describe. Design to cope with these issues is increasingly effective because the variables are understood, there is adequate technology to cope and perhaps more important, the availability of cheap, reliable communication and control systems can provide flexibility and adaptability in the design process and the product. For example, the concept of *Intelligent buildings* has recently developed. These depend on computers and communications networks. At the design and construction stage these facilities support effective management control and the integration and phasing of all the complex processes and products which need to be brought together. The product will have energy management, full environmental control including lighting, heating and ventilation, fire prevention, security and so on, all managed automatically by one control system. There will be elaborate facilities for data banks, computation and communication systems between people possibly within the same network or possibly in an independent network. Overall system failure would be catastrophic but the probability of failure is very low. There would be a serious problem if electric power was lost although there may be limited emergency systems. The approach could in principle be extended to larger and larger building complexes and even to whole cities. Geneva has made a tentative start in rationalising all the different services: water, gas, electricity and communications in the way they are channelled under streets and in paying more attention than is usually the case to the integration of public transport. In common with every other municipality they have yet to find a way of coping successfully with the private car.

Increased attention to the needs of users extends from public spaces and buildings to all products used by the consumer.

7.1.3 Consumer ergonomics

The strategy of applying ergonomics to environments such as hotels, hospitals, schools, homes and the equipment used in them relies on the same concepts as those developed for military and industrial ergonomics, but there are some differences:

- the complete age range must be considered from children to old people. Thus the range of any relevant parameters from body size to behaviour norms is much larger
- the systematic approach has to be largely through design. No training requirements can be expected, although there is some scope for design of instructions. It cannot be assumed of course that the user will read the instructions
- the objectives are not so clear. Aesthetic as well as ergonomic criteria apply although fortunately these usually reinforce each other. Indeed there is a school of thought that if the function is right the appearance will take care of itself, but this underestimates the total contribution of industrial designers and architects. Safety remains important, productivity may not be critical. 'Comfort' becomes the dominant criterion for some situations and products. Details of the application of consumer ergonomics are given in Kirk and Ridgway, (1970, 1971) and Wilson and Whittington, (1981).

Comfort, like health, is easier to define by its absence rather than by its presence. In spite of a number of gallant attempts the measurement of comfort does not seem feasible, although measures of discomfort have attained some success. The evidence is usually based on opinions, although some contribution is possible from electromyography and from principles of good posture. Short-term comfort assessment based on the immediate impression of the first few minutes of experience may be different from the view after hours or months of exposure. Hence the difficulty of selecting satisfactory chairs. Comfort is one of those important but frustrating concepts, widely used and apparently mutually understood in ordinary life, but not susceptible to precise definition leading to measurement. The association between comfort and arousal is not clear, if comfort is intended to imply relaxation it may not be a suitable criterion for some situations. If, on the other hand, it is identified with healthy posture this may suggest different objectives and measures. Healthy posture is particularly important for those with motor disabilities, the disabled in general are a separate topic of study overlapping into consumer ergonomics but also into industrial ergonomics.

7.1.4   Disabled individuals

The concept of disability is on the borderline between medical, psychological and socio-economic models. There is further complexity in that any bodily impairment is bound to have mental consequences and vice versa. Neglecting the interaction of body and mind is convenient in the interests of simplicity, but it is not ultimately sustainable in relation to any topic and least of all in relation to disability. Individuals can suffer from multiple disabilities and the consequences for the person, for others, and for society generally are different depending on the age of onset.

In all ergonomic practice there are underlying issues of ethics and human dignity on which are superimposed the more measurable criteria of economics, productivity, safety, and efficiency generally. This remains true of disability studies but for these latter the humanistic aspects are more generally obvious. Treatment of the disabled is an indicator of the quality of a civilised society and this requirement is sufficiently fundamental to be written into constitutions. For example, the European Charter has a clause about equal opportunities for the disabled. The same sentiment is expressed in more detail by the International Labour Office in the form of three principles (ILO, 1973):

- disabled persons should be afforded an equal opportunity with the non-disabled to perform work for which they are qualified
- disabled persons should have full opportunity to accept suitable work with employers of their own choice

 – emphasis should be placed on the abilities and work capacities of disabled persons and not on their disabilities

Note the emphasis on persons. For all the reasons mentioned above disability can only be fully described in relation to individuals. Nevertheless, if the objectives are to be met it is necessary to clarify concepts, generate taxonomies and proceed as far as possible towards measurement.

The terminology used is ambiguous, for example disability and handicap are often used interchangeably but there is now some consensus. *Impairment* refers to a residual consequence of disease, injury or genetic endowment; description and minimisation of impairment are within the province of medicine. There are curative and therapeutic aspects. *Disability* is a functional term, the consequences of impairment described so as to indicate the limitation on the 'normal' range of possible activity. *Handicap* is the consequence in the context of the individual's interaction with society, his needs and aspirations, his potentiality for work in the sense of activity with personal and monetary rewards. *Invalidity* refers to state support in the form of pensions, allowances and services (W.H.O. 1980, Duckworth, 1983). These distinctions which are partially taxonomic and partially descriptive of overlapping stages in the rehabilitation processes are summarised in Fig. 7.1. Each is descriptive not just of the individual but also of his interaction with society. Impairment changes occur as medicine advances, disability can be changed by training, handicap depends on the socio-economic conditions at a given time, e.g. degree of demand for labour, and invalidity is a matter of political policy. For these reasons a disabled individual often feels some grievance in that, from one point of view, his disablement is due to community achievements and attitudes rather than to him. For example, a person who uses a wheelchair for mobility is disabled by the environment rather than by his impairment if there are no facilities for ramps in parallel with steps.

Policies and facilities vary widely even within European countries. The Scandinavian countries pay more attention than do others to the design of the environment including domestic situations. All countries have rehabilitation centres, but some countries such as Germany tend to have large centres where the complete range of facilities including expertise can be made available, other countries such as Italy have smaller centres on the grounds of less travel and maintenance of closer contact with families. Available facilities are not just a function of national wealth, although clearly this is an important parameter, some poorer countries such as Poland have facilities which are much better than would be expected.

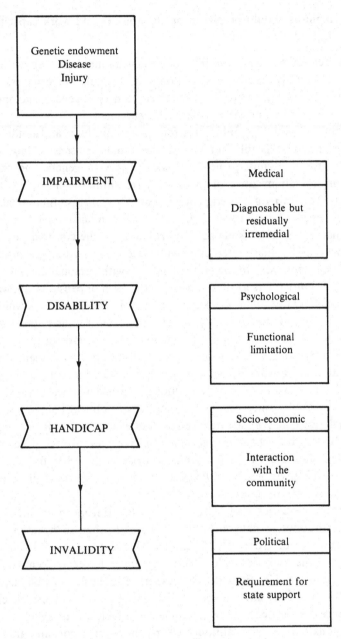

Fig. 7.1. Disablement terminology and the rehabilitation process.

7.2   Knowledge

There is little established knowledge relevant to this area which has not already been reviewed in earlier chapters.

On the issue of total population and available resources opinion is still divided. Barney (1980) concludes that there are already too many people for the world to support effectively, Simon and Kahn (1984) predict that it could easily support twice the current population. Even on relatively straightforward questions such as supplies of air, water, food and fuel, it is not possible to anticipate how the ingenuity of the human race will result in better means of coping. On social questions such as the quality of life within high density populations there is plenty of room for speculation which can be optimistic or pessimistic. Some demographic data are given in Chapter 1. Estimates of increases in population up to 2025 are shown in Fig. 7.2. The population of Europe is expected to change relatively little, but at the other end of the range the population of Africa is expected to treble over forty years. In 2025 the population of the world could be over 8 billion. One general tendency throughout the world is the drift to larger and larger population centres. This drift increases with standard of living. For example, Norway has to make consider-

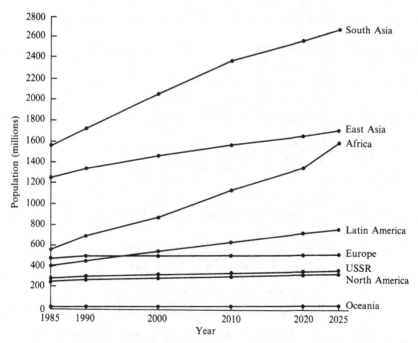

Fig. 7.2. Estimates of population increases. (*Demographic Year Book*)

able government effort, particularly farming subsidies, to keep the countryside occupied. The urban proportion of the population for an arbitrary selection of countries is shown in Fig. 7.3. Numerical data is one foundation for consideration of societal issues, but it is never sufficient in isolation.

Knowing the proportion of young or old people for example does not change the requirement that in societal or environmental design their special

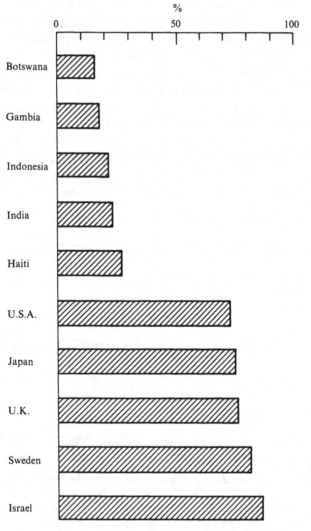

Fig. 7.3. Urban proportion of total population (live in towns of at least 1000 inhabitants) (*Demographic Year Book*).

needs should be considered. This is not a technical or economic kind of choice based on evidence, it is a moral requirement. Correspondingly, facilities and services for disabled individuals are not dictated by economic criteria, although there are in fact considerable economic benefits in reducing disability and handicap for each individual as much as possible.

Surprisingly little is known about numbers of disabled people. The only way to find out would be to have a precise set of definitions and to 'knock on every door' to ask questions. Governmental statistics on invalidity and disability registers are indicators only. Individuals have their own reasons for not registering even when a need is clear or registering when a need is not clear. Harris *et al.* (1971) conducted a survey of people over 15 years living at home in Great Britain (i.e. excluding those in institutions) and attempted to detect those with physical handicaps. Between one quarter and one third had appreciable disability, and about half of this group were severely or very severely disabled. These data are relevant to provision of invalidity allowances and design of domestic and public spaces. The proportion of disabled starts to accelerate from about 45 years onwards and is about 40% for those over 65 years.

For the population of working age the proportion of disabled in European countries seems to be between 5% and 10% depending on the definition of disability (Rouault, 1978). It should be emphasised that numerical answers to questions about disability and handicap vary widely with the reasons for the survey, sample sources, and with definitions. Nevertheless, it is clear that there is a considerable proportion of the population and a very large number of individuals to be considered.

7.3   Principles, methods and procedures
7.3.1   *Control for ill-defined issues*

It has been emphasised throughout this book that complete understanding is not essential for effective action and adaptive reaction. Incomplete information is the natural state. The skilled operator copes by generating hypotheses and confirming, expanding or rejecting them on the basis of new evidence which he creates by the action–feedback process. The process control room is part of a larger but analogous system in which a team of operators monitor a situation, select potentially ameliorative strategies, take related action and observe the consequences. In both cases there is a background of knowledge and theory which guides the tentative hypotheses and the search for confirmatory evidence. The so-called scientific method is a formalised special case of the same process. There is therefore no great precedent and there can be no objection to taking action in situations where theory and understanding generally are incomplete. The intelligent strategy is always to proceed tentatively on the basis of what is known, but to continue to seek for further evidence. In larger systems the feedback following action and the search for new data require consideration as an essential part of the design process. The less well-established the theory and knowledge the more important it is to ensure that these development and confirmatory mechanisms are available.

It was suggested in the previous chapter that this method is appropriate for safety and accident studies. It is also appropriate for the whole range of issues which arise in the context of this chapter. Academics are properly concerned with development of theory, but, for practitioners, the priority is ameliorative action now with theoretical advances as a useful by-product. The practitioner proceeding on the basis of limited understanding is not a charlatan unless he pretends that his knowledge is better than it actually is.

7.3.2   *User preference studies*

Given that the environment and its contents can be designed to suit the user, the problem is what is best for him and the system and what his preferences are. User requirement and user preference studies are fraught with difficulties.

It is usually impossible to define alternatives in simple terms so that people can be asked to make a choice. To take an absurd example, there would be no point in asking whether television or radio is preferred. For blind or deaf individuals the answer is obvious, for those with complete and effective sensory mechanisms television is suitable for some purposes and radio for others. In any case it depends on the programmes not the existence of the medium. Situations involve many variables; in the environment and contained items, in the kind and quality of services provided, in the objectives and tasks of the users and in personality differences for example, questions such as the urban versus the rural environment, private versus open office systems and public versus private transport systems. The answer is always somewhere between the extremes and the design art is to provide as many as possible of the advantages of both extremes whilst avoiding the disadvantages.

There is a pervading dilemma in that people cannot comment on products with which they have no experience and when they have some experience their opinions will be dominated by those features to which they are accustomed. This is not to suggest that such studies have no value, merely that all such data should always be regarded as a tentative indication rather than as firm evidence.

These studies are usually conducted by the standard survey methods described in Chapter 2. The key problems are the selection of and the communication with the sample. There is a great deal of specialist expertise and knowledge in this market research field, most of it not published openly because it is of some commercial value. The extensive use of computer data banks and the generation of glossy reports too readily disguise the weakness of the basic data.

7.3.3   The rehabilitation of the disabled

Given that rehabilitation requires two closely related sets of processes concerned respectively with assessment and resettlement, many disciplines have a contribution to make, these processes are currently conducted in most countries by using a team approach. The individual attends a rehabilitation centre either on a residential or a daily attendance basis. The centre usually provides treatment and training as well as assessment. One of their more important functions is to build up individual self-confidence, which can be assisted by the habit of successfully attending the centre ('going to work') on a routine basis. The core of the team will consist of a physician, a psychologist and training supervisor, although others such as psychiatrists, physio-therapists and resettlement officers can have contributions to make. Each must get to know the individual quite well and this process together with many case conferences means that the total procedure is very expensive.

From the administrative point of view the ideal outcome of an assessment would be a number (percentage disablement) used for an invalidity pension and a description of the optimal avenue towards employment. This is a *fata morgana*. Even attempts to use a multi-digit number incorporating categories and degrees of severity for each category lose the essence of the individual case, although they can be useful for statistical purposes such as epidemiology and planning of services. The International Classification of Impairment, Disease and Handicap is summarised in Table 7.1. These taxonomies clearly have been strongly influenced by medical thinking and are oriented towards ease of diagnosis rather than either scientific theory or occupational needs. The WHO (1980) report does point out that the physicians' judgements, performance measures and legal definitions should not be treated as equivalent.

The ergonomist is interested in the contribution he can make to features such as quality of life (design of domestic arrangements, wheelchairs and so on) and employability (jobs design and training). For these purposes we need taxonomies based on available occupations, work demands and matching human resources (Singleton, 1979). Table 7.2 shows a structure of job de-mands and human functions. Taxonomies of skills which essentially mediate between capacities, aspirations, and job demands are illustrated in Tables 2.1 and 2.10. Job demand catalogues require job taxonomies with associated

Table 7.1. *International classification of impairment, disability and handicap* (W.H.O., 1980)

Impairments (I code)	1. Intellectual
	2. Other psychological
	3. Language
	4. Aural
	5. Ocular
	6. Visceral
	7. Skeletal
	8. Disfiguring
	9. Others
Disabilities (D code)	1. Behaviour
	2. Communication
	3. Personal care
	4. Locomotion
	5. Body disposition
	6. Dexterity
	7. Situational
	8. Particular skill
	9. Others
Handicaps (H code)	1. Orientation
	2. Physical independence
	3. Mobility
	4. Occupational
	5. Social integration
	6. Economic self-sufficiency
	7. Others

Table 7.2. *Job demands and human functions* (from Singleton, 1979)

Resource	*Physiological support systems subject to malfunction*
Energy	Circulatory, respiratory, digestive
Locomotion } Manipulation }	Skeletal, muscular
Co-ordination	Special senses
Cognitive	Central nervous system
Conative	CNS and endocrine

descriptions (Chapter 3). The most important aspect in terms of the individual for which we currently have no useful taxonomies is aspirations and conative aspects generally. Factors described colloquially by terms such as self-image, self-confidence, drive and the will to work are not yet susceptible to taxonomic definition or measurement. Such assessment has to be impressionistic, but is none the less important. Some factors which determine aspiration can be described reasonably precisely, these are age, sex, personality, interests and abilities. The relationship of these various factors is shown in Fig. 7.4.

The different avenues towards an occupation are: school to work, return to previous occupation, return to employer and change from old to new employer. Returning to the previous occupation is comparatively the easiest option. If it is feasible considerable efforts in terms of retraining and job modification are justified. Most employers feel some responsibility for employees who become disabled, the more so if the disability has some possible connection with work such as an accident or a stress-related disease. Finding a new employer is difficult because all industry is competitive. National laws such as the U.K. requirement that, with the exception of very small companies, all companies should employ disabled people up to at least 3% of their workforce is a useful persuader, although more at the moral rather than the legalistic level because of the difficulty of defining who is disabled. For the transition from school to work there are many difficulties including assessment. Most tests for young people take some account of age, and this distorts the picture because the consensus amongst specialists in this area is that a young disabled person is, on average, about two years behind his fully fit contemporaries in both social and intellectual development. This can easily

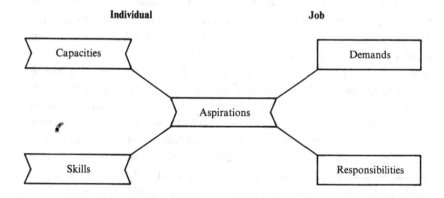

Fig. 7.4. Factors relevant to occupational rehabilitation.

lead to measures of ability being used to underestimate true capacity. Assessment and resettlement methodology is reviewed in Singleton and Debney (1982).

7.4 Applications
7.4.1 *Office design*

Increased data processing facilities and other technological aids have not yet reduced office staffs in the way that automation has reduced workers employed in manufacturing. In spite of fanciful predictions about the 'paperless office' the amount of paper used continues to increase, partly because of the perhaps too readily available facilities from printing, photocopying and fax machines, and the universal preference for hard copy as opposed to screened information.

An office is essentially an information processing system and can be analysed as such. That is, by examining inputs, outputs, processing and storage (Chapter 1), offices always involve people as operators and customers and there is, therefore, a need to look at social as well as informational and commercial aspects of transactions. These can be analysed as tasks and considered in the context of required skills. The design of office spaces also requires consideration of more elusive aspects such as power, politics and prestige.

The consequences for office ergonomics which follow from the widespread introduction of computers are described in detail in Grandjean (1986), The higher technology in office buildings and in office equipment, including synthetic furniture fabrics and floor covers, has resulted in many more potential health hazards (Hedge, 1987). Some of these, such as contact dermatitis and 'humidifier fever' are essentially biological, the two main sources suspected of psychological effects are air ionization and indoor air quality more generally. The consequences are known collectively as the 'sick-building syndrome', indicated not only by specific health problems from eye, nose and throat symptoms, but also by unexpectedly low productivity, absenteeism, low morale, lethargy and general absence of well-being. Atmospheric molecules can carry positive or negative electric charges. In large air-conditioned buildings the concentration of these air ions may vary 'unnaturally'. There are indications from research on mice and rats that high concentrations of negative ions are beneficial, and positive ions are detrimental. Research on people is still producing conflicting results. This has not inhibited the sale of ionizing machines which generate negative ions. Indoor air quality is a loosely defined term usually referring to the presence of pollutants such as radon, formaldehyde and the products of smoking, or more simply inadequate ventilation for spaces containing high densities of people. The origin and extent of this as a serious issue for office workers is still not clear. The broad remedy would seem to be better ventilation in terms not only of total air change, but air flow across all the work spaces. There is a nice borderline between the stuffy and the draughty environment.

The standard ergonomics issues of chair, desk and work-space design, lighting and so on are described in the previous volume *The Body at Work*. Each office space and worker is a miniature communication centre using interfaces such as computers, telephones, paper-based channels and direct verbal communication. The design of the work-space should incorporate these considerations. In particular talking to others is rarely taken into account as an important component of many tasks. All office workers follow procedures, their primary design and requirement for continuous updating can benefit from formal analysis. This is not to suggest that office work, any more than factory work, should reduce the operators to automata. Nevertheless, in all cases the scope for individual initiatives and strategies is embedded in the requirement at least for guidelines. This is often neglected as too vague an issue for systematic study with consequences in errors and in the need for further communication which would have been much reduced had there been more forethought. Grievances develop because operators are blamed for mistakes which they know intuitively are due to system design inadequacies.

The factors to be considered are the same for office design as for any other man–machine information handling system from control rooms to car driving (Table 7.3). At the job satisfaction end of the spectrum it is not adequate to rely on questionnaire-based inquiries, even when there are facilities available to manipulate various aspects and compare 'before' and 'after' collective opinions. There are large individual differences: some people resist change but others enjoy novelty, some are more influenced for better or worse by the investigator rather than the investigation, opinions can be biased in favour of what will suit the establishment rather than the task. It is difficult to distinguish long-term from short-term effects in everything from chair design through consequences of learning and fatigue, to potential health hazards. Job satisfaction parameters can be isolated and assessed in terms of relative importance by preliminary studies of operator opinions based on previous extensive experience, of morbidity data and of performance records. Sanders and McCormick (1987) consider the design of offices in terms of cognitive, social, procedural and physical tasks.

It is extremely difficult to develop norms or bench-marks for performance in offices. The situation is confused by several features:

Table 7.3. *Check-list – the design of an information processing centre*
(Control Rooms, Offices, Driver work-stations, etc.)

Resources for the study
– what resources are available in terms of:
  – budget?
  – time window?
  – skilled man-hours?
  – available skill repertoire?
– are there facilities to generate and codify the required range of documentation?
– is the organisational climate suitable in terms of:
  – management support?
  – perceived need?
  – receptivity of associated staff?
  – possibility of implementation?

Environment work space
  – size and location of space
  – accessibility
  – heating/ventilation
  – fire hazards
  – security requirements
  – lighting/colour
  – layout
  – furniture

Staffing
– numbers and roles of operators
– relationship with operators outside information centre
– locations of work-spaces relative to each other and to information interfaces
– working conditions:
  – hours
  – rest pauses
  – subsistence facilities
  – work layout
  – work demand cycle
  – stressors

Information system
– interface with environment
  – real display
  – communication network (including data processing system)
– internal consoles
– displays
– controls
– personal data banks, e.g. files, procedures
– conversational interactions

Table 7.3. (*cont.*)

- management
- colleagues
- customers
- mass-media
- general public
- self-learning and skill development facilities

Support systems
- selection of staff
- training and re-training
- operating instructions
- briefing, debriefing and updating
- personnel aspects:
  - pay
  - recognition
- motivational aspects (Effort–Achievement–Reward relationships)
- satisfaction aspects
  - enlargement
  - enrichment
  - dedication
- other morale aspects

- office staffs can be increased for political reasons which are quite separate from performance requirements. An office manager can assume that his role is enhanced by a bigger office rather than a more efficient one
- efficiency within an office (or indeed any other service organisation) can be increased at the expense of a poorer service to the users or customers. An understaffed office may not have time to complete necessary tasks. An overstaffed office can increase the work of others they should be serving within the same organisation by asking for more and more data (often called 'returns') which they can process to keep themselves occupied
- it is easier to start processes than it is to terminate them. Routines can be continued far beyond their useful life because no one has the responsibility of questioning their effectiveness. Boards or other supervisory committees are always tempted to suggest new processes, e.g. to collect more statistics, but these are assessed solely in terms of value but not in the context of their cost
- there are cyclical fashion aspects, for ten or twenty years centralisation is the vogue and this is followed by a similar period of

decentralisation and distributed decision-making. The size, location and functions of offices follow this cycle
– there are prestige aspects such as having a headquarters office in the capital city. This is not only an unnecessary overhead but an interference with the productive parts of the organisation which must supply returns and adapt to insensitive policy decisions. These offices are sometimes justified on the grounds of the need to be close to financial markets but the worldwide stock market crash of 1987 demonstrated that changes in the value of shares can take place in a way which is totally disconnected from the industrial performance of the organisation either before or after the event
– the design of independent or non-interactive office tasks is difficult, sometimes impossible, and when tasks are separated the increase in productivity is not linear because the operators must spend time interacting with each other. It is quite usual to find that when the load of one operator rises to the point where two are required, in fact four must be deployed because they need to spend half their time interacting with each other. To suggest that as the load increases linearly the personnel numbers increase geometrically is perhaps an exaggeration, but there is an effect of this kind
– the weekly, monthly or annual cycle of work-load may be such that staff are seriously underemployed during some phases because they are needed at peak loads

For all these reasons it is desirable, if possible, to start an office analysis by looking at the overall inputs and outputs with close examination of the necessity or value of each item. As in other kinds of system analysis it is not appropriate to start with the detail even when there are obvious potentialities for considerable improvement in some details. A top–down rather than a bottom–up study is the more apposite. Information technology accentuates the tendency to increase the information flow and processing beyond the real requirements. The requirements or objectives need to be separated into parts for objective assessment. For example, the broad title 'financial control' obscures a number of quite separate functions: the need to avoid leakage due to dishonesty or carelessness, the need to employ a scarce resource efficiently, and the use of financial data for management purposes.

7.4.2   Car design
Cars provide people with wheels which are intended to carry them

speedily, comfortably and safely along roads. From a Human Factors view-point, the key person is the driver, although others such as the passenger and the maintenance engineer need consideration.

To meet the human requirements, the design of cars has developed slowly from a concentration on mechanisms (engines, suspensions and the like) to a more systems orientation of the car as an extension of the driver. He controls the system on the basis of mainly visual information and executes his commands by hand and foot actions. This last is unusual, in most systems other than vehicles only the hands are involved. As a human operator the driver is also unusual in that he often remains in a restricted seated position for several hours. In other task situations there is greater flexibility of posture and the opportunity to move around, at least within the work-space. There is task variety in that the environment changes continually, not always predictably, and sometimes radically when, for example, the car moves from a motorway to a city street. The task is dangerous, much more so than working in a factory or an office, and many of the hazards are created by the driver.

Car manufacture is the epitome of mass production, large numbers of identical products are made although there is inevitably quite large variation in driver attributes, such as size, strength, resilience, visual capability and skill. The driver's opinion matters in the choice of car. For all these reasons, human factors aspects of driver-space design are important but difficult.

Design procedure

The driver-space of a new car evolves from previous cars made by the same company. This maintains the company image, it also reduces the need for production changes and problems for drivers transferring from older vehicles. In any case, given the restrictions of the orthodox control layout and the various international standards to do with dials and controls, there is only a limited design envelope within which innovation is possible. There is restriction also by regulations developed in the interests of safety in many countries. Within the E.E.C. these regulations have been standardised although they are administered nationally. For example, in the U.K. the Department of Transport is responsible for type approval.

Designers in particular companies take note of any innovations by other car manufacturers within the same market but these are not often surprising or disconcerting. The industry is still engineering-based although the instigating technology now comes from instrumentation, computers and electronics generally as well as from mechanics. Styling also remains a strong influence although the excesses of dramatic changes in body shape on an annual basis have given way to longer design cycles and a more sober approach to function in parallel with style in the fashion/appearance sense.

The Human Factors specialist occupies the middle ground between creative thinking in front of a blank sheet of paper and minor changes in the control surface for newly installed functions such as electric window control. Ideally this middle ground should develop on the basis of greater understanding of the attributes and requirements of specific driver populations. In recent years car manufacturers have paid much greater attention to the description of their customers and their reaction to particular products, but, to date, this has not gone very much beyond anthropometric data, opinion of styling and experience of reliability. It would be feasible to conduct studies of driver populations engaged in access, egress, driving in different conditions and generally using the car, but, at present, these tend to be carried out only on drivers employed by the particular company. These expert drivers have specific insights but their reactions and opinions are unlikely to be identical to those of customers. The same is true for the opinions of motoring correspondents employed by the mass media.

Some information from customers is fed back through marketing and sales activities, but this is random rather than systematic. In general there do seem to be gaps in the information network supplying those responsible for design which could be filled by systematic ergonomics investigations. This applies not only to car designers but also to the designers employed by suppliers of components such as seats, controls, displays and other driver–car interface elements. Most current work of this kind is done under the heading of 'clinics' in which samples of users are asked their opinions of features such as appearance, comfort and layout. Surveys of recent customers are also carried out by written questionnaire or by telephone.

Thus the design procedure has moved on from the traditional reliance on the flair of one enthusiast to guidance from many regulations, standards and opinions. The result is better design in terms of fitness for ordinary purposes, but some loss of more elusive qualities such as car personality and uniqueness of particular marques. Modern cars accurately convey the impression of having been designed by committees.

Computer-aided design and manufacture

Within the last five years there has been a radical change in moving designers from the drawing-board to the screen and keyboard. This not only provides greater flexibility in innovation but also greatly improves the storage of data and decisions and communication with procurement and production.

It also eases the introduction of ergonomic requirements in that questions of reliability, control reach, seat posture, headroom and so on can be assessed by the manipulation of three-dimensional spaces and surfaces.

Designing skills change accordingly but do not diminish because all the traditional trade-offs and compromises still have to be made. Obviously the interior space interacts with the external shape and size and the requirements of the mechanical components.

Computer-based simulation is used to assess safety features such as what happens if the car hits a fixed surface, another car, or a pedestrian.

The technological push

Developments in materials and mechanisms continue to drive design changes in the car. Engines are becoming more efficient, the greater use of plastic materials and improvements in metal alloys and lubricants lead to better designs including the reduced need for regular maintenance. However, from the driver's viewpoint, superior performance, ride and handling accentuate his demands so that he expects the system to be faster but otherwise equally safe and comfortable. Car advertisement tries to present the image of high performance on empty roads and landscapes, but the reality is the crowded motorway and the slow or stationary urban traffic.

New aids for the driver can be divided into two categories – those to do with car control and those to do with car habitation, that is the need to be inside for quite long periods.

Car control systems now include power-assisted brakes and steering, anti-locking devices on brakes, automatic choke and gear-boxes, central locking, cruise control, electrically controlled windows and mirrors, and greater variety in seat and steering adjustments. Four-wheel drive systems, either selected or permanent, are also available. For the next generation more of these facilities will spread to cheaper cars. Innovation is currently centred on computer driven devices including screen displays of car and engine performance, better warning systems, systems for controlling economy and navigation systems. Safety which began with seat belts has extended into collapsible steering wheels and crumpling extensions around a rigid cabin shell. There is some potential here for more automatic control of deceleration in emergencies although there are serious problems if such devices malfunction.

Car habitation support started with heaters, ventilators and radios. Environmental control is now quite sophisticated and the limitations are not in technology directly but in the cost/benefit aspects e.g. for air conditioning. In-car entertainment from radio and tapes is elaborate, quite small cars may now be equipped with four speakers so that there is little scope for extension. Car telephones and other communication devices are coming into increasing use, especially in big cities. Driver facilities when the car is stationary have not been widely developed even for activities such as reading and writing. Storage for paper, drink and food is poor.

Continuity and change

The variety of available technology, particularly that stemming from electronics, results in problems of selectivity rather than creativity.

The designer has to consider what the customer might welcome, what he might accept and what he might reject as technological gimmickry. The optimal choice varies with the market for the particular vehicle. There are a few small car-making companies where the customer appeal is based on no change, others which are always at the frontiers of change. The mass-market car has a model change cycle of four to six years, the customer expects advances at this rate but not faster, otherwise depreciation will be too high. The luxury car will change on a much slower cycle, nine to twelve years. When a model is changed the initiating feature is the exterior styling which the interior must follow although there is some iteration.

Authorities such as governments and standards institutions do not encourage radical innovation and nor does the customer. The control-space is unlikely to change from the basic layout of windscreen, steering-wheel, seat, a few hand and foot controls and a few displays. The habitat-space also seems to be reaching a plateau in terms of environmental control, entertainment and some external communication.

Partly by tradition and partly because of the dominance of engineering technology few companies employ specialist ergonomists. This fact conceals the tremendous change in attitude and activity which has occurred over the past decade. Human factors are taken into consideration mainly by personnel who are basically automobile engineers and have titles such as interior designer or interior stylist. They use the basic concepts of ergonomics and integrate them with technology and styling to produce design solutions which, superficially at least, are quite reasonable from an ergonomics view-point.

The customer–designer loop

One way to leaven the tyranny of the technological dominance would be to increase the weighting on customer requirements. This would not be easy because there are considerable individual differences and people are often not clear in their own minds about what they would like, let alone what they need. Most people prefer to react rather than to speculate without guidance.

Nevertheless this is a fair challenge to the ergonomist who should be able to devise techniques which provide potential choices to which the customer might assign priorities or, to add other dimensions, provide a needs and requirements space including costs, benefits and pleasures through which the customer might define a path. In effect, this is done at present by design committees within companies, but they contain customer representation only indirectly through evidence from clinics and other expressions of opinion. Correspondingly one could expect companies to conduct or obtain independent ergonomics audits on products nearing design completion.

Competition and fashion
Since car designers keep in very close touch with the work of their competitors any manifestly beneficial innovation is very quickly copied into other cars in the same class. This applies generally to styling (the most sensitive indicator of the age of a film or photograph is the appearance of cars) and to ergonomics aspects. Almost all cars have kept in step in changes such as putting numbers horizontally instead of around the radius of the dial, substituting black for chrome bezels, reversing contrast to provide light coloured numbers on dark coloured dials, placing instruments in front of the driver instead of symmetrically across the dashboard, designing steering-wheel spokes which do not interfere with vision, shading instruments from windscreen reflections, and supplying stalks which carry multiple switches.

Continuing problems
The topics on which ergonomics ought to be able to make a contribution have been accepted since the 1950s. They include:

- posture; the dimensions of the work-space to cater for the particular driver population in terms of display and control positions and seat design. There has been a considerable contribution here particularly with the advent of computer-aided design already mentioned. Nevertheless there are many unresolved issues in relation to the details of optimal support. For example, the wide seat-back which allows variety of posture versus the moulded seat-back which maintains positions during manoeuvres such as fast cornering. Little is known about optimal density of seating support and the relationship between seat dynamic response and suspension response
- fatigue; it is universal personal experience that driving for several hours is tiring but the measurement of this phenomenon has proved highly elusive. Early work on fatigue *per se* was replaced by extensive work on related concepts such as stress and mental work-load but still without a very clear contribution to the real problem

- attention/arousal; except perhaps in the case of the novice the full attention of the driver is not required. In common with many other monitoring tasks the optimal set seems to be to scan the changing situation and adjust arousal and attention according to the demand as it is and as it seems likely to develop. There seems to be no general answer to questions such as whether in-car entertainment is a good thing in maintaining overall arousal or a bad thing in distracting attention, there are large differences within and between individuals as well as between situations
- safety; engineered safety has concentrated on improved packaging by seat-belts, collapsing steering columns and avoidance of rigid edges but provision of a rigid cabin inside a collapsing exterior. Design to avoid accidents has not proved to be very productive. This is mainly because drivers tend to utilise performance improvements as such rather than as sources of reduced risk

This negative list indicates that ergonomists and supporting biological and behavioural scientists have not been able to deal with some of the obvious problems. However the car is a good illustration of the way in which ergonomics often does not happen directly as a result of experiments or theories. Rather the gradually increasing sensitivity to the needs of people coupled with the increasing flexibility provided by technology provides the fertile ground in which ergonomics principles can be successfully applied.

The rapid change in the utilisation of ergonomics over the past decade and the public awareness expressed by common aphorisms such as 'ergonomically-designed' and 'user-friendly' augurs well for the future.

7.4.3   Ergonomics and disability

Visit car factories across Europe and the most striking impression is that all are making the same product by the same methods. Most such factories have rehabilitation workshops attached, and if the observer walks away from the design offices and production lines to this workshop it will be immediately obvious which country he is in.

Rehabilitation centres not attached to particular companies show even more clearly the very considerable differences which reflect national characteristics. This is not to suggest that some countries do this job better than do others. Each country applies assessment and rehabilitation procedures developed to suit its own national and migrant workers.

There seem to be disproportionately high numbers of migrant workers in rehabilitation centres. There are a range of reasons why this is so. Prosaically it is because disabled migrant workers don't have homes and families to rely on.

More elusively but equally importantly it is because a person's identity is a function of where he comes from, where he lives and who he lives with as well as how he works. For a migrant worker there is unusually high dependence on work as a source of identity, together with the associated physical strength and manual skills. If all this is diminished by disease or accident the effects are more profound than those following similar physical damage to a person who has other sources of identity which remain intact.

There are also disproportionately high numbers of males. This seems to be because, in Europe at least, going to work is still regarded as a more significant attribute of men rather than of women. Disabled females are assumed to be best coped with within the home environment where the degree and kind of domestic work can be adjusted to suit their disabilities.

These points reinforce the view that the underlying purpose of rehabilitation is the restoration of identity and self-confidence and that there remain considerable national and cultural differences. Such a view is necessary to understand what happens and why to individuals in rehabilitation centres. Having accepted this, the techniques used are largely the same as in other areas of ergonomics.

There is considerable scope for the application of training, job design and specifically designed support for sensory, central and effector processes. The consideration of work-space design for disabled persons can lead to solutions which are equally applicable to other workers with the same tasks. Training requires particular emphasis on accentuation of motivation because the restoration of self-image and the building up of self-confidence are such key aspects. A positive consequence of this is that when a disabled individual finds by experience that he can cope successfully with a task or job his consistency and enthusiasm readily become very high. Task design may require the introduction of additional sensory cues, e.g. more tactile guidance for the partially sighted, and changes in machine orientation to make tasks easier for those with postural limitations, e.g. tilting a machine tool or providing sliding seats along a work-bench. There is still a tendency, however, to regard employment as restricted to manufacturing industry, many disabilities do not interfere with service occupations, particularly those requiring social interaction where specialist facilities may be required only in location of stored materials, keyboards, telephones and so on.

A system approach to resettlement is essential because some disabilities do not restrict job performance as such, but access to and egress from the work-space require facilitation. This also applies to hazards, particularly in terms of what happens if incidents such as fires occur.

All rehabilitation work is man-power intensive and therefore increasingly expensive as technology advances. Yet it is essential that considerable professional resources are focussed on each individual. The use of rehabilitation teams has obvious advantages in the provision of the appropriate range of skills in diagnosis, training and job design, but there are also advantages in one person, a rehabilitation counsellor, getting to know the disabled individual very well and having access to more specific expertise when this is required. Interestingly enough, when this is attempted e.g. Singleton and Papworth (1980), it is relatively straightforward to develop adequate counsellor skills, but there is greater difficulty in developing adequate self-confidence so that the counsellor can make independent decisions and set objectives for other professionals such as medical doctors, psychologists and ergonomists.

As mentioned in the first chapter, it is necessary when dealing with workforces of a hundred million or more, and with large-scale technologically based industries, to develop overall concepts of taxonomies of kinds of occupation, tasks and skills, of the human operator with his generalised advantages and limitations, and of the man within man–machine, socio-technical and fiscal-economic systems. Work with the disabled is a salutary reminder that although many policies and concepts have to be rigorously defined and applied on a large scale, the task of the student of the mind at work ultimately comes down to utilising ill-defined concepts such as identity, self-image and self-confidence, and coping with vulnerable individuals, healthy or otherwise, each of which is just trying to make a living and establish a place in a community.

References

Ardrey, R. (1966). *The Territorial Imperative*. New York: Athenaeum.
Barney, G.O. (ed.). (1980). *The Global 2000 Report to the President*. Washington: Government Printing Office.
Canter, D. (1975). *Environmental Interaction*. Surrey: University Press.
Duckworth, D. (1983). *The Classification and Measurement of Disability*. London: H.M.S.O.
Forrester, J.W. (1970). *World Dynamics*. Cambridge: Wright-Allen Press.
Grandjean, E. (1986). *Ergonomics in Computerized Offices*. London: Taylor Francis.
Harris, A.I., Cox, E. and Smith, C.R.W. (1971). *Handicapped and Impaired in Great Britain. Part. I*. London: H.M.S.O.
Hedge, A. (1987). Office health hazards: an annotated bibliography. *Ergonomics*, **30.5**. 733–72.
I.L.O. (1973). *Basic Principles of the Vocational Rehabilitation of the Disabled*. 3rd. edition. Geneva: International Labour Office.
Kirk, N.S. and Ridgway, S. (1970, 1971). Ergonomics testing of consumer products. *Applied Ergonomics*, **1.5**. 295–300, **2.1**. 12–18.
Meadows, D.H. (1972). *Limits to Growth*. Washington: Earth Island.
Mesarovic, M. and Pestel, E. (1975). *Mankind at the Turning Point*. London: Hutchinson.

Newman, O. (1972). *Defensible Space*. New York: Macmillan.

Peccei, A. (1977). *The Human Quality*. London: Pergamon.

Rouault, G.Y. (1978). *The Handicapped and their Employment. A Statistical Study of the Situation in the Member States of the European Communities*. Brussels: Office for Official Publications of the European Communities.

Sanders, M.S. and McCormick, E.J. (1987). *Human Factors in Engineering and Design*. New York: McGraw Hill.

Simon, J. and Kahn, H. (1984). *The Resourceful Earth*. Oxford: Blackwell.

Singleton, W.T. (1967). Macro-ergonomics. *Universities Quarterly*. **21.2**. 199–204

Singleton, W.T. (1979). Occupational disability. In Singleton W.T. (ed.). *The Study of Real Skills. Vol.2. Compliance* and *Excellence*. Lancaster: M.T. Press.

Singleton, W.T. and Debney, L.M. (eds.). (1982). *Occupational Disability*. Lancaster: M.T. Press.

Singleton, W.T. and Papworth, C. (1980). *Rehabilitation and the Occupational Health Nurse*. Aston University, Applied Psychology Report 92.

W.H.O. (1980). *International Classification of Impairments, Disabilities and Handicaps*. Geneva: World Health Organisation.

Wilson, J. and Whittington (eds.). (1981). Consumer ergonomics. Special issue, *Applied Ergonomics*. **12.3**.

Author Index

Page numbers in roman type refer to the text and those in *italic type* refer to the lists of references.

Albers, W.A., 261, *305*, *306*
Altman, J.W., 195, *303*
Alvey, J., 239, 240, *256*
Anastasi, A., 148, *157*
Andersen, R.S., 298, *303*
Annett, J. 66, *78*, 110, *131*
ANPAT, 267, *303*
Anthony, R.D., *258*
Appley, M.H., *131*, *192*
Ardrey, R., 311. 336
Argyle, M., 113, *131*, 140, 141, *157*, *304*
Attneave, F., 96, *131*
Austin, G.A., *131*
Avery, A.W., *132*

Baddeley, A.D., 96, *131*
Baker, E., 75, *78*
Barber, J.W., 122, *131*
Barnes, N., 122, *133*
Barney, G.O., 317, 336
Baron, S., 204, *256*
Barroquet, A., *192*
Bartlett, F.C., 97, 98, *131*, 142, *157*, 161, *191*, 198, *256*
Bartley, S.H., 160, *191*
Bates, J.A.V., 2, *79*
Battersby, A., 59, *78*
Belbin, E.M., 91, *131*
Bennett, J., *258*
Berg, G.G., 261, *303*
Bergquist, U.O.V., 189, *191*
Bernotat, R.K., 202, *256*, *258*
Berry, J.W., 92, *132*, *134*
Bide, A., 240, 241, *257*
Biderman, A.D., 113, *131*
Bignell, V., 274, *303*
Bilodeau, E.A., 110, *131*

Birren, J.E., 90, *131*
Blum., M.L., 110, *131*, 143, *157*
Bohn, M.J., 106, 120, *134*
Bohr, E. 287, *304*
Bons, P.M., *157*
Bourne, P.G., 164, *191*
Brehmer, B., 262, 271, *304*
Brislin, R., *134*
Broadbent, D.E., 166, *191*
Brock, G.W., *132*
Brogger, A., 261, 265, *305*, *306*
Brown, R., 143, *157*
Bruner, J.S., 98, *131*
Bytheway, C.W., 61, *78*

Campbell, R.N., 99, *131*
Canter, D., 312, *336*
Carbonell, J.R., 204, *257*
Carmichael, L., 109, *131*
Case, D., *258*
Cassie, A., 106, *132*
Chadwick-Jones, J., 151, *157*
Chapanis, A., 53, *78*, 102, *131*, 177, 180, *181*, *257*
Charles, G.W.F., 252, *258*
Cherns, A.B., 33, *78*, 181, *191*, 265, *304*
Cherry, C., 202, *257*
Child, J., 144, *157*
Chomsky, N., 99, *131*
Churchman, C.W., *78*
Chute, E., 160, *191*
Colquhoun, W.P., 168, *191*
Conrad, R., 97, *131*
Cook, J.S., *257*
Cooper, C.L., 164, *191*
Cooper, M.G., 261, *304*
Corlett, N., 188, *191*

Cornford, F.M., 155, *157*
Coufal, J.D., *132*
Cox, E., *336*
Craik, K.J.W., 98, *131*
Crawley, R.C., 28, 34, 66, *78, 79*
Cresswell, C.W., 266, *304*
Crombach, L.S., 92, 93, *131*
Crossman, E.R.F.W., 203, *257*

Das, J.P., *131*
Davies, D.R., 166, 167, *191*, 199, *257*
Davis, D.R., *131*, 161, *191*, 270, *306*
Davis, L.E., 33, *78*, 112, 181, *191*
Dearborn, W.F., 109, *131*
Debney, L.M., 324, *337*
De Greene, K.B., 273, *303, 304*
Dodd, B., *132*
Draguns, J., *134*
Drasdo, M., 114, *131*
Drenth, P.J.D., 93, 106, *131*
Drucker, P., 144, *157*
Drury, C.G., 112, *131*, 187, *191*
Duckworth, D., 315, *336*
Duncan, K.D., 66, *78, 79, 134*, 145, *157*, 183, *191*, 288, *304, 305, 306, 307*

Easterby, R.S., 74, *78, 79, 134*, 211, *257*, *259*, 287, *304, 307*
Edholm, O.G., 75, *78*, 254, 255, *257*
Edwards, E., 2, *78*, 96, *131*, 252, *257*
Embrey, D., 299, *304*
Emery, F.E., 33, *78*
Eysenck, H.J., 89, *131*

Ferrell, W.R., 205, *258*
Fiedler, F.E., 143, *157*
Fischhoff, B., *306*
Fisher, R.A., 202
Fitts, P.M., 35, *78*, 207, *257, 295, 304*
Flowers, B., 274, *304*
Floyd, W.F., 160, *191, 192*
Fogel, L.J., 205, 252, *257*
Folkard, S., 188, *191*
Forrester, J.W., 310, *336*
Forsyth, R., 234, *257*
Fox, J.G., 112, *131*, 187, *191, 192, 193*
Freud, S., 270, *304*
Friedman, M.P., 89, *131*, 164
Froggatt, P., 266, *304*
Furnham, A., 141, *157*

Gabor, D., 202

Gagne, R.M., *79*, 93, 94, 129, *132, 133*, 288, *304, 305*
Garner, W.R., *131*, 197, 205, *257*
Gartner, K.-P., 202, *256, 258*
Gerver, D., 99, *132*
Gibson, J.J., 197, *257*
Giles, W.J., 70, *79*
Glaser, R., 124, *132*
Glass, D.V., *304*
Goddard, G., 281, *304*
Goodnow, J.J., *131*
Grandjean, E., 188, *192*, 324, *336*
Gray, M.J., *78*
Green, A.E., 261, *304*
Greenwood, M., 266, *304*
Gregory, R.L., 170, *192*
Gruneberg, M.M., *79, 157, 191*
Gunderson, E.K.E., 164, *192*
Guilford, J.P., 89, *132*
Guttman, H.E., 299, *306*

Hale, A.R., 262, 288, *304*
Hale, M., *305*
Harre, H., *192*
Harri-Augstein, E.G., 94, *134*
Harris, A.I., 319, *336*
Hastings, L.L., *157*
Haugeland, J., 234, *257*
Hawkins, F., 253, *257*
Head, H., 83, *132*
Hedge, A., 275, *304*, 324, *336*
Heim, A., 106, *132*
Hellesoy, O.H., 181, *192*
Heron, A., *134*
Herriot, P., 99, *132*
Herzberg, F.B., 145, *157*
Hick, W.E., 2, *79*, 207, *257*
Hilgard, E.R., 93, *132*
Hoffman, B., 276, *304*
Hoiberg, A., 92, *132*
Holding, D.H., 110, *132, 133*
Hovden, J., *133*, 261, *304, 306*
Hudson, R.A., *257*
Hull, C.L., 93
Humphrey, G., 98, *132*
Hutchinson, P., 273, *305*
Hyman, R., 207, *257*

I.L.O., 24, 26, 27, 51, *79*, 265, *304*, 314, *336*
I.P.M., 70, *79*
Irvine, S.H., 92, *132*

Jacobs, G.O., 273, *305*
Jessup, G., 106, *132*
Jessup, H., 106, *132*
Joanning, H., 112, *132*
Johannsen, G., 2, 40, 79, 202, *258*
Johnson, R.A., 144, *157*
Johnson-Laird, P.N., 99, *132*
Jones, R.E., 295, *304*
Jordan, N., 35, *79*
Jung, C.A., 162, *192*

Kahn, H., 317, *337*
Kahneman, D., 262, *305*
Kast, F.E., *157*
Kay, H., 124, *132*
Kelley, C.R., 202, 207, *257*
Kelly, G.A., 95, *132*
Kidd, J.S., 270, 293, *305*
Killcross, M.C., 106, *132*
King, D., 110, *132*
Kirk, N.S., 313, *336*
Kjellen, U., 297, *305, 306*
Klein, L., 33, *79*
Kleinman, D.L., 204, *256*
Kline, P., 90, *132*
Knight, M.A.G., *134*
Koch, S., *307*
Kraiss, K-F., 129, *133*
Krendel, E., 207, 208
Kubr, M., 155, *157*
Kurppa, K., 175, *192*

Lacy, B.A., 114, *132*
Lagerlof, E., 268, *305*
Lamb, R., *192*
Lambert, W.W., *134*
Lazarus, R.S., 165, *192*
Le Bon, G., 141, *157*
Lees, F.B., 2, *78*
Leplat, J., 297, *304, 305, 306, 307*
Levi, L., 170, *192*
Lewin, K., 93, 99, *132*, 140, *157*, 269, *305*
Lichtenstein, S., *306*
Licklider, J.C.R., 242, *257*
Lindsley, D.B., *193*
Lippit, R., *157*
Lischeron, J.A., 181, *193*
Lloyd, P., 160, *192*
Lonner, W.J., *134*
Lowrance, W.W., 260, *305*
Lund, M.W., *257*
Lupton, T., 34, *79*

MacCurdy, J.T., 143, *157*
MacKay, D.M., 202, *257*
Mackworth, N.H., 109, *132*, 166, *192*
Maillie, H.D., 261, *303*
Manenica, I., *191*
Marquis, D.G., 93, *132*
Martin, J., *305*
Maslow, A.H., 145, *157*
Mason, A.E., 274, *306*
Mausner, M., *157*
Mayes, A., 160, *192*
Maynard, H.B., 55, *79*
Mayo, E., 143, *157*
McCormick, E.J., 150, *157*, 325, *337*
McFarland, D.J., 168, *192*
McFarland, R.A., 264, 266, 280, *305*
McGregor, D., 143, *157*
McNemar, Q., 178, *192*
McRuer, D.T., 207, 208
Meadows, D.H., 310, *336*
Meetham, A.R., *257*
Meister, D., 293, *305*
Melhuish, E.C., 112, *132*
Melton, A.W., 93, *132*
Mesarovic, M., 310, *336*
Metz, B.G., 256, *257*
Meyer, J.J., 170, *192*
Michie, D., 234, *257*
Miller, G.A., 96, 110, *132, 133*
Miller, R.B., 110, *133*
Moore, A.K., 150, *158*
Moore, R.C., 265, *305*
Moraal, J., 129, *133*
Moray, N., 171, *192*
Morgan, C.T., *131*, 209, *257*
Morgan, D.G., 240, *257*
Morris, J.N., *304*
M.S.C., *132*
Murray, H., 32, *79*
Murrell, K.F.H., 186, *192*, 254, *257*
Muscio, B., 160, *192*

Naylor, J.C., 110, *131*, 143, *157*
Nedzynski, S., 189, *192*
Neisser, E., 198, *257*
Nelson-Jones, R., 90, *133*
Newell, A., 198, *257*
Newman, J.H., 139, *157*
Newman, O., 312, *337*
Noro, K., 238, *258*
N.U.R.E.G., 262, 274, *305*
N.U.R.E.G./CR1270, 285, *305*

O'Connor, N., *131*
Oftedal, P., 261, 265, *305, 306*
O'Shaughnessy, J., 145, *158*

Page, M., 113, *133*
Papworth, C., 336, *337*
Parasuraman, R., 166, 167, *191*, 199, 257
Parkinson, N., 174
Parry, M.H., 113, *133*, 270, *305*
Parsons, H.M., 129, *133*
Patrick, J., 150, *158*
Patten, T.H., Jr., 70, *79*
Payne, R.L., 144, *158*, 164, *191*
Peccei, A., 310, *337*
Perrow, C., 227, *258*, 274, *305*
Pestel, E., 310, *336*
Peters, G., *303*
Piaget, J., 99, *133*
Pittard, J., *192*
Pochin, E.E., 300, *305*
Poulton, E.C., 207, *258*
Powell, P., 266, *305*
Pugh, D.S., 144, *158*
Pym, C., *303*

Rabideau, G.F., 293, *305*
Rahe, R.H., 164, *192*
Ramsden, J., 110, *133*
Randell, G.A., 104, *133*
Rasmussen, J., 175, *192*, 271, *304, 305, 306, 307*
Reason, J., 271, *306*
Rey, P., 170, *192*
Rich, E., 234, *258*
Ridgway, S., 313, *336*
Rivers, W.H.R., 155, *158*
Robens Committee, 264, 266, *306*
Robinson, J., 122, *133*
Robinson, P.F., 70, *79*
Rogers, C.R., 95, *133*
Roscoe, S.N., 252, *258*
Rosenman, R.H., 164
Rosenzweig, J.E., *157*
R.O.S.P.A., 280, *306*
Rouault, G.Y., 319, *337*
Rouse, W.B., 175, *192*, 205, *258*
Rowe, W.D., 260, 298, *306*
Rubinstein, T., 274, *306*
Rutter, D.R., 105, 112, *133*

Saari, J., 297, *306*
Sage, A.P., 245, *258*

Sandelin, J., *258*
Sanders, M.S., 325, *337*
Schaie, K.W., 90, *131*
Schwab, J.L., *79*
Schwing, R.C., 261, *305, 306*
Sell, R.G., *78, 79*, 181, *192*
Selye, H., 163, *192*
Sen, R.N., 155, *158*
Seymour, W.D., 83, 110, *133*
Shackel, B., 235, *258*
Shackleton, V.J., 112, *131*
Shannon, C.E., 201, 202, *258*
Shapiro, S.C., 234, *258*
Shaws, A.G., 55, *79*
Shepherd, D.A., 66, *79*
Sheridan, T.B., 2, 40, *79*, 202, 205, *258*
Sherif, M., 99, *133*, 140, *158*
Shipley, P., *78, 79*, 181, *192*
Shorter, D.N., *257*
Siegel, S., 178, *192*
Sime, M., *132*
Simister, R., 152, *158*
Simon, H.A., 198, *257*
Simon, J., 317, *337*
Simon, M., *305*
Skinner, B.F., 93
Sinaiko, H.W., 99, *132, 304*
Singer, E.J., 110, *133*
Singleton, W.T., 8, 13, 14, 15, 28, 34, 35, 41, 56, *78, 79*, 81, 83, 91, 99, 110, 112, 113, 114, 115, 120, *131, 132, 133, 134*, 143, 147, 152, 156, *157, 158*, 160, 163, 165, 168, 174, *192, 193*, 195, 206, 208, 214, 221, 232, 243, 246, *257, 258, 259*, 261, 263, 265, 268, 269, 270, 271, 281, 282, 288, 294, 295, 297, 300, *304, 306, 307*, 310, 321, 322, 324, 336, *337*
Slovic, P., 262, *305, 306*
Sluckin, W., 160, *193*
Smallwood, R., 204, *258*
Smith, C.R.W., *336*
Smith, M., *258*
Smith, P.J., 99, *131*
Smith, P.S., 141, *158*
Snyderman, B.B., *157*
Spurgeon, P., 66, *78, 132, 133, 134, 157*
Stammers, R.B., *78*, 129, *132, 133, 134*, 253, *259*
Stegmerton, G.J., *79*
Stevens, S.S., *78*, 195, *258*
Storr, A., 270, *306*
Story, D.T., 129, *134*

Super, D.E., 106, 120, *134*
Swain, A.D., 38, *79*, 299, *306*

Tainsh, M., 67, *79*, *257*
Tanner, I., 34, *79*
Taylor, A., 160, *193*
Taylor, D.H., 271, *307*
Taylor, F.V., 270, *307*
Taylor, J.C., 33, *78*, 181, *191*
Thomas, L.F.T., 94, *134*
Thorndike, E.L., 83, 93, *134*
Thorne, R.G., 252, *258*
Tilley, K.W., 112, *134*
Tolman, E.C., 93
Triandis, H.C., 92, *134*
Trist, E.L., 32, 33, *78*, *79*
Trotter, W., 141, *158*
Trumbull, R., *131*, *192*
Tustin, A., 207
Tversky, A., *305*
Tye, W., 273, 276, *307*

Vandenberg, J.P., 287, *307*
Verhulst, M., *78*
Vigotsky, L.S., 198, *258*

Walker, J., *258*
Wall, T.D., 181, *193*
Wallis, D., *79*, 124, 125, *134*, *157*, *191*
War Manpower Commission, 122, *134*

Warr, P.B., *131*, *133*, 145, *158*, 181, *193*
Wason, P.C., 99, *132*
Weaver, D.R., *258*
Weaver, W., 201, *258*
Welford, A.T., 90, 91, 110, *134*, 160, *191*, *192*, 206, 209, *258*, *259*, *304*
Wheeler, R.H., 93
White, P.K., *157*
Whitfield, D., *79*, *134*, 156, *158*, *192*, *193*, 253, *259*, *307*
Whittington, A., 313, *337*
W.H.O., 315, 321, 322, *337*
Wickens, C.D., 97, *134*, 199, 208, *259*
Wiener, N., 199, *259*
Williams, J.C., 129, *134*
Williams, S.B., 165, *193*
Williges, R.C. 242, *259*
Wilson, J., *191*, 313, *337*
Winston, P., 234, *259*
Wisner, A., 155, *158*
Wohl, T.G., 38, *79*, 245, *259*
Wolfle, D., 122, *134*
Woods, H.M., 266, *304*
Woodworth, R.S., 96, *134*
Wulfeck, J.W., 35, *79*

Yates, F., 107, *134*

Zeitlin, L.R., 35, *79*
Zwaga, H., 74, *78*, *257*, *259*, 287, *304*

Subject Index

abilities, 88
absolute judgment, 203
accidents, 265
  aircraft, 276
  data, 277
  data interpretation, 277
  data sources, 276
  fatalities, 278–83
  maximum credible, 274
  nuclear, 262
  proneness, 266
  rail, 276
  reduction, 284
  research, 268, 302
  road, 176, 261
  Acts of God, 265, 269
age differences, 90
agriculture, 25
A.I., 234
alarm
  architecture, 228
  context, 221
  interfaces, 227
  operator aids, 232
  recipient, 229
  systems, 225
allocation of function, 35–42
Alma Ata declaration, 156
ambiguity, 201
amenities, 25
anticipation, 207
apprenticeship, 113
aptitudes, 88
arousal, 161, 334
A.S.M.E. symbols, 51, 53
aspirations, 137
astronauts, 272
A.T.C., 251, 253
attitudes, 113, 138, 288
auditory system, 194, 195, 206

authority gradient, 252
autonomous groups, 33
aviation psychology, 250

bandwidth, 204
batch production, 151
belief, 139
Bhopal chemical plant, 274
Birmingham map, 210
blink rate, 170
BLS, 264, 289
B.S., 256

CAD, 330
CAI, 124, 127
capacities, 88
car design, 328
catastrophes, 261, 274
CBT, 127
Central Training Council, 122
centralised control systems, 220
checklists, 74, 254, 291, 326
Chernobyl, 274
choice responses, 203
chronocyclograph, 56
circadian rhythms, 162, 167, 187
climatic differences, 92
Club of Rome, 310
coding, 211
CODOT, 119
cognition, 89, 138, 198
cognitive ergonomics, 138
cognitive map, 138
combinatorial explosion, 234
comfort, 313
command and control, 87
committees, 146
composite group, 33
computers, 233
conation, 89, 138

construction, 153
consumer ergonomics, 313
control for ill-defined issues, 319
control centres
  military, 243
  process, 246
controls, 217
  acceleration, 219
  cranks and levers, 219
  displacement, 219
  jerk, 219
  keys, 219
  knobs, 219
  pedals, 219
  pressure, 219
  rate aided, 219
  selectors, 219
  stereotypes, 218
  switches, 219
  velocity, 219
cultural differences, 92
culture, 139
cybernetics, 199

data acquisition, 205
decision-making, 208
defence in depth, 275
defensible space, 311
demographic data, 21
Department of Employment, 122
Department of Transport, 308, 329
depth interviews, 150
design
  for maintenance, 184
  for operation, 183
  team organisation, 15
developing countries, 30, 155
dials, 211
D.I.N., 256
disability, 315, 322
disabled individuals, 314, 319
disasters, 273
display/control stereotypes, 220
displays, 208
  analogue, 212
  command, 212
  compatibility, 216
  computer-driven, 213
  hard-wired, 213
  design, 214
  digital, 212
  hybrid, 212

legibility, 214
pictorial, 212
predictor, 212, 252
qualitative, 212
quantitative, 212
quickened, 212, 252
real/artificial, 212
static/dynamic, 212
stereotypes, 213
storage, 212
unburdened, 212
DOT, 119
drive, 138
dyad, 140

E.A.R. theory, 145
E.C.G., 169
economic differences, 92
education, 31
E.E.G., 169
E.M.G., 169
environment, 310
equivocation, 201
ergograph, 160
error rates, 102
ESPRIT, 240
ETA, 299
ethnic differences, 92
EUREKA, 240
experiments, 176
expert systems, 234

F.A.S.T. chart, 62
fatigue, 160, 333
feedback, 110
fishing, 25
Fitts' Law, 207
Fitts' List, 35, 36
flair, 245
flatlands, 309
flicker fusion frequency, 170
formats, 211, 242, 252
FTA, 299
function control, 49

GAS, 163
Gaussian curve, 179
Gestalt principles, 209
Gestalt psychology, 93
group dynamics, 99
groups, 312

G.S.R. 169
guidance, 115

H.2000, 156
handicap, 315, 322
haptic system, 197
Hawthorne experiments, 143
hazard reduction, 290, 298
HCI, 127, 235, 239, 240, 241
Health and Safety at Work etc. Act, 264, 289
hearing, 195, 197
heat stress, 163
herds, 141
hermeneutics, 271
HI, 127
Hick's Law, 207
HRA, 299
HSC, 264
HSE, 264
human dynamics, 202
human errors, 222, 269, 271, 290, 293, 294
human limitations, 223
human resources, 25, 27, 29
humanising work, 33, 34
hygiene factors, 145

I.E.A., 75, 254
I.F.F., 225
IKBS, 239
ILO, 24, 51, 156, 262, 265, 276
immediate memory, 203
impairment, 315, 322
individual differences, 88
industrial stressors, 172
industrial training, 109
industrial training boards, 122
information acceptance, 194, 211
information theory, 96, 201
    bits versus chunks, 96
information transmission, 199, 205
inspection, 186
instinct, 138
intelligence, 89
intelligent buildings, 312
interface design, 218
interface network diagram, 65
internal noise, 209
interview board 117
interviewing, 102
introspection, 198
introversion/extraversion, 162

invalidity, 315
ISO, 256
IT 239

job, 42
    analysis, 43, 44, 148
    demands, 4, 322
    description, 44, 117
    design, 180
    design movement, 33
    satisfaction, 325
JSP, 150

Kalman filter, 204
kinaesthetic system, 194, 195, 206
knowledge of results, 109
knowledge texts, 75

labour law, 263
laisse-faire group, 140
language, 99, 203
large groups, 141
LCUs, 164
leadership, 142
learning, 93, 100
Le Chatilier's principle, 84
leisure, 31
life expectation, 22
London *Times*, 310

macro-systems, 20
maintenance, 86
management consultant, 154
man–computer communication, 236
man–computer system, 233
man–machine communication, 236
man–machine systems, 32, 34, 233
manpower planning, 70
manual control, 202, 207
manuals, 76
M.C.I., 67
McRuer and Krendel's equation, 208
meaning, 196, 197
memory, 96, 100
    episodic/semantic, 96
    iconic/echoic, 97
    short-term/long-term, 97
mental load, 164, 171
mental models, 85, 270
mimicking, 204
mind-set, 98, 222
MMI, 41, 127, 239

MMI chart, 63
mobs, 141
motion detection, 195
motivation theory, 144
motivators, 145
motives, 138
motor control, 203

NATO, 242
need, 138
needs hierarchy, 145
N.F., 256
NGOs, 157
NIMBY, 260
NIOSH, 264
NSC, 276
nuclear power, 261, 274

occupation, 43
office design, 324
offices, 9
off-line information, 59
on-line information, 59
operator description, 117
operator training, 109
opinion, 139
organisation theory, 143
OSHA, 263

PAQ, 150
pedals, 217
perception, 196, 197, 203
perceptual anchors, 205
performance shaping factors, 299
personality, 89
PIACT, 156
pilot, 4, 250, 251
placement, 120
planning, 310
population density, 317
posture, 333
power station, 9, 10
PRA, 299
President Lincoln, 25
procedures, 40, 72, 74
programmed instruction, 123
psycholinguistics, 198
psychological refractory period, 205
psychophysics, 211

questionnaires, 107
queuing, 204

QWOL, 33

RACE, 240
rationalisation, 139
reaction times, 205
rehabilitation, 321
rehabilitation centres, 334
reliability, 105, 271
reliability analysis, 273, 299
REM, 163
repertory grid, 95
repetitive strain injuries, 189
responsibility charts, 66
risk, 260
risk analysis, 298
robotics, 237
role analysis, 147, 221, 251
role playing, 148
role reversal, 148
ROSPA, 276, 278, 280
routines, 75

safety, 262, 334
  climate, 289
  codes of practice, 301
  compliance, 300
  genesis, 297
  inspectors, 263
  law, 263, 301
  management, 288
  occupational, 264
  organisation, 297
  procedures, 286
  standards, 301
  systems, 265, 294, 295
  training, 287
scales, 178
scanning, 204
SCs, 256
schema, 82, 97, 99
SE, 239
selection, 115
sensation, 194
set, 138
sex differences, 91
Shannon–Wiener equation, 201
shift systems, 187
sick building syndrome, 324
signal detection theory, 199
signal/noise ratio, 209
signification, 197
simulators, 15, 128

Single European Act, 263
sinus arrythmia, 169
skills, 81
  analysis, 42, 112, 113
  basic, 82
  description, 43
  key features, 115
  management, 114
  motor/perceptual, 83
  social, 114
  training, 111
SLIM, 299
small groups, 139
smell, 194
social contract, 8
social distance, 311
socio-technical systems, 32
somaesthetic system, 194, 195, 197
standards, 254
status, 139
strain, 169
stress, 31, 163, 166
structure, 197, 209
supervisory control, 2, 40
surveys, 106, 108
system
  concept, 8
  design process, 11
  malfunctions, 223

tactile system, 194, 195
tailored testing, 106
task, 42, 237
task analysis, 41, 43, 237, 251
  algorithm charts, 59
  block diagrams, 57, 58
  by discussion, 61
  control room operator, 47
  diagnosis, 49
  diagnostic, 47
  F.A.S.T. diagram, 61
  flow charts, 56
  hierarchical analysis, 66
  job process analysis, 67
  link design charts, 56
  machine tool, 47
  observation, 50
  procedural, 45
  process charts, 50
  protocol analysis, 67
  responsibility charts, 65
  talk-through, 45

  sequence charts, 55
  time-line diagrams, 61
  walk-through, 45
taste, 194
TC, 256
Technical Support Centre, 222
territory, 140, 311
TES, 126
T-group, 140
Theory X/Y, 143
THERP, 299
thinking, 96
Three Mile Island, 227, 274
time-line diagram, 64
TOTE, 110
toxic plume, 275
tracking, 202, 203
training
  aids, 123
  attitude, 113
  conceptual, 123
  design, 121
  diagnostic, 288
  expert system, 126
  military, 124
  part/whole, 110
  programmed, 123
  progressive-part, 110
  safety, 287
  shell, 126
  skill, 111
  strategic, 112
  task, 108
  taxonomies, 125
transactional analysis, 251
transfer effects, 177
transfer theory, 202
travel office, 10
trials, 176
tunnel vision, 161
Tustin's equation, 207
TWI, 122
Type A/B behaviour, 164

unemployment, 29
United Kingdom, 25
user preference studies, 320

validity, 105
VDUs, 188, 190, 228, 236, 241, 247, 252
vestibular system, 194, 195
vibration detection, 195
vigilance, 165, 167

vision, 194, 195, 197, 205, 206
VLSI, 239

W.H.O., 156
work motivation, 34

world population, 22, 317

Youth Training Schemes, 122

zero defect programmes, 273